NEUROTOXINS
IN CLINICAL PRACTICE

Neurologic Illness:
DIAGNOSIS & TREATMENT

EDITOR-IN-CHIEF
Michael I. Weintraub, M.D.
New York Medical College
Valhalla, NY

EDITORIAL BOARD

D. Frank Benson, M.D.
University of California
Los Angeles, CA

Noble J. David, M.D.
University of Miami
Miami, FL

Simon Horenstein, M.D.
St. Louis School of Medicine
St. Louis, MO

Jonathan H. Pincus, M.D.
Yale University
New Haven, CT

Clinical Evaluation and Diagnosis of Speech Disorders
E. Jeffrey Metter, M.D.

Diagnosis and Management of Muscle Disease
Albert P. Galdi, M.D.

Infectious Diseases of the Central Nervous System
Richard A. Thompson, M.D. and John R. Green, M.D., eds.

Neurotoxins in Clinical Practice
Christopher G. Goetz, M.D.

Hysterical Conversion Reactions
Michael I. Weintraub, M.D.

NEUROTOXINS IN CLINICAL PRACTICE

Christopher G. Goetz
Department of Neurological Sciences
Rush-Presbyterian-St. Luke's Medical Center
Chicago, Illinois

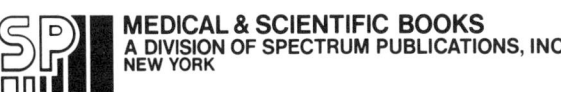
MEDICAL & SCIENTIFIC BOOKS
A DIVISION OF SPECTRUM PUBLICATIONS, INC
NEW YORK

Copyright © 1985 by Spectrum Publications, Inc.

All rights reserved. No part of this book may be reproduced in any form, by photostat, microform, retrieval system, or any other means without prior written permission of the copyright holder or his licensee.

SPECTRUM PUBLICATIONS, INC.
175-20 Wexford Terrace
Jamaica, NY 11432

Library of Congress Cataloging in Publication Data

Goetz, Christopher, G.
  Neurotoxins in clinical practice.

  (Neurologic illness)
  Includes bibliographies and index.
  1. Nervous system–Diseases. 2. Neurotoxic agents.
I. Title. II. Series. [DNLM: 1. Neurotoxins–poisoning.
2. Nervous System Diseases–chemically induced.
QW 630 G611n]
RC347.G63   1985   616.8   85-2107
ISBN 0-89335-224-1

Printed in the United States of America

To my colleagues, teachers, and friends:
Harold L. Klawans, M.D., and Caroline M. Tanner, M.D.

Contents

Preface	ix
Introduction: General Considerations	xi
Charts of Clinical Syndromes Produced by Various Toxins	xv

I. METALS

1. Lead	3
2. Mercury	19
3. Arsenic	36
4. Other Metals	45

II. INDUSTRIAL TOXINS

5. Organic Solvents	65
6. Gases	91
7. Pesticides and Other Environmental Toxins	107

III. BIOLOGICAL TOXINS

8. Bacterial Toxins	135
9. Animal Poisons and Venoms	148
10. Botanical Toxins	161

IV. IATROGENIC AND MEDICINAL TOXINS

11. Neurological Drugs	185
12. Psychiatric Drugs	211
13. Narcotics and Hypnosedatives	232
14. Stimulants and Hallucinogens	251
15. Antibiotics	275
16. Antineoplastic Agents	293
17. Dietary Toxins and Miscellaneous Drugs	313
Index	341

Preface

THIS book is an outgrowth of a chapter on neurotoxicology in Baker and Baker's *Clinical Neurology*. The format is similar with more detail on three areas: the mechanism of action of various toxins, their clinical presentations, and the management of intoxicated patients. Even with the extensive clinical literature on neurotoxicology, the biochemical foundations of toxic reactions are often not understood. Even when specific effects can be identified on neuronal tissue in the laboratory, it is not always clear that these changes relate to any human dysfunction.

As the title indicates, the book is a clinical discussion of neurotoxicology. I have organized it in two ways: clinical presentations and chemical categories. A series of charts at the beginning of the book lists toxins by the clinical syndromes they provoke. If the clinician is faced with a syndrome (cerebrovascular accident, myopathy, motor neuron disease), and a toxic source is entertained, these lists will assist in the patient's evaluation. They do not always include a clinical presentation for a toxin if only rare clinical reports exist. In contrast the text discusses toxins by chemical divisions with four sections based on convenient, if not always scientific, subcategories. The first focuses on metals, emphasizing that these toxins are clinically applicable, especially with recent reports of chronic cumulative effects on the nervous system. The second section concentrates on biological toxins from bacterial exotoxins to animal venoms and poisonous plants. Some of these chemicals are not frequently encountered in the United States, but because they often have relatively pure neurochemical properties, they serve increasingly as models for the study of neurologic diseases. Two large sections follow, the first devoted to industrial toxins, a burgeoning field of interest, since each year new products fumigate, spill into or otherwise contaminate the environment. Gases and solvents are often mixed products, so that the identification of the causative toxin can often be difficult. Finally, the last section discusses a number of drugs with prominent and often dose limiting neurologic side effects. These drugs are not usually considered neurotoxins in the strict sense of the agents in the first three sections, but because drugs are widely used and prescribed specifically by clinicians, it is appropriate to be aware of the inadvertent neurotoxicity associated with regular therapy or overdose.

Since the text is designed to be practical, many topics are not discussed. Those readers who are motivated to read in more detail are referred to the bibliography and to three significant sources that I have used extensively in the compilation of this volume:

Experimental and Clinical Neurotoxicology, ed. by P. S. Spencer and H. H. Schaumburg, Williams & Wilkins, Baltimore, 1980.

Handbook of Clinical Neurology, vols. 36 and 37. *Intoxications of the Nervous System,* ed. P. J. Vinken, G. W. Bruyn, M. M. Cohen, H. L. Klawans, North Holland Publishing Company, Amsterdam, 1979.

Neurological Complications of Therapy: Selected Topics, ed. by A. Silverstein, Futura, Mt. Kisco, New York, 1982.

I am greatful to my neurologist colleagues who encouraged this project and to the neurology residents in the Rush-Presbyterian-St. Luke's Medical Center neurology training program whose suggestions and comments during a neuropharmacology seminar helped to focus this text.

Introduction: General Considerations

THREE themes recur throughout this book. The first is the concept of selective vulnerability applicable at the subcellular, cellular, nuclear and regional levels of nervous system organization. Figure 1 shows a model alpha motor neuron with its cell body and dendritic tree, its long axons covered with myelin sheaths that protect electrical conductive efficiency, and its synaptic terminal where neurotransmitter release occurs. Toxins have been identified that selectively alter activity at each of these subcellular divisions, precipitating different syndromes of neurologic dysfunction. Cellular differences in susceptibility to neurotoxins also exist. Small, poorly myelinated fibers may be affected by one toxin where large well-myelinated fibers are left relatively spared. The vulnerability of cell groups or larger areas of the nervous system are equally variable; where one region may be devastated by a toxin (carbon monoxide and the globus pallidus), nearby regions are minimally altered. The explanation for such selective differences are multiple and include the basic chemical structure of the poison and the target organ, as well as the presence or absence of multiple protective mechanisms. One fundamental difference between the central nervous system and the peripheral nervous system is the presence in the former of the blood–brain barrier that protects the spinal cord, brain stem and cortex from indiscriminate exposure to exogenous and endogenous circulating products. Throughout this text the concept of selective vulnerability—anatomically, physiologically, and pharmacologically—is reiterated.

The second recurring theme is that neurologic signs in a patient always relate to both the area of the damaged nervous system and to the structures left functioning. In the normal, healthy state there is constant balance between

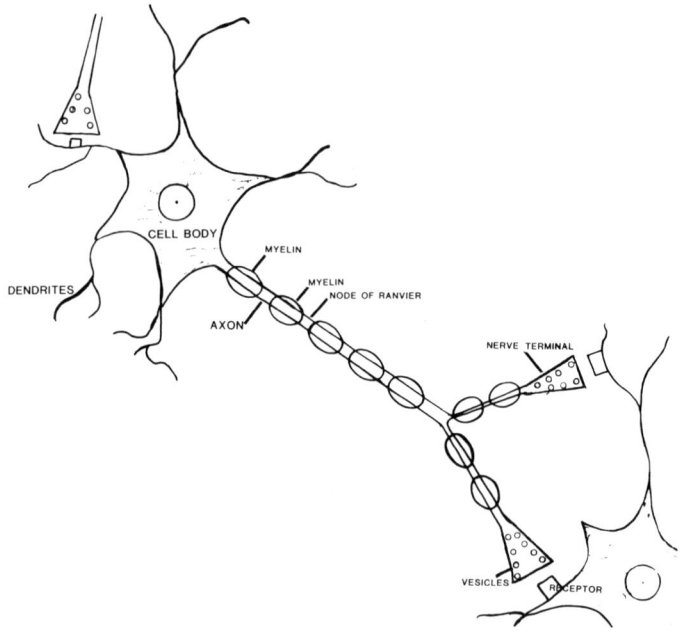

Figure 1. Schematic drawing of a typical motor neuron.

opposing muscle groups and between mutually antagonistic neurotransmitter systems; when one group or system is damaged, the opposing forces predominate and can provoke secondary dysfunction. For example, after a patient experiences a cerebrovascular accident, he is not only weak from the damaged neuronal tissue, but he may also have intense flexor spasms because of the overactive and now unopposed flexor muscle responses. Whether a toxin induces its primary symptoms and signs through direct neuronal damage or through the indirect overactivity of an unopposed neuronal system is usually not determined. In neurotoxicology, as in all of neurology, the neuronal systems left functioning may be equally disabling to the areas left damaged.

The third theme is that a dead neuron is not replaced. When cells in the nervous system are killed, they will not be replenished, in contrast to most other cellular systems in the body. Aberrant regrowth in damaged cells, however, does occur and the most prominent examples are axonal distal regeneration. In the peripheral nervous system, when an axon is severed but the cell body is left intact, there is a progressive growth of the axon that may innervate the normal tissue or direct itself to an aberrant location. Peculiar reinnervation syndromes after damage to an axon can plague patients chronically long after a toxin or other source of axonal damage has been removed.

Charts of Clinical Syndromes Produced by Various Toxins

NEUROTOXINS: A CLINICAL APPROACH

Cerebellar Dysfunction

	Chapter
Metals	
Mercury	2
Bismuth, bromides, manganese, zinc, thallium	4
Industrial toxins	
Solvents: mixed solvents, isopropyl alcohol, benzene, toluene, aniline, trichloroethylene	5
Gases: carbon monoxide, methyl chloride, halothane	6
Pesticides and other environmental toxins: organophosphates, hydrocarbons, methyl bromide, acrylamide, triorthocresyl phosphate	7
Biological toxins	
Plant: mushrooms, ackee, cyanide	10
Iatrogenic toxins and drugs	
Neurology: phenytoin, phenobarbital, primidone, carbamazepine, valproate, anticholinergics, centrally active cholinesterase inhibitors	11
Psychiatry: lithium, mebrobamate, benzodiazepines	12
Hypnosedatives/narcotics: ethclorvynol, barbiturates, chloral hydrate, narcotics	13
Antibiotics: isoniazid	15
Antineoplastics: methotrexate, 5-FU, cytarabine, hexamethylmelamine	16
Dietary and miscellaneous: alcohol (nutrition), indomethacin	17

Cerebrovascular Accidents

	Chapter
Metals	
Mercury (possibly)	2
Industrial toxins	
Solvents: benzene, carbon tetrachloride	5
Gases: carbon monoxide	6
Biological toxins	
Bacteria: diphtheria	8
Animal: scorpion stings	9
Plant: ergots, cyanide, rapeseed oil	10
Iatrogenic toxins and drugs	
Psychiatry: MAO inhibitors	12
Hypnosedatives/narcotics: narcotics (with amphetamines) "Ts and Blues"	13
Stimulants/hallucinogens: amphetamine, over-the-counter stimulants	14
Antibiotics: sulfonamides	15
Antineoplastic: alkylating agents, methotrexate, asparaginase	16
Dietary and miscellaneous: alcohol (subdural hematoma), oral contraceptives, quinidine	17

Clinical Syndromes

Cranial Neuropathies

	Chapter
Metals	
Lead	1
Thallium, gold, bismuth, bromides	4
Industrial toxins	
Solvents: methyl alcohol, ethylene glycol, trichlorethylene, hexane, MBK	5
Gases: carbon disulfide	6
Pesticides and other environmental toxins: tetrachlorethane, dioxin	7
Biological toxins	
Bacteria: diphtheria, tetanus, botulism	8
Animal: tick paralysis, fish toxins, snake venoms, gila monsters	9
Plant: cyanide, rapeseed oil, ackee	10
Iatrogenic toxins and drugs	
Antibiotics: (ototoxicity) aminoglycosides, chloramphenicol, chloroquine, erythromycin, polymixins, minocycline, tetracyclines; (other cranial neuropathy) chloroquine	15
Antineoplastics: alkylating agents, vinca alkaloids, cis-platinum	16
Dietary and miscellaneous: alcohol (nutrition/trauma), salicylates, digitalis, quinidine, penicillamine	17

NEUROTOXINS: A CLINICAL APPROACH

Encephalopathy

	Chapter
Metals	
Lead	1
Mercury	2
Aluminum, antimony, bismuth, bromides, manganese, silicon	4
Industrial toxins	
Solvents: mixed, methyl alcohol, ethylene glycol, amyl alcohol, isopropyl alcohol, acetone, benzene, toluene, aniline, carbon tetrachloride, trichlorethylene	5
Gases: carbon monoxide, hydrogen sulfide, carbon disulfide, ethylene oxide, nitrous oxide, methyl chloride, halothane	6
Pesticides and other environmental toxins: organophosphates, picrotoxin, hydrocarbons, methylbromide, hexachlorophene, dioxin, styrene, camphor, hydrazine, acrylamide, tetrachlorethane, chlordecone	7
Biological toxins	
Bacteria: diphtheria (anoxic)	8
Plant: mushrooms, anticholinergic plants, ackee, rapeseed oil, khat, ergot plants, cyanide, convulsant and depressant plants	10
Iatrogenic drugs and toxins	
Neurology: phenytoin, phenobarbital, primidone, carbamazepine, valproate, anticholinergic drugs, dopaminergic drugs, steroids, baclofen, centrally active cholinesterase inhibitors	11
Psychiatry: neuroleptics, antidepressants, lithium, benzodiazepines, MAO inhibitors, meprobamate	12
Hypnosedatives/narcotics: all narcotics, barbiturates, and other hypnosedatives	13
Stimulants/hallucinogens: amphetamine, methylphenidate, cocaine, marijuana, phencyclidine, all hallucinogens and over-the-counter stimulants	14
Antibiotics: miconazole, cycloserine, ethionamide, nalidixic acid, sulfonamides, metronizadole, chloramphenicol	15
Antineoplastics: alkylating agents, methotrexate, 5-FU, azacytidine, vinca alkaloids, nitrosoureas, hexamethylmelamine, asparaginase, procarbazine	16
Dietary and miscellaneous: alcohol, salicylics, indomethacin, naproxen, sulidac, digitalis, methyldopa, clonidine, reserpine, propranolol, lidocaine, BAL, disulfiram, vitamin D, monosodium glutamate	17

Clinical Syndromes

Extrapyramidal and Involuntary Movement Disorders

	Chapter
Metals	
Lead (T)	1
Mercury (T, C, MC)	2
Bismuth (MC, T); manganese (P); thallium (C, T, MC); bromide (T); zinc (T)	4
Industrial toxins	
Solvents: methyl alcohol (P); toluene (T); trichlorethane (T); carbon tetrachloride (P)	5
Gases: carbon monoxide (P); carbon disulfide (P); hydrogen sulfide (T); methyl chloride (T)	6
Pesticides and other environmental toxins: organophosphates (T); DDT and hydrocarbons (T, MC); chlordane (T); picrotoxin (T); methylbromide (T, MC); dioxin (T); chlordecone (T)	7
Biological toxins	
Bacteria: diphtheria (C)	8
Animal: black widow spider (T); scorpion (T)	9
Plant: mushrooms, especially *A. muscaria* (MC); *Lathyrus sativus* and *Lathyrus cicera* (T); anticholinergic plants (MC), ergot drugs (C)	10
Iatrogenic toxins and drugs	
Neurology: phenytoin (T, C, MC, D); barbiturates (withdrawal, T); primidone (withdrawal, T); carbamazepine (C, D, MC); valproate (T, MC); anticholinergic drugs (T, MC); dopaminergics (C, MC, D)	11
Psychiatry: neuroleptics (P, T, C, D); antidepressants (T, MC); lithium (T, C); reserpine (P, T)	12
Hypnosedatives/narcotics: (all agents, withdrawal, T); MPTP (P, T, MC); narcotics (MC); methaqualone (MC)	13
Stimulants/hallucinogens; amphetamine (T, C); methylphenidate (T, C); cocaine (T); caffeine (T); nicotine (T); over-the-counter stimulants (T); hallucinogens (T); marijuana (T); PCP (D)	14
Antibiotics: chloroquine (D); penicillin (MC); cyclosine (T, MC), ethionamide (T)	15
Antineoplastics: hexamethylmelamine (T); methotrexate (T); 5-FU (P, T)	16
Dietary and miscellaneous: alcohol (T, MC, C); salicylates (T); methyldopa (P); lidocaine (T); metoclopramide (D, T, P, C); oral contraceptives (C)	17

Key: T = tremor; D = dystonia; C = chorea; MC = myoclonus; P = parkinsonism

NEUROTOXINS: A CLINICAL APPROACH

Motor Neuron Disease

	Chapter
Metals	
Lead	1
Mercury	2
Selenium, manganese	4
Industrial toxins	
Solvents: triorthocresylphosphate, organophosphates, trichlorethylene	5
Biological toxins	
Plant: *Lathyrus sativus, Lathyrus cicera*	10

Myalgia, Muscle Spasm, and/or Trismus

	Chapter
Metals	
Zinc	4
Industrial toxins	
Solvents: ethylene glycol	5
Gases: halothane	6
Pesticides and other environmental toxins: organophosphates, strychnine, picrotoxin, hydrocarbons, hexachlorophene	7
Biological toxins	
Bacteria: tetanus	8
Animal: snake bites, scorpion, spider bites	9
Plant: mushrooms, rapeseed oil	10
Iatrogenic toxins and drugs	
Neurology: dantrolene	11
Antibiotics: isoniazid	15
Antineoplastic: cis-platinum	16
Dietary and miscellaneous: lidocaine, BAL, EDTA	17

Clinical Syndromes

Myelopathy

	Chapter
Metals	
Arsenic	3
Bismuth	4
Industrial toxins	
Solvents: N-hexane	5
Pesticides and other environmental toxins: TOCP, organophosphates, acrylamide	7
Biological toxins	
Animal: bee stings	9
Plant: *Lathyrus sativus, Lathyrus cicera,* cyanide	10
Iatrogenic toxins and drugs	
Hypnosedatives/narcotics: opiates	13
Antibiotics: amphotericin B, sulfonamides	15
Antineoplastics: alkylating agents, methotrexate	16

Myopathy (M), Neuromuscular Blockage (NM), and Myotonia (MT)

	Chapter
Metals	
Barium (M)	4
Industrial toxins	
Solvents: mixed solvent (M), trichlorethylene (NM)	5
Gases: halothane (malignant hyperthermia) (M), carbon monoxide (M)	6
Pesticides and other environmental toxins: chlordane (M), organophosphates (NM), hydrocarbons (NM), chlordecone (M)	7
Biological toxins	
Bacteria: diphtheria (M), botulism (NM), tetanus (M)	8
Animal: snake venoms (M, NM), fish venoms (M, NM), gila monsters (M)	9
Plant: rapeseed oil (M), curare (NM)	10
Iatrogenic toxins and drugs	
Neurology: baclofen (weakness), dantrolene (weakness), steroids (M), cholinesterase inhibitors (NM)	11
Hypnosedatives/narcotics: opiates (secondary M)	13
Antibiotics: chloroquine (M), aminoglycosides (NM), clindamycin (NM), lincomycin (NM), polymixins (NM), tetracyclines (NM)	15
Antineoplastics: azacytidine (M), vinca alkaloids (M), procarbazine (M)	16
Dietary and miscellaneous: alcohol (M), penicillamine (N, NM), DAC (MT); clofibrate (MT), propranolol (MT)	17

NEUROTOXINS: A CLINICAL APPROACH

Ocular Abnormalities

	Chapter
Metals	
Lead: ON, P, EOM	1
Mercury: ON, CB	2
Arsenic: ON, EOM	3
Others: thallium (ON, PUP), bromides (PUP, EOM), gold (EOM)	4
Industrial toxins	
Solvents: methyl alcohol (ON, EOM), benzene (ON, RN), acetone (PUP), toluene (ON), carbon tetrachloride (ON), trichlorethylene (ON, RN, EOM)	5
Gases: nitrous oxide (ON), carbon monoxide (CB), carbon disulfide (ON, PUP)	6
Pesticides and other environmental toxins: DDT and other insecticides (ON), organophosphates (PUP), picrotoxin (PUP, ON), chlordecone (P, EOM)	7
Biological toxins	
Bacteria: botulism (PUP, EOM), diphtheria (EOM)	8
Animal: scorpion sting (PUP), bee sting (ON, PUP), snake venoms (PUP, EOM), tick (EOM)	9
Plant: cyanide (ON), rapeseed oil (P), anticholinergics, plants (PUP, EOM), mushrooms, especially a. muscaria (PUP)	10
Iatrogenic toxins and drugs	
Neurology: carbamazepine (EOM), valproate (PUP), phenobarbital (PUP), primidone (PUP), anticholinergic drugs (PUP, EOM), steroids (PC)	11
Psychiatry: neuroleptics (PUP), antidepressants (PUP), MAO inhibitors (PUP), benzodiazepines (PUP)	12
Hypnosedatives/narcotics: ethclorvynol (ON), chloral hydrate (ON, PUP), opiates (PUP), barbiturates (PUP), glutethimide (PUP)	13
Stimulants/hallucinogens: nicotine (ON), amphetamine (PUP), cocaine (PUP), hallucinogens (PUP), phencyclidine (PUP), methylphenidate (PUP), caffeine (PUP)	14
Antibiotics: aminoglycosides (EOM), ampicillin (PC), nalidixic acid (PC), tetracycline (PC), chloramphenicol (ON), ethambutol (ON), INH (ON), chloroquine (EOM, ON), nitrofurantoin (EOM, RN)	15
Antineoplastics: methotrexate (ON), cytosine arabinoside (ON), vinca alkaloids (EOM, ON), cis-platinum (ON)	16
Miscellaneous and dietary: salicylates (PUP), quinidine (P, ON), disulfiram (RN), oral contraceptives (PC, RN, ON), alcohol (ON, EOM), [nutrition]), vitamin A (PC, EOM), digitalis ([blurred vision], PUP, ON, EOM), lidocaine (EOM), penicillamine (ON, EOM)	17

Key: ON = optic neuropathy; RN = retrobulbar neuropathy; P = papilledema; CB = cortical or cerebral blindness; PC = pseudotumor cerebri, PUP = pupillary changes, EOM = extraocular muscle palsies.

Clinical Syndromes

Peripheral Neuropathy

	Chapter
Metals	
Lead	1
Mercury	2
Arsenic	3
Other metals: gold, thallium	4
Industrial toxins	
Solvents: mixed solvents, benzene, toluene, N-hexane, MBK, trichlorethylene, carbon tetrachloride	5
Gases: carbon monoxide, nitrous oxide, carbon disulfide, ethylene oxide	6
Pesticides and other environmental toxins: organophosphates (esp. TOCP, DDT, and hydrocarbons); PNU pesticides, dioxin, styrene, acrylamide, tetrachlorethane, chlordecone	7
Biological toxins	
Bacteria: diphtheria	8
Animal: bee stings, tick paralysis, fish toxins	9
Plant: *Lathyrus sativus* and *Lathyrus cicera,* cyanide, rapeseed oil	10
Iatrogenic toxins and drugs	
Neurology: phenytoin	11
Psychiatry: lithium	12
Hypnosedatives/narcotics: narcotics, methaqualone	13
Stimulants/hallucinogens: nicotine	14
Antibiotics: aminoglycosides, amphotericin, chloramphenicol, ethambutol, INH, nitrofurantoin, sulfonamides, polymyxins, chloroquine, metronidazole, penicillins	15
Antineoplastics: vincristine, vinblastine, vindesine, cis-platinum, alkylating agents, procarbazine, hexamethylmelamine	16
Dietary and miscellaneous: alcohol (trauma), hydralazine, disulfiram, oral contraceptives, sulindac, vitamin D (secondary), Vitamin B_6	17

NEUROTOXINS: A CLINICAL APPROACH

Seizures

	Chapter
Metals	
Lead	1
Mercury	2
Arsenic	3
Aluminum, thallium, antimony	4
Industrial toxins	
Solvents: methyl alcohol, ethylene glycol, benzene, carbon tetrachloride	5
Gases: hydrogen sulfide, carbon monoxide, methyl chloride, halothane	6
Pesticides and other environmental toxins: organophosphates, strychnine, picrotoxin, hexachlorophene, hexachlorocyclohexane, camphor, hydrazine, chlordane	7
Biological toxins	
Bacteria: diphtheria (anoxic), tetanus (anoxic)	8
Animal: scorpion (anoxic), snake venom (anoxic)	9
Plant: ackee (Jamaican vomiting illness), cyanide, mushrooms, anticholinergic plants, convulsant plants, ergots	10
Iatrogenic toxins and drugs	
Neurology: barbiturates (withdrawal), primidone (withdrawal), valproate, carbamazepine, phenytoin, steroids, baclofen, centrally active cholinesterase inhibitors	11
Psychiatry: neuroleptics, reserpine, benzodiapines (withdrawal), meprobamate, antidepressants, MAO inhibitors, lithium	12
Hypnosedatives/narcotics: "Ts and Blues," hypnosedatives, barbiturates (withdrawal), meperidine, methaqualone	13
Stimulants/hallucinogens: xanthine, nicotine, over-the-counter stimulants, phencyclidine, amphetamine	14
Antibiotics: penicillin, cephalosporin, INH, nalidixic acid, cycloserine, ethionamide, polymixins	15
Antineoplastics: alkylating agents, methotrexate, vinca alkaloids, asparaginase, nitrosoureas, hexamethylmelamine	16
Dietary and miscellaneous: alcohol, salicylates, indomethacin, digitalis, lidocaine, BAL, oral contraceptives, quinidine	17

I.
Metals

CHAPTER 1

Lead

LEAD toxicity has haunted man since the beginning of recorded history. Lead sulfate cosmetic pastes have been found in Egyptian caves and may well have been a toxic product for ancient people. The Greeks, Chinese, and Mexicans used lead for jewelry and construction tools. Rome's ruling class may have poisoned itself by drinking tainted wine and water from lead-lined vessels or pipe systems [12]. Although its use declined after the fall of Rome, lead became a popular metal again during the Middle Ages and later lead sources included pewter products and glazed earthen ware. Tanquerel Des Planches' treatise of 1839 describes 72 cases of chronic lead encephalopathy, and indicates that virtually all the great ancient physicians, including Hippocrates, Nicander, Celsus, Galen, and Aretaeus were familiar with lead colic and the often associated paralysis and pain [28]. Today, the major sources of lead exposure include batteries, battery oxides, and lead alkyls. Because of these industrial products, man has added sufficient lead to the atmosphere of the northern hemisphere to increase its concentration to approximately 1,000 times the estimated natural level [25]. Although mortality for children and adults has significantly declined, lead toxicity remains a serious source of morbidity.

In 1977 the U.S. Environmental Protection Agency published extensive studies on blood levels of lead in remote, rural, suburban and urban populations [29]. These studies as a whole indicate that mean blood level values for lead are highest for urban dwellers, intermediate for suburbanites, and lowest for rural residents. Three other epidemiologic/demographic conclusions are possible. Children demonstrate higher mean blood level values than adults in the same environmental setting, a distinction most pronounced for children under five years of age. This difference may reflect the enhanced rate of lead absorption in young children and also the common practice in toddlers of ingesting potentially toxic non-food products (pica). Second, in adults, males appear to

METALS

Table 1.1. Occupations Associated with Potential Lead Toxicity and Various Job-Related Sources of Lead

Automobile manufacture and repair	Brass and bronze
Bottle capping	Dyes
Bookbinding	Enamels
Brick making	Explosives
Cement, plastic mixing	Fuel (airplane, auto)
Dentistry	Insecticides
Etching	Leather, tannery goods
Gardening	Linoleum
Glass manufacture	Paints
Paper production	Pharmaceuticals
Plumbing	Photography equipment
Painting, lithography	Pottery
Shoe manufacture and repair	Plastics
Tree and crop spraying	Refineries (petroleum)
	Rubber
Artificial flowers	Storage batteries
Artificial pearls	

have a greater mean blood level than females and third, black subjects in the United States demonstrate higher mean blood lead values than whites.

High risk occupations include jobs where workers are exposed to automobile exhaust fumes, lead fumes or lead powder (Table 1.1). In those persons not occupationally exposed to lead, dietary lead intake comprises a significant source of lead exposure, through ceramic vessels, "moonshine" whiskey in lead-containing stills, or the ingestion of numerous Chinese herbal remedies. Calculations indicate that a sustained dietary intake of 100 micrograms of lead translates to a blood lead level of 6 micrograms lead/dl blood. Approximately one-third of the lead assimilated by a normal healthy adult is absorbed through the lungs from atmospheric or vaporized metal [8]. Because ingested but unabsorbed lead is excreted by the intestinal tract, fecal excretion is a sensitive index of lead entering the body by ingestion. Animals excrete 90 percent of orally administered lead within eight days. Once absorbed, lead is eliminated through urine and sweat. It may also be reexcreted into the intestinal tract through the bile. The rate of lead absorption may be influenced by diet and appears to be increased by a high fat, low mineral diet, and decreased by a high mineral diet [2]. Regular alcohol consumption may be an exogenous factor predisposing to lead poisoning [9].

Numerous other sources of intoxication have been noted, including the illegal distillation of alcohol using leaded pipes and the use of rain water passing through leaded containers or conduits. Lead may be absorbed from lead pellets

following gunshot wounds, and even from lead shot lodged in the appendix. Lead intoxication of virtual epidemic proportions has resulted from burning salvaged lead-containing batteries as fuel by low-income families. Intoxication has also occurred when medication containing lead was applied to ulcers and to breast fissures of nursing mothers, as well as after the use of cosmetics. An epidemic of lead poisoning was noted in Gurkha soldiers in Hong Kong following the use of contaminated curry powder. The picture is more complex in children five years of age and younger, since lead-contaminated soil and paint are often ingested by toddlers (pica). The deterioration of American urban dwellings, formerly painted with lead paint, as well as the urban proximity to car exhaust fumes and industrial sources of lead increases the risk to the young poor [32]. Nonurban air-lead concentrations are on the average 0.1 micrograms lead/m^3 air, while the corresponding mean urban level for lead in U.S. cities is estimated to be ten fold higher (1 microgram lead/m^3). Christian et al. noted that 79 percent of accidental deaths in children treated at the Chicago Poison Control Center resulted from lead poisoning [7].

Lead absorption from the gastrointestinal tract appears to differ with age. In adults, approximately ten percent of ingested lead is absorbed; however, in children GI absorption is considerably higher and estimated to range from 40 to 50 percent [21]. If the exposure is from lead in beverages, the absorption may be even greater. Five hundred cases of lead intoxication were reported in New York City alone in 1965. Blanksma and his associates carried out mass screening of infants of excessive blood lead concentrations using atomic absorption spectroscopy [3]. Of 68,744 children tested over a two-year period, 5.7 percent exhibited blood lead concentrations in the potentially toxic levels of over 49 μg/dl of blood.

Safety limits for lead in the work place have been determined and are reported as an exposure concentration weighted for chronic work in an average 8 hour workday, 40 hour workweek (threshold limit value-time weighted average, TLV-TWA). For inorganic lead dust or lead arsenate, this value is 0.15 mg/m^3. A second safety determination for toxic products is the threshold limit value-short term exposure limit (TLV-STEL), representing the maximal safe exposure over 15 minutes. For lead, this value is 0.45 mg/m^3.

Maximal susceptibility to lead toxicity occurs in the child below the age of three with decreasing impact afterwards [15]. It is said that children over the age of six should be considered as adults in terms of the clinical pattern of lead toxicity since toxic exposure in older children does not induce the usual dramatic form of childhood encephalopathy. Little information is available on the newborn infant. Once absorbed, lead travels bound by erythrocytes. There are three lead compartments in man: circulating blood, a labile soft tissue fraction, and bone. The half-life of bone lead in man is estimated at ten years, while the half-life of blood may be as short as two weeks. Lead passes the placenta and the fetus may suffer the consequences of maternal lead exposure.

Biochemical Effects

Lead intoxication diminishes cerebral glucose supplies, and overall metabolism is retarded because of enzyme inhibition at several sites. Since lead reacts with sulfhydryl groups, enzymes and other compounds containing that group are primarily affected.

Glyceraldehyde phosphate dehydrogenase, a sulfhydryl-containing enzyme essential to glycolysis, is inhibited by lead. There is, however, simultaneous inhibition of the S-H enzymes in the tricarboxylic acid cycle so that serum concentrations of lactate and pyruvate are increased. Additionally, compounds in the electron transport system may be affected. Some molecules of cytochrome c, isolated from lead-intoxicated rats were found to be synthesized without iron [30]. It was suggested that some symptoms of lead intoxication may be reversed by supplementation of the diet with iron. Conversely, an iron-deficient diet in rats fed subtoxic doses of lead (200 μg/dl in drinking water) for 10 weeks resulted in increasing organ retention of lead and augmented urinary excretion of delta-aminolevulinic acid (ALA) [27]. Reactions related to the oxidation of glucose are further depressed by the interactions of lead with the sulhydryl groups of lipoic acid, coenzyme A, and pantotheine.

Porphyrin metabolism is considerably deranged in lead intoxication [20]. Figure 1 indicates sites where lead interferes with the ultimate synthesis of heme from coenzyme A and glycine.

Although patients with lead poisoning and those with acute intermittent porphyria often exhibit similar biochemical findings, the two conditions can be distinguished biochemically. In acute porphyria, urinary uroporphyrin and porphobilinogen levels are increased to a greater extent than coproporphyrin III or ALA. In lead poisoning the opposite is true, with concentrations of coproporphyrin III often increased to 500 mg/dl. Erythrocyte protoporphyrins may be increased to 150 mg/dl.

Lead forms mercaptides with the sulfhydryl group of cysteine and stable complexes with side chains of such amino acids as serine and threonine. Lead reacts also with a number of compounds that contain phosphate groups. In vitro, the addition of lead to adenosine monophosphate results in a precipitant of lead adenylate.

Significant alterations have been noted in the brain of developing animals. The administration of lead acetate to the diet of nursing rats scarcely affected concentrations of RNA, DNA, and protein in the brains of the offspring despite cerebellar and cerebral concentrations of 70 and 30 ppm, respectively. There was, however, a 15-20% diminution in cell number, suggesting retardation of

LEAD

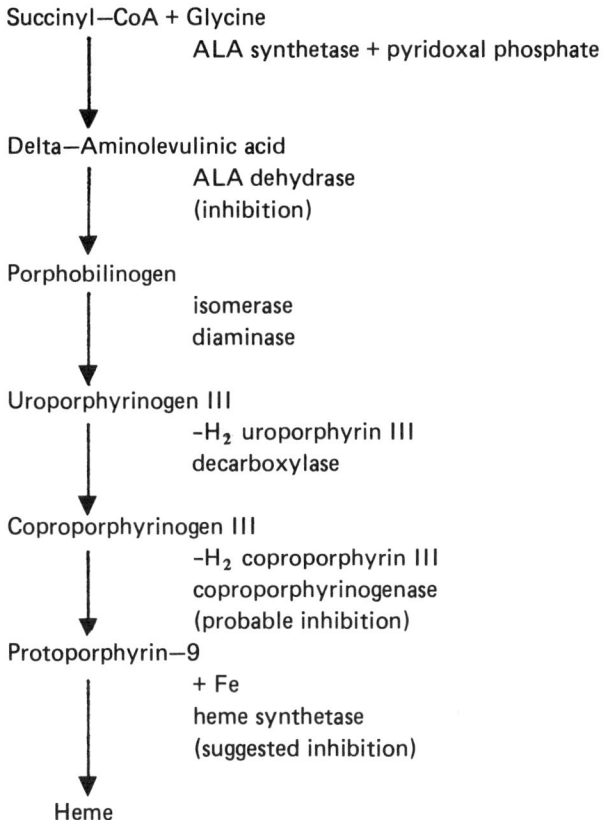

Figure 1.1. Parentheses indicate sites where lead interferes with the ultimate synthetase of heme from co-enzyme A and glycine.

new cell formation [23]. Krigman et al. employed lead carbonate similarly and noted that by the thirtieth day, fetal cerebral concentrations were nearly four times the maternal [22]. The immature animals exhibited retarded growth, decreased cerebral cell population and apparently deficient myelination.

Animals administered lead compounds during development have also exhibited alterations in certain neurotransmitters. Sauerhoff and Michaelson noted dopamine to be significantly decreased at 21 and 29 days of maternal administration of lead acetate, while norepinephrine to dopamine ratios decreased approximately 20% [26]. It is known that lead inhibits adenyl cyclase activity which may be related directly to its effects on neurotransmitter function.

Intoxication due to organic lead compounds has been documented following exposure to tetraethyl lead. Although the toxicity of this material has been attributed to its decomposition to inorganic lead, the solubility, absorption characteristics, and clinical manifestations of tetraethyl lead differ from those observed in inorganic lead intoxication. Tetraethyl lead is absorbed rapidly from the skin as well as lungs and gastrointestinal tract, passes the blood-brain barrier readily and is soluble in CNS structures. It is converted by liver microsomes to triethyl lead, the form which seems responsible for the toxic effects. Conversion to triethyl lead also occurs in the brain and kidneys [4]. Cerebral concentrations of triethyl lead are not as high as those in other organs; however, the compound is extremely stable and remains for extended periods within the nervous system. The brain is also unusually sensitive to the effects of triethyl lead. Oxidative phosphorylation is inhibited by the compound in vitro resulting in a lowering of concentrations of phosphocreatinine in cerebral preparations. Oxygen consumption is decreased as is the output of carbon dioxide from glucose [10]. Experimentally, triethyl lead chloride intoxication has been noted to decrease the incorporation of labeled sulfate into sulfatides, indicating inhibition of myelin synthesis, and possibly demyelination [18].

Pathology

With lead encephalopathy the brain is soft and may exhibit flattened convolutions. A pressure cone may be present along the base of the cerebellum. Occasionally, there are punctate hemorrhages, dilation of the vessels, and even dilation of the ventricular system, especially in the frontal portions.

Histologically, the most striking finding is extensive involvement of the ganglion cells. In some cortical areas these cells are swollen and appear homogeneous, glossy, and rounded. Chromatolysis may be complete and slight neuronophagia can be observed. Occasionally, there is a mild focal or diffuse glial increase. Hemorrhages may be present, often in the region of the fourth ventricle. Some perivascular spaces seem to be filled with a homogeneous material, and the presence of a so-called serous inflammation has been emphasized as characteristic for lead encephalopathy.

Spinal cord lesions are less frequent than is cerebral involvement. The cord damage may be extensive; it is most marked in the white matter. Often, there is an almost complete demyelination of the posterior columns and a partial involvement of the spinal cerebellar and cortical spinal tracts. Glial reaction is minimal. The nerve cells show both pyknosis and swelling and the peripheral nerves may exhibit some demyelination. In experimental animals, prominent demyelination and remyelination in different segments of the same involved nerve are seen. Minute hemorrhages may also be seen in the peripheral nerves. Involvement of other organs occurs in lead intoxication, including hepatic disease as well as renal involvement and myocardial damage (in both cases occurring with intrastitial fibrosis) [13].

LEAD

Clinical Syndromes

Encephalopathy

Acute, subacute, and chronic encephalopathy occurs and may follow either inorganic or organic lead exposure. Although controversies exist over the toxic threshold of lead at different age groups, all observers agree that the developing brain is the most susceptible target for its impact. Encephalopathy seen in childhood will be considered separately from that seen in adult patients since the severity and prognosis of the two are rather distinct. In adults, acute lead encephalopathy due to industrial lead exposure is now rare. When it occurs, a severe delirium develops, often with combative irrational behavior and seizures. Transient paresis and aphasias have been described in the older literature and may well have represented post-ictal phenomena. Increasing attention to the subacute forms of encephalopathy in childhood has suggested a possibly similar form in adults which may be more widespread than previously assumed. This view is supported by early observations that, prior to the severe encephalopathic picture of lead encephalopathy, lead workers developed subtle and often nonspecific symptoms such as sleep disturbance, increased distractability, and memory dysfunction [1]. The hallmark of chronic lead exposure in adults is psychomotor disturbance and dementia. This clinical syndrome may relate to the primary effects on brain cells of chronic lead exposure, and also to the complicating features of lead-induced hepatic cirrhosis, nephropathy, and secondary hypertension [16]. Optic atrophy may also be present, as well as mild facial or ocular motor nerve paresis, and aphonia due to laryngeal paralysis.

In the adult encephalopathy, seizures are usually generalized, although 35 percent of patients in one study had lateralizing neurologic signs most related to recurrent focal motor seizures. The mental picture may be one of global confusion or frank psychosis with hallucinations and belligerent paranoia [34]. In the study population mentioned above, the cerebral spinal fluid was abnormal in 32 percent of patients including mild pleocytosis and protein elevation; glucose was normal in all but one patient.

In children, the early signs of encephalopathy are a change in behavior from the active and happy affect of childhood to listlessness and drowsiness with clumsiness and ataxia. Often the gravity of the encephalopathy is not appreciated until convulsions, coma, or even respiratory arrest occurs. This sudden and unpredictable decline may well relate to rapid increases in intracranial pressure. Those children with the worse prognosis have significant increases in intracranial pressure with papilledema, brainstem compression, and respiratory compromise.

Since the neurologic manifestations of lead encephalopathy are protean and the decline in neurologic function may be precipitous, the treating physician should consider this diagnosis in any child with a change in mental status, gait disorder, or history of seizures. The index of suspicion is, of course, heightened if there is a history of exposure to industrial fumes or lead tainted products. The sequelae after acute encephalopathy are multiple and often devastating. In one report, half the patients showed manifestations of severe permanent brain damage, including mental retardation, recurrent seizures, and optic atrophy [6].

Because the clinical course of lead intoxicated patients has traditionally focused on the symptomatic and rapidly progressive case, the concept of chronic lead encephalopathy in children has not been studied extensively. It has, however, been suggested that such a diagnosis be considered when evaluating a pediatric patient for schizophrenia, behavioral management difficulties, or unexplained neurodegenerative syndromes [33]. To support this, one can refer to the 1943 study of twenty children who were exposed to lead from infancy but who never developed acute encephalopathic signs. When they were evaluated at school age, nineteen of twenty were in fact failing in school. A more recent study [11] demonstrated significant differences in psychomotor testing between unexposed children and children exposed to high lead concentration when tested at preschool and school ages.

Bornschein et al. reviewed 22 studies of behavioral and intelligence differences in children with clinical encephalopathy who were exposed to moderate lead levels. These studies are in summary contradictory and no clear statement can be made regarding the relative health hazard of moderate lead exposure to children. The effects of low or moderate chronic lead could be subtle (involving primarily impulse control and attention span, both difficult disabilities to measure on the scales used) or small (2-3 points decrease in I.Q.) and therefore difficult to demonstrate unequivocally [5].

The mechanism whereby lead actually induces an encephalopathy appears to relate to two complementary mechanisms: a direct lead effect on neurons and a lead-induced alteration in the blood-brain barrier. Structural changes in blood vessels have been seen with lead toxicity both in large and small vessels. A serous meningitis has been induced with lead exposure that may be related directly to increased permeability. In addition to such vascular changes, the direct toxic effect of lead on neurons has been studied in guinea pigs where encephalopathy develops without vasculopathy.

Peripheral Neuropathy

Peripheral nerve involvement is characteristic of chronic lead intoxication in adults. Both sensory and motor components are often present, although motor components are usually more pronounced. The sensory complaints are usually paresthesias and spontaneous pain. The motor components include local weakness, atrophy, and fasciculations. A number of specific mononeuropathies have been described in relation to lead intoxication. For example, a wrist drop, usually beginning in the right hand, is seen in painters using lead products. Paralysis does not appear to be related directly to the length of exposure and can develop during the first month of work or after many years exposure. Weakness begins most distally and gradually progresses to involve the long extensors of the wrist. The resultant wasting over the posterior aspect of the forearm throws into relief the supinator longus muscle. An associated tremor saturninus, a fine and irregular tremor of the fingers sometimes associated with lip tremor, is well described and indistinguishable from the more widely appreciated tremor associated with mercury toxicity [19].

A more extensive bilateral neuropathy involving the hands, fingers and deltoid, biceps and triceps muscles also occurs. A third form of lead neuropathy (file cutters paralysis) was traditionally seen more in the left hand than in the right, and appeared to relate to direct lead particle exposure of the involved muscles. Marked thenar, hypothenar, and interossei wasting is characteristic of this neuropathy [14].

A fourth neuropathy is that of foot drop, historically most associated with cabaret dancers who drank alcohol distilled in lead pipes, and also seen in children. Progressive atrophy and fasciculations with pyramidal signs have also been described, and in these cases the toxicity would resemble amyotrophic lateral sclerosis. In those patients with predominantly motor findings, nerve conduction velocities may not be altered even after significant occupational exposure. This may be explained by the fact that conduction velocities measure only the fastest conducting fibers which may not be affected by axonal toxicity of lead. In animals, lead induces demyelinating neuropathy, but in man the degeneration is primarily axonal. The resultant electromyographic studies often show active denervation and fibrillations, but nerve conduction velocities within the normal range.

The cellular basis of lead neuropathy has also been studied. It is unclear whether lead is actually accumulated in nerves and, if so, where subcellular distribution would be. Multiple factors may be important and include vascular damage, Schwann cell disruption, and stromal and neuronal toxicity. Lead may alter myelin composition by binding with membranes or altering the synthesis of lipids and proteins. It may also act indirectly to induce perineural edema that leads to myelin damage and ischemia [24]. A bilateral distal polyneuropathy may also occur which has no characteristics to distinguish it from other metabolic or toxin related neuropathies.

Diagnosis

The clinical picture in children or adults of either encephalopathy or neuropathy is insufficiently distinct for a diagnosis of lead poisoning. Other evidence must be obtained to establish the diagnosis and institute proper therapy. Among the additional findings are (1) lead line in the gingiva near the border of the teeth; (2) lead colic; (3) secondary anemia with the red cells characteristically showing basophilic stippling; (4) lead in the urine, stools, and cerebrospinal fluid; (5) roentgenograms of long bones showing dense bands at the growing margins of the bones [31]; (6) a black discolorizing of the skin after scarification of the forearm with 25% sodium sulfite solution.

The specific evaluation of encephalopathy is difficult since a patient with increased intracranial pressure is at high risk for a lumbar puncture. Lumbar puncture, when performed, should be done only with extreme caution; a small gauge lumbar puncture needle should be used and no more than one milliliter of fluid removed. Adjunctive tests such as electroencephalogram and computerized tomography, while sometimes abnormal, are not specific.

The most important tests to order for the biochemical diagnosis are: whole blood lead levels, erythrocyte protophorphyrins, and the urinary coprophoryrins.

Ten to twenty-five percent of inner city children have lead levels greater than 40 micrograms percent. Current recommendations regarding the urgency of care for children with abnormal lead levels are based on the following classes of cases:

Blood lead (micrograms/dl blood)		Free erythrocyte protoporphyrin level (micrograms/dl blood)
Normal	< 29	< 59
Mild	30–49	60–109
Moderate	50–79	110–189
Severe	> 80	> 190

Chelation is presently the treatment of choice; the therapy is varied according to acuteness and form of involvement. Because of the extreme toxicity of circulating lead, it is essential that there be an adequate ratio of chelating agents to lead ion concentration. A short discussion of the principles of chelation therapy follows, and since it is applicable to other metals, it will be referred to in other chapters. More specific therapeutic recommendations are discussed separately.

General Principles of Chelation

Chelating agents hold metallic ions within the molecule. Naturally occurring chelators include vitamin B_{12} (for cobalt), hemoglobin (for iron), and chlorophyll (for magnesium). Exogenously administered chelators reverse or prevent the attachment of heavy metals to various essential body chemicals. In order to be effective, however, chelating agents should possess other properties as well: high water solubility, resistance to metabolic degradation, ability to reach those

LEAD

organs where metals are concentrated, and the ability to form complexes which are less toxic than the metal itself. With such principles in mind, dimercaprol (BAL) was developed through logical research. Originally developed to treat arsenic toxicity, its use has now been expanded to treat also mercury and cadmium intoxication and occasionally gold and bismuth. It does not fulfill all the desired qualities, because it is not stable in aqueous solution and must be given intramuscularly in an oil vehicle. Dimercaprol has its own set of neurotoxic effects, including convulsions due to brain capillary injury, hypertension, headache, and a strange burning sensation of the genitals. In spite of increased blood pressure associated with the medication, the drug is generally considered worth giving in patients even with cardiac or cerebrovascular disease since metal intoxication can be life threatening [17].

Calcium disodium-EDTA is useful as a chelator since calcium displaces other metals. Although rapid infusion of sodium-EDTA causes hypocalcemic tetany, $CaNa_2$-EDTA quickly given even in large doses is considered safe. EDTA has a great affinity for lead and with lead toxicity, dramatic excretion rates can be effected with this drug. Having even greater affinity for zinc and calcium, EDTA will expectedly increase dramatically the zinc urinary excretion rate. Other metals like manganese and iron are poorly mobilized so that EDTA is primarily used only for lead intoxication. Although an oral form is available, intravenous treatment is recommended. Neurotoxicity is low, although myalgias and headaches are reported. Penicillamine is an amino acid that is effective in metal toxicity because it forms water soluble metal chelators. It is reportedly effective in combating lead, mercury, copper, and zinc overload. Well absorbed from the gastrointestinal tract, this agent is more easy to administer than BAL or EDTA. It is excreted unmetabolized in the urine. The d-isomer is considered safest since B_6-dependent enzymes are much less affected by D-penicillamine than the L- form. Potential side effects of chelators are discussed in Chapter 17.

Practical Management

In children and adults with mild elevations in blood lead levels, outpatient chelation therapy with EDTA may be instituted. A single dose of 50 mg/kg up to 1 gram intramuscularly may be given daily for a series of five days with appropriate urine and blood monitoring. (Good hydration should be maintained and blood urea nitrogen, calcium, creatinine, and lead excretion should be monitored.)

In patients who are symptomatic, or in whom the lead level is found to be in the moderate to severe range indicated above, inpatient chelation should be instituted. Renal toxicity is reversible but significant, and good hydration must be maintained. EDTA dosage should not exceed 50 mg/kg body weight/

24 hours or greater than 1.5 grams/day in adults. Therapy should be undertaken for 3-5 days at a time under most conditions with a respite of at least 48 hours between chelation cycles.

BAL is an effective chelating agent, but is currently used predominantly in severe cases of lead toxicity as an adjunct to EDTA. BAL enhances excretion through fecal as well as urinary routes. BAL cannot be used in patients receiving iron therapy since it forms a toxic complex with the iron molecule. The usual recommended dose is 12 mg/kg/day up to 24 mg/kg/day in 3-6 divided doses. When the blood lead has dropped to mild or moderate levels, BAL is discontinued and EDTA administered alone.

Penicillamine has the advantage of being an oral agent which can be given over a long period of time to enhance lead excretion from bone. It cannot be given when the patient is actively ingesting lead since it enhances absorption of ingested lead through the gastrointestinal tract. Penicillamine is approved for the treatment of Wilson's disease, cystinuria, and severe active rheumatoid arthritis. It is not approved for the treatment of lead poisoning or other metal toxicity so that physicians using this drug at the present time should operate under an approved investigational drug protocol. Penicillamine has been used in conjunction with EDTA therapy.

If the patient with encephalopathy develops seizures, they are treated with traditional anticonvulsants. Paraldehyde may be more effective than phenytoin or phenobarbital. It is especially important to monitor fluid balances in such patients since hydration must be maintained to reduce medication toxicity, but overhydration must be avoided to minimize increased intracranial pressure.

Chelating agents remove other metals as well as lead so that after chelation, iron replacement is mandatory for six months, and iron levels should be assessed for at least one year.

The most important aspects of treatment are preventive. Children should be removed from the environment where pica products are available. In industrial workers exposed to organic lead, protective clothing is essential since tetraethyl lead is absorbed through the skin to a significant degree. Calcium deficiency is a potential risk factor for children exposed to lead since low calcium diets are associated with increased lead absorption.

■ STUDY QUESTIONS

In an adult suspected of chronic lead intoxication, which test should be performed?

1. X-rays of the long bone.
2. Lead blood levels.
3. Free erythrocyte protoporphyrin.

LEAD

4. Blood delta amino-levulinic acid level.
5. Urine coproporphyrin.
6. Urine lead.

Answers: 2, 3, 5

Long bone x-rays are significant only in children who are actively growing. Whole blood level is useful as well as free erythrocyte protoporphyrin levels which may be the earliest and most sensitive index compared to function. D-ALA when assayed in the urine is useful. Another yielding urinary test is the coproporphyrin. Urine lead levels without whole blood levels are too variable and alone are not usually helpful.

What factors affect increased lead absorption?

1. Sunlight.
2. Iron deficiency.
3. Fever and acidosis.
4. Calcium deficiency.

Answers: All of the above

Since most childhood cases of lead encephalopathy occur between spring and fall, the effect of ultraviolet light on lead absorption has been suggested. Children with significant iron deficiency absorb up to 50 percent of ingested lead. In addition to the other two correct answers, more lead toxicity is seen in blacks than whites, and in alcoholics than in nonalcoholics; whether these differences relate to genetic, metabolic, or social differences has not been determined.

Lead toxicity in children differs from that in adults because:

1. Encephalopathy is rare.
2. Elevated free erythrocyte protoporphyrins do not occur.
3. Severe anemia is prominent.
4. Seizures are more common.
5. Painful neuropathy is quite typical.

Answer: 4

Encephalopathy is the hallmark of childhood lead intoxication, with listless or hyperactive behavior that can proceed to seizures and coma. The biochemical markers typical of adult disease are also seen with children, and anemia is not a prominent feature of either. Neuropathy is seen primarily in adults and is predominantly motor and not sensory.

Lead poisoning is the proper diagnosis in which of the following?

1. An eight-year-old child with progressive irritability and two confirmed lead levels of 75 micrograms percent whole blood.
2. An asymptomatic child with a free erythrocyte protoporphyrin level of 110 micrograms percent whole blood.

3. A one-year-old child with lead level of 20 micrograms percent whole blood, and free erythrocyte protoporphyrin 50 micrograms percent, and with new onset of nystagmus and wrist drop.

Answer: 1

The chart in the text (p. 12) helps as a reference for this question. Blood level of lead is highly indicative of toxicity; importantly, free erythrocyte protoporphyrin levels may be elevated in iron deficiency without lead intoxication, so FEP cannot be used in isolation. The third patient has neither the clinical presentation nor the blood abnormalities to suggest plumbism.

True statements regarding chelation include:

1. Penicillamine is the preferred drug for children who are currently consuming lead at the time of diagnosis.
2. BAL is not stable in water solution and must be given as a deep injection.
3. EDTA is highly active for lead, but is less powerful for many other metals.
4. BAL can remove lead from erythrocytes but has little effect on bone stores.

Answers: 2, 3, 4

Penicillamine is not recommended for the patient actively ingesting lead. EDTA is the preferred treatment for lead toxicity. BAL, because of its oil base, requires injection that can be quite painful and is associated with sterile abcess formation. EDTA, a potent chelator for lead and zinc, is not significantly useful for such metals as manganese. Bone stores of lead are poorly mobilized by all chelators.

■ REFERENCES

1. Aub JC: Lead poisoning. Medicine Monographs, Vol. 7. Williams and Wilkins, Baltimore, MD, 1926.
2. Barltrop D, Khoo HE: The influence of nutritional factors on lead absorption. Postgrad. Med. 51:795–800, 1975.
3. Blanksma LA, Sachs HK, Murray EF, O'Connell MJ: Blood lead levels in Chicago children. Pediatrics 44:661, 1969.
4. Bolanowska W, Wisniewska-Knypl B: Dealkylation of tetraethyl lead in homogenate of rat and rabbit tissue. Biochem. Pharmacol. 20:2108-2110, 1971.
5. Bornschein B, Pearson D, Reiter L: Behavioral effects of moderate lead exposure in children and animals. CRC Crit. Rev. Toxicol., 1980.
6. Chisolm JJ, Jr, Harrison HE: The exposure of children to lead. Pediatrics 18:943, 1956.
7. Christian JR, Celewyz BS, Andelman SL: A three year study of lead poisoning in Chicago: II. Case findings in asymptomatic children using urinary coproporphyrin as a screening test. Amer. J. Public Health 54:1245, 1964.

8. Cohen MM: Biochemical aspects of lead neurotoxicity. In PJ Vinken and GW Bruyn, eds., Handbook of Clinical Neurology, Vol. 36, pp. 65-72, North-Holland Publishing Co., Amsterdam, 1979.
9. Cramer K: Predisposing factor for lead poisoning. Acta Med. Scand. 445 (suppl): 56, 1966.
10. Cremer JE: The action of triethyl tin, triethyl lead, ethylmercury and other inhibitors of the metabolism of brain and kidney slices in vitro using substrates labelled with ^{14}C. J. Neurochem. 9:289-298, 1962.
11. De La Burde B, Choate MS: Does asymptomatic lead exposure in children have latent sequelae? Pediatrics 81:1088-1091, 1972.
12. Gilfillan SC: Lead poisoning and the fall of Rome. J. Occup. Med. 7:53, 1966.
13. Goetz CG, Klawans HL, Cohen MM: Neurotoxic agents. In AB Baker and CH Baker, eds., Clinical Neurology, pp. 1-84. Harper and Row, Philadelphia, 1981.
14. Goldstein NP, McCall JT, Dyck PJ: Metal neuropathy. In PJ Dyck, PK Thomas, EH Lambert, eds., Peripheral Neuropathy, pp. 1227-1262. WB Saunders, Philadelphia, 1975.
15. Graef JW: Clinical aspects of lead poisoning. In PJ Vinken and GW Bruyn, eds., Handbook of Clinical Neurology, pp. 1-34. North-Holland Pub. Co., Amsterdam, 1979.
16. Graff J: Lead poisoning. In, Harvard Child Health Project: Children's Medical Care, Needs and Treatments, pp. 121-141. Ballinger, Cambridge, MA, 1977.
17. Greenhouse AH: Heavy metals and the nervous system. Clinical Neuropharm. 5:45-92, 1982.
18. Grundt I, Offner LT, Konat G, Clausen J: The effect of methyl-mercury chloride and triethyl lead chloride on sulphate incorporation into sulphatides of rat cerebellum slices during myelination. Environ. Physiol. Biochem. 4:166-171, 1974.
19. Hunter D: The Diseases of Occupations. Hodder and Stoughton, London, 1978.
20. Kreimer-Birnbaum M, Grinstein M: Porphyrin biosynthesis. 3: Porphyrin metabolism in experimental lead poisoning. Biochem. Biophys. Acta (Amst.) 1965:110-123.
21. Krigman MR, Bouldin TW, Mushak P: Lead. In PS Spencer, HH Schaumburg, eds., Experimental and Clinical Neurotoxicology, pp. 490-507, Williams and Wilkins, Baltimore, 1980.
22. Krigman MR, Druse MJ, Traylor TD, Wilson MH, Newell LR, Hogan EL: Lead encephalopathy in the developing rat: effect upon myelination. J. Neuropath. Exp. Neurol. 33:58-73, 1974.
23. Michaelson IA: Effects of inorganic lead on RNA, DNA and protein content in the developing neonatal rat brain. Toxicol. Appl. Pharmacol. 26: 539-548, 1973.
24. Ohnishi A, Schilling K, Brimijoin WS, Lambert EH, Fairbanks VG, Dyck

PJ: Lead neuropathy: 1. Morphometry, nerve conduction, and choline acetyltransferase transport: New finding of edema associated with segmental demyelination. J. Neuropath. Exp. Neurol. 36:499, 1977.
25. Patterson CC: Contaminated and natural lead environment of man. Arch. Environ. Health 2:344–360, 1966.
26. Sauerhoff M, Michaelson W: Hyperactivity and brain catecholamines in lead exposed developing rats. Science 182:1022–1024, 1973.
27. Six KH, Goyer RA: The influence of iron deficiency on tissue content and toxicity of ingested lead in the rat. J. Lab. Clin. Med. 79:128–136, 1972.
28. Tanquerel des Planches J: Traite des maladies de plomb aux saturnines. Ferra, Paris, 1839.
29. U. S. Environmental Protection Agency: Air Quality Criteria for Lead. Office of Research and Development, Washington, D.C., EPA-600/8-77-107, 1977.
30. Van Der Kool JM, Landeberg R: In vivo synthesis of iron-free cytochrome C during lead intoxication. FEBS Lett. 73:254–256, 1977.
31. Vogt EC: Roentgenologic diagnosis of lead poisoning in infants and children. JAMA 98:125, 1932.
32. Waldron HA: Lead, In, Metals in the Environment, pp. 155–198. Academic Press, London, 1980.
33. White HH, Fowler FD: Chronic lead encephalopathy. Pediatrics 25:309, 1960.
34. Whitefield CL, Ch'ien LT, Whitehead JD: Lead encephalopathy in adults. Amer. J. Med. 52:289-298, 1972.

CHAPTER 2

Mercury

HUMAN mercurial intoxication results from exposure to the metal, its inorganic salts, and organic compounds that are freely degraded to the inorganic state. Another form of mercurialism with potentially different chemical and clinical manifestations results from intoxication with alkyl compounds, particularly methyl and ethyl mercury.

Mercury was most likely first used by man in the form of cinnabar as a red pigment for painting and coloring. Ancient Egyptian and Pakistani ruins contain examples of art work in cinnabar pigment. During the Roman era, mercuric amalgams were in popular use, and Dioscorides later recorded that cinnabar was excellent for healing burns and pustules. The Hindus felt mercury had aphrodisiacal properties and the Chinese thought it had immortalizing qualities. The metal gained wider acceptance during the 1800s when it was used to control smut growth in grain fields, and to control maggots and other pests. The inorganic mercury compounds have been used as antiseptics, disinfectants and purgatives in both human and veterinary medicine, although today most have been replaced by safer products. Mercurialism was once a significant problem in hat factories, but since mercuric nitrate has been replaced by hydrogen peroxide in processing felt, this toxic source is now obsolete [1]. Current sources (estimated in 1970) are: electrical apparatus (25.9 percent), chlorine production (24.4 percent), paint (16.8 percent), dental preparation and pharmaceuticals (4.8 percent), agricultural pesticides (2.9 percent), and paper and pulp production (0.4 percent) (Table 2.1). Since only minor amounts of mercury-containing products are recycled, most is finally returned into the atmosphere, or into surface waters, soil or various land fills or refuse dumps. Additional cases of toxicity followed the uses of mercuric chloride as a local antiseptic and calomel, in excess, as a diuretic. Organic mercury sources are mainly contaminated food products, either seafood or grain treated with mercuric compounds [9].

TABLE 2.1. Occupations with Significant Risk of Mercury Intoxication, and Other Job-Related Sources of Mercury

Alcohol distillation and brewing	Disinfectants
Chlorine production for antiseptics	Dyes
Dentistry	Furs
Electrical apparatus production	Leather-tanning goods
Etching and lithography	Paints
Farming	Pharmaceuticals and medical compounds
Millinery	(e.g., teething powder, ammoniated mer-
Metal workers in factories (fumes of	cury ointments, calomel, and anti-
melted metals or metal dust)	septics
Paper production	Photographic equipment
Taxidermy	Pottery
Welding	Pesticides
	Storage batteries
Artificial flowers	
Cosmetics	

Metallic mercury, the shiny liquid found in thermometers, can be safely ingested in quantities up to 100 grams, so that the major danger of biting a thermometer is broken glass [8].

From large epidemiologic studies, it appears that not all patients equally exposed to mercury in fact develop signs of mercury toxicity. Hygiene, diet, and intrinsic differences in mercury metabolism may account for some of these differences. Workers who neglect to wash their hands before eating, and who forget to have work clothes and gloves cleaned frequently appear to be at significantly higher risk for inorganic mercury toxicity. In addition, miners who roll cigarettes with dirty hands appear to be more susceptible to the toxic effects of mercury. Similarly, from early reports of patients with scurvy, vitamin deficiency may increase susceptibility to mercury intoxication. Animal studies with two other metals, cobalt and selenium, toxic in themselves, appear in their normal doses to protect against the effects of mercury. These studies in animals may have future therapeutic importance. (See the section on practical management in this chapter.)

INORGANIC MERCURY TOXICITY

Since metallic mercury volatilizes at room temperature, it readily contaminates the air, condenses on skin and respiratory membranes and is swallowed with saliva. It is absorbed from skin and gastrointestinal and respiratory tracts. Elemental, nonionized mercury is transported in the blood bound to plasma proteins and hemoglobin. Cerebral uptake varies depending on chemical form; however, under appropriate conditions the brain incorporates mercury rapidly.

MERCURY

During incorporation the blood-brain barrier is damaged and becomes more permeable to materials which may not pass the barrier ordinarily. Once incorporated, mercury is retained in the body for extended periods. It has been found in the urine as long as six years after cessation of exposure. Renal excretion is tubular rather than glomerular, and lower amounts are eliminated in the feces as mercury ions.

Biochemistry and Pathology

Inorganic mercury has a remarkable affinity for the kidney and as a result, symptoms of intoxication relate predominantly to that organ, and can lead to death rapidly after acute ingestion of mercuric compounds. Although neural concentrations are markedly less than renal, they still approximate 10 times the plasma level after experimental administration of a single dose of mercuric nitrate. Once incorporated into the nervous system, mercury is very slowly eliminated. Concentrations vary in different areas in the CNS. In rabbits examined 96 hours after a single dose of mercuric chloride, the highest neural concentration of inorganic mercury was discerned in the brain stem followed in decreasing order by cerebellum, cerebral cortex and hippocampus. However, the variations were within a relatively narrow range. Despite this, there may be marked differences in cellular mercury concentrations. Certain cells, particularly in the brain stem, eliminate inorganic mercury very slowly and contain concentrations as high as 16 times the magnitude of neighboring cells [5].

Serum concentrations are unreliable indicators of inorganic mercury toxicity. Blood levels vary markedly among individuals with the same exposure and often vary on different days in the same individual. The majority of uninvolved subjects have serum concentrations usually below 3 μg/liter. Only 5% exhibited concentrations above 20 μg/liter. Toxic symptoms are usually present when concentrations exceed 500 μg/liter, and blood concentrations below 100 μg/liter are considered to be safe. Urinary excretion is similarly an untrustworthy measure of toxicity, since symptoms have been noted in patients excreting 200 μg/liter of urine and are absent in others with excretion as high as 1000 μg/liter [4].

Inorganic mercury produces its toxic effects by altering membranes, particularly through combination with S-H, S-S and other groups. Like lead, mercury inhibits glucose oxidation by affinity for S-H groups in enzymes as well as in lipoic acid, coenzyme A and pantetheine. Unlike lead, however, mercury forms complexes with amino groups of proteins. The affinity for the S-H group of proteins results in change of conformation with possible pathophysiologic results. An example is the effect on muscle phosphorylase. When exposed to mercury there is no immediate inactivation of the enzyme, but a slow change occurs, indicating alteration in the protein composition.

Mercuric salts also bind indoles and, in vitro, have been demonstrated to cleave some disulfide linkages. In addition, mercury binds and interferes with the activity of reduced nicotinamide-adenine diphosphate (NADH). Urinary coproporphyrin levels are elevated in patients with mercury intoxication, but unlike lead poisoning there is no correlation with delta aminolevulinic acid concentrations [11].

Little information is available concerning the pathologic alterations resulting from inorganic mercury intoxication [9]. Only few post mortem examinations have been reported, and the findings have varied from normal to slight neuronal damage with evidence of intracellular mercury.

Clinical Features (See Table 2.2)

Acute poisoning usually manifests itself by an inflammation of the mouth, salivation, and severe gastrointestinal disturbances, such as colic and diarrhea. The breath has a fetid odor, often described as "metallic." A brownish mercurial linear streak may be visible along the margin of the teeth. In many cases, there is a marked irritability and a rapid onset of weakness in the lower limbs. Acute psychotic episodes with delirium, hallucinations, and marked motor activity may occur. If death occurs from acute intoxication, the cause is usually loss of blood and fluid from gastrointestinal routes within the first 24 hours; after 24 hours, the cause of death may be renal failure due to necrosis of the proximal tubules and basement membrane. If the patient survives the first days, a membranous colitis due to mercuric ion excretion into the large intestine develops and can lead to additional fluid loss and death.

Clinically, when patients become acutely intoxicated with inorganic mercury, they may have inadvertently ingested an antiseptic kept in the medicine cabinet. Alternatively, a child may accidentally drink the antiseptic, attracted by its pleasing color. If a patient arrives at an emergency room with massive vomiting and bloody diarrhea, brownish lesions in the mouth may be the significant clue of inorganic mercury toxicity. As indicated above, in such patients, the major initial threat is one of gastrointestinal hemorrhage, but after 24 hours, renal failure becomes the predominant cause of morbidity.

The chronic form of mercurialism is more common. It is prevalent in industries using mercury. Onset of the illness may be subtle, manifesting itself in a tremor and weakness of the limbs or in a progressive personality change. Other dyskinetic movements, pareses, and even convulsions may be present. Clonic spasms may involve the entire body and may be very severe. Occasionally a typical picture of parkinsonism with rigidity predominates.

The mercurial tremor, also known as "hatters' shakes" or "Danbury shakes," is generally a fine and regular tremor that can be interrupted by much coarser, myoclonic jerks. It may be seen at rest, and in the early stages often diminishes with activity, although with progression, gait and balance can be altered by the

MERCURY

TABLE 2.2. Mercury Toxicity: Clinical Forms

Acute inorganic
  Massive gastrointestinal vomiting and colitis with renal failure

Chronic inorganic
1. Coarse tremor with progressive mental irritability
2. Acrodynia in children

Organic
1. Dysarthria, ataxia, polyneuropathy and cortical blindness with constrictive vision
2. Upper and lower motor neuron signs (amyotrophic lateral sclerosis picture)
3. Cerebrovascular accidents?

Note: Although these clinical pictures are classically associated with toxic exposure, there is growing evidence that significant clinical overlap exists.

---

continuous trembling. Alcoholism may predispose to the development of tremor, and it is claimed that abstainers do not develop this toxic sign to a severe degree [6].

Personality changes generally accompany or precede the motor phenomena. Marked tiredness, irritability, insomnia, and depression appear early. This picture may persist for weeks or months and is referred to as "mercurial neurasthenia." These symptoms may be interrupted or accompanied by periods of excitability and irritability which often become marked when the patient is exposed to emotional tension (erethism). Many are forced to discontinue their work because they are no longer able to take orders without losing their tempers. The hyperirritability becomes extremely violent, assaultive or even homicidal, and some cases terminate in a severe psychosis. In the more severe cases, the apathy progresses to extreme lethargy, the patient falling asleep as soon as he sits down [6].

Neurologically there is often a wide variety of findings, such as vertigo, nystagmus, blurred vision, narrowing of the visual fields, optic neuritis, optic atrophy, ataxia with a positive Romberg sign, seizures, and vegetative disturbances. There may be paresthesias and extreme pain or peripheral neuropathy with muscle atrophy.

An elderly patient with chronic mercury intoxication who has progressive and unusual shaking and mental alterations may at first be thought to have Parkinson's disease. The tremor, however, is not solely a rest tremor, and is usually coarser than that of Parkinson's disease. Nevertheless, if a patient has an occupational exposure to chronic mercurial fumes as well as the unusual behavior and irritability described above, an examination of the patient's blood, urine, and hair mercury would be indicated [12].

The major form of chronic mercurialism in children is acrodynia [9], a syndrome of painful neuropathy involving significant autonomic changes. The characteristic features include hands and feet that are red and cold, painful limbs, profuse sweating of the trunk, severe constipation and weakness. There may be an associated tremor that recalls adult mercury intoxication, and personality changes suggestive of erethism also occur. The frequency of childhood mercury toxicity is not established; Warkany estimated that only one in 500 children with significant mercury exposure suffered acrodynia [17]. The condition can be reversed with removal from exposure and treatment, although recovery is slow.

The major exposure for chronic intoxication with mercury in children is from teething powders. Other sources of inorganic mercury to which a child might be exposed would cause usually acute intoxication with the same massive gastrointestinal and renal failure as adults. Since chronic oral mercury intoxication from inorganic compounds would be most unusual in adults, this difference in exposure may explain the difference in clinical presentation between children (acrodynia) and adults (tremor with progressive mental alterations).

ORGANIC MERCURY TOXICITY

Organic mercury products include both aryl and alkyl compounds; the aryl derivatives are primarily salts of phenyl mercury hydrochloride; the alkyl agents are various methyl, ethyl and diethyl compounds. The organic mercury products with hydrocarbon groups of low molecular weight appear to be most toxic.

Alkyl mercury poisoning has followed ingestion of contaminated sea food or exposure to alkyl mercury employed in antifungal treatment of seed grain. Massive intoxication has occurred in individuals living in the vicinity of Minamata Bay, Japan, as a result of ingestion of fish and shell-fish containing methyl mercury. Similar problems have occurred to a lesser degree in Scandinavia. Involvement in the Minamata Bay area resulted in at least 111 cases of organic mercurialism with 42 known deaths. Since mercury crosses the placental barrier, fetal injury was particularly severe. During the involvement, 42 of 400 live births exhibited evidence of brain damage despite lack of clinical symptoms in all but one mother.

The contamination resulted from discharge of an effluent containing inorganic mercury from an adjacent chemical plant. The mercury was then methylated by microorganisms in the sediment of the bay. Methylation occurred both enzymatically and nonenzymatically, and partly involved B_{12} compounds. The methyl mercury so formed was incorporated into the protein of fish and shell fish, and the alkyl mercury remained bound to the protein for long periods, since the half-life is several years [3].

MERCURY

The literature prior to 1972 documented several thousand instances of alkyl mercury intoxication following consumption of mercury-treated grain in Pakistan, Iraq and Guatemala.

Organic mercury is an effective agent in the prevention of such seed-borne diseases of cereals as bunt for wheat, smut for barley and leaf stripe for oats and barley. In 1972 the most catastrophic epidemic of organic mercury poisoning occurred in Iraq. A total of 6,530 patients were hospitalized for treatment and 459 known fatalities occurred, principally as a result of eating homemade bread prepared from seed treated with a methyl mercury fungicide. Alkyl mercury entered the body following ingestion as well as through inhalation or skin contact in those handling the grain [2].

Additional toxic sources included ingested animal products from livestock fed treated grain, vegetation either stored in sacks previously containing treated grain or grown on contaminated soil, game birds that had consumed the treated grains sown in the fields, fish from rivers where treated grain had been dumped or where drainage occurred from treated fields, and maternal milk consumed by infants whose mothers were exposed to the toxin. Although most cases of organic mercury toxicity have been reported outside of the United States, New Mexican farmers have experienced toxicity related to eating livestock that has been fed grain treated with mercury-containing fungicides [10].

Following exposure to organic mercury 90% of the metal within the bloodstream remains in organic form related to red blood cells. In plasma, milk, urine, cerebrospinal fluid and amniotic fluid, however, concentrations of mercury are lower than in whole blood and the proportion of mercury degraded to the inorganic form is higher. Although the mercury content of plasma and milk correlates closely with that of whole blood, the amount of mercury excreted in the urine is an inaccurate indication of blood concentration. Organic mercury is slowly excreted through the kidneys with a half-life in the body reported to vary from 40 to 105 days. Mercury in organic form crosses the placenta, resulting in blood concentrations in the fetus equal to or greater than in maternal blood.

The WHO (1976) report suggested that long-term daily intake of approximately five micrograms/kilogram body weight of total mercury as methyl mercury after steady state results in a blood mercury concentration of 20-50 micrograms/dl and a hair mercury concentration between 50-120 micrograms/gram [18]. These levels would correspond to the earliest adverse signs. These figures are for adults and could be entirely different for children and especially for the fetus. Importantly, methyl mercury compounds are selectively absorbed by the fetus and numerous reports have demonstrated fetal methyl mercury poisoning when mothers showed no clinical evidence of toxicity. Methyl mercury is also secreted into breast milk; thus the infant is exposed to its prior fetal burden plus a continuing supply of mercury from the mother's milk. In the Iraq outbreak, blood levels in the infants correlated with mercury levels in the mother's milk [2].

Biochemistry and Pathology

Alkyl mercury compounds share many of the biochemical effects of their inorganic counterparts since they also complex with sulfhydryl radicals. The blood-brain barrier provides little impediment to the crossing of alkyl mercurials and once reaching the brain, turnover is slower than in other organs. After chronic exposure, about 10% of the total body burden of alkyl phosphates localizes in the brain. There is a strong affinity for the sulfhydryl group of amino acids. Thus, the alkyl mercury is quickly bound to protein or polypeptides and tends to remain in bound organic form. Less than 3% of the total is degraded to inorganic mercury.

In experimental animals, the calcarine fissure appears to be the cerebral site with highest mercury affinity. In a single human fatality owing to organic mercurial intoxication, histologic changes as well as a high mercurial content were noted in the corpus callosum. Excretion is principally through the gastrointestinal tract, mostly through biliary secretion, although there is evidence of secretion from the intestinal mucosa. Gastrointestinal trace reabsorption into the bloodstream is almost immediate [15].

Shiraki has published extensive neuropathologic descriptions of the findings in fatal cases of methyl mercury intoxication stemming from the Minamata epidemic, based on 10 cases of his own and over sixty additional examinations [14]. He reported damage to peripheral neurons and the myelin sheath accompanied by glial proliferation and mobilization of phagocytes. The most severe damage was noted in the calcarine cortex (primary visual cortex), followed by the cerebellar cortex, particularly in the granule cells, the pre- and post-central gyri, the transverse gyrus and the putamen.

These findings correlate well with the clinical features of the syndrome of organic mercury toxicity described below. They also correlate with the mercury distribution studies obtained in laboratory animals. When methyl mercury was given to animals, maximal mercury concentrations occurred in the calcarine cortex and cerebellum [19]. Subchronic and continuous administration of methyl mercuric hydroxide to rats induced high concentrations of mercury in the spinal dorsal root ganglion, with the spinal cord and peripheral nerves containing significantly less mercury.

Clinical Features (See Tables 2.2 and 2.3)

The clinical triad of organic mercury toxicity is peripheral neuropathy, ataxia and cortical blindness. No earlier warning signs may occur until the patient has already been exposed to toxic, sometimes even fatal, doses of alkyl mercury. There is then a latent period of two weeks to several months before neural symptoms appear. The clinical evidence of neural involvement also correlates with

TABLE 2.3 Frequency of Clinical Signs and Symptoms in Methyl Mercury Poisoning

Symptoms and signs	Frequency (percent)
Constriction of visual fields	100
Sensory disturbance	100
Ataxia	94
Impairment of speech	88
Impairment of hearing	85
Impairment of gait	82
Tremor	76
Mental disturbance	71
Exaggerated tendon reflexes	38
Hypersalivation	24
Hyperhydrosis	24
Muscular rigidity	21
Ballism	15
Chorea	15
Pathological reflexes (increased or decreased)	12
Athetosis	9
Contractures	9

From Takeuchi and co-workers [15].

biochemical findings [4]. The most frequent initial manifestations are paresthesias of the extremities, beginning in the fingers and toes and extending to a glove stocking distribution. Touch and pain are the modalities most impaired. However, vibration and joint position sensation may also be involved later. Visual fields may be concentrically constricted, and this alteration appears as the initial symptom in almost half the cases. The visual defects take primarily the form of cortical blindness, where the patient does not see well, but the pupillary reaction is left unimpaired. Excellent pathologic correlation has been established between the degree of visual impairment and the degree of striate (visual) cortex damage [14]. As the condition progresses, almost all patients demonstrate evidence of cerebellar involvement with ataxia, a diadochokinesia, dysarthria and nystagmus. Neurogenic deafness is another commonly observed finding. A number of less common manifestations such as resting or postural tremor, chorea, athetosis, myoclonus, rigidity, decerebrate posturing, lability of affect, mental deterioration, comatose states, akinetic mutism, contractions, and excessive sweating have also been observed (see Table 2.3; also [13]).

Signs of brain damage including retardation and "cerebral palsy" may result in infants born of intoxicated mothers. In addition, behavioral changes have been noted in the offspring of mice treated with methyl mercury in doses insufficient to affect the brain weight, protein or acetylcholinesterase [16].

A second prominent clinical pattern has been described in patients exposed to chronic mercury—motor neuron disease, resembling amyotrophic lateral sclerosis (ALS). In these patients, a gradual weakness develops and the combined features of both upper motor neuron disease (increased reflexes and prominent jaw jerk) and lower motor neuron disease (fasciculations and atrophy) can be seen. The sensory examination in these patients is normal. They often may complain of a sore mouth, a metallic taste in the mouth, and have systemic complaints, including epigastric discomfort, diarrhea, and insomnia. There may be tremor and irritability reminiscent of signs of inorganic toxicity described earlier. The prominent features here, however, are confined to the motor system only and atrophy of muscles in association with hyperreflexia distinguishes this presentation of mercury intoxication.

Further toxic effects of organic mercury have been suggested but not well established. A curious early cerebrovascular atherosclerosis has been seen in infants and young adults with organic mercury intoxication suggesting a possible relation. Many adults studied in the Minamata region also suffered with such lesions, although their age made it difficult to make direct inferences; the vascular lesions extend beyond the nervous system and involve the renal, cardiac and systemic circulations.

The Minamata Bay incident, now well established as related to organic mercury toxicity, was a clinical mystery in the 1950s. The triad of findings in the patient was described as above: polyneuropathy, cortical blindness, and prominent ataxia. In the absence of fever, viral encephalopathy was considered unlikely. The observation that cats were dying of the disease suggested that poisoned fish might be a vehicle; later, the disease was experimentally reproduced in cats by feeding them sea products from Minamata Bay. The identification of lenticular nucleus destruction found in one autopsy victim from the Minamata Bay region suggested manganese toxicity and this observation further led to the investigation of multiple potentially toxic metals. In 1968 Dr. D. McAlpine returned to the picture of polyneuropathy, ataxia, and cortical blindness, stressing the triad as typical of alkyl mercury toxicity, which led rapidly to the definitive diagnosis [13].

Although the presenting clinical signs seen in chronic inorganic mercury intoxication are usually different from those seen with organic mercury intoxication, there is undoubtedly significant overlap. Kark has described an instance where a patient with clear-cut elemental mercury poisoning presented with signs of dysarthria, ataxia and constrictive visual fields. The converse has also been reported, in that patients with clear-cut organic mercury intoxication present with the usual tremor and mental alterations of elemental mercury poisoning. As such, the clinical presentation predicts, but does not establish unequivocally the type of mercury poisoning [10].

There is no adequate physiologic or biochemical explanation for the various

MERCURY

clinical presentations of mercury intoxication. Clearly, the routes of exposure are different for inorganic (usually skin or pulmonary absorption) and organic (usually oral exposure). Also, organic mercury poisoning is usually documented after a single heavy exposure and clinical signs usually develop precipitously within two months. This temporal difference may in some way explain varied clinical presentations. If the chronicity of exposure is an important differentiating factor for the clinical presentation of mercury toxicity, low level chronic exposure to organic mercury may in the future be associated with the usual tremor and mental alterations that typify inorganic toxicity.

Diagnosis of Inorganic or Organic Mercury Intoxication

Mercury toxicity is difficult to diagnose through laboratory data. Urinary excretion can vary tenfold without apparent explanation in a patient chronically exposed to mercury. As a generally accepted role, however, excretion of mercury greater than 150 micrograms/liter is considered toxic. This estimate is based on the calculation that the threshold limit value for safety in the air of 0.6 mg/m^3 generally renders urinary mercury excretion of less than 150 micrograms/liter. (See Table 2.4.)

Blood and hair concentrations do not show so much variance, but again they may not be absolutely indicative of mercury toxicity. Mercury is analyzed on whole blood samples in heparinized venous tubes by selective cold vapor absorption spectrometry (inorganic) and by gas chromatography (methyl mercury). Toxic blood levels are in excess of fifty micrograms/100 ml. The hair samples must be collected in a specific manner. Hair must be cut close to the scalp and then washed to remove contaminants that are often in hair dyes or hair treatments. Afterwards, hair may be analyzed, although various reports differ in their protocols. It is estimated that the hair level is usually 300 times that seen in the blood, so that the appropriate calculations may be made to establish toxicity. The advantage of hair over blood or urine is that hair grows at a rate of about 1 cm/month. Hence, a 12-cm hair sample, if it is selectively analyzed, provides data over the past year. For temporal analysis, large crops of hair must be cut simultaneously and bound, then sliced in sections of 1 cm.

The systemic toxicity of phenyl mercury was recently studied in an epidemic outbreak of Argentinean children exposed to mercuric fungicide in their diaper disinfectant. Three developed acrodynia. Elevated levels of gamma-glutamyl transpeptidase, an enzyme in the brush borders of the renal tubular cells, occurred at toxic mercury levels, suggesting that there is a threshold for mercury toxicity at this organ. This has not been extrapolated to the nervous system, but suggests that enzyme alterations may become future indices of end-organ damage [5a].

TABLE 2.4. Safe and Toxic Levels Determined for Mercury

Threshold limit value of non-alkyl mercury concentration: short term maximal exposure limit (TLV-STEL) = 0.15 mg/m^3 : alkyl mercury 0.03 mg/m^3
Threshold limit value of non-alkyl mercury: time weighted average (TLV-TWA) = 0.05 mg/m^3 : alkyl mercury 0.01 mg/m^3
Toxic levels:
    Urine: greater than 150 micrograms/liter (unreliable)
    Blood: greater than 50 micrograms/100 ml.
    Hair: usually 300 times that of blood.

Practical Management

The first step in management is to end mercury exposure. The clearance rate of mercury varies greatly, and in the case of methyl mercury the clearance half-life may range from forty to over one hundred days. In patients with debilitating disease or malnutrition, these rates may be altered.

If acute exposure has occurred, lavage with egg white solution, 2-5% sodium bicarbonate, or a 5% solution of sodium formaldehyde sulfoxalate is recommended. The protein in the egg whites precipitates the mercury, while the sodium formaldehyde sulfoxylate converts mercuric ions to mercurous ions, which are much less rapidly and completely absorbed.

Mercury-binding chelators augment excretion of the metal in patients intoxicated with either organic or inorganic mercurials but the effects are irregular. The agents employed include D-penicillamine, n-acetyl DL penicillamine, thiol resins and BAL [5,7]. The last-named compound is no longer used in most settings, since it is reported to increase cerebral mercury concentrations in animals experimentally receiving the methyl form. Furthermore although BAL may be an excellent antidote in acute mercury poisoning, it appears signficantly less effective for the more common chronic form. EDTA is contraindicated in all forms of mercurialism for two reasons: first, it is ineffective in displacing mercury from its tight binding to sulfhydryl enzymes; and second, its toxicity relates primarily to proximal renal tubular damage, the site of mercury-induced renal disease.

D-Penicillamine in a daily dose of 2 grams for an adult can be administered for hastening the removal of metal. Mercury levels in the blood may decrease dramatically, although in severely affected patients, clinical deficits may not change.

When chelating agents are administered, mercury concentrations of blood increase for 1-3 days, presumably as a result of rapid mobilization from the tissues with a slower rate of urinary and fecal excretion. After this period blood concentrations decline. Thiol resins are not absorbed from the gastrointestinal tract; they are administered orally to bind mercury in bile and other fluids within the intestine. Fecal excretion is then enhanced by preventing reabsorption of methyl mercury so that redistribution of mercury in the body will not occur. Since thiol resins cannot reenter the body, they do not have potentially adverse systemic effects.

Spironolactone has also been employed in the experimental treatment of inorganic mercury poisoning. The protective effect appears related to increasing stool excretion through an as yet unknown mechanism.

Thioacetamide administration to rats intoxicated with mercuric chloride or phenyl mercury acetate results in augmented urinary excretion. Although thioacetamide appears to be the most effective of the experimental drugs for mercury release, it is not recommended for therapeutic use because it produces renal cellular damage.

Because some individuals may have increased blood concentrations of mercury and yet be free of symptoms, certain agents have been suggested to modify the toxic expression of mercury. Two such agents have been selenium and vitamin E. In experimental studies, the coadministration of mercury and selenium results in decreased toxicity for both agents. Most of these studies employ rather high, nonnutritional doses of selenium, typically 5ppm or more. Biochemical analysis demonstrates that when selenium is coadministered in the nervous system, the accumulation of mercury is not diminished but seemingly toxic levels of mercury are not correlative with toxic effects. Hence, selenium is not simply chelating the bulk of the brain mercury. It has been suggested that selenium molecules induce the formation of large protein complexes which in turn bind to multiple molecules of mercury. In this way, mercury could be potentially inactivated by the smaller amounts of selenium [3].

Vitamin E stabilizes plasma membranes in hepatocytes, erythrocytes and leukocytes as well as lysosmal membranes. In animal studies, vitamin E has been shown to offer a protective effect against the behavioral manifestations of methyl mercury toxicity. Such studies have not been extended to humans.

Physical therapy can aid those patients with persisting deficits, especially those who have mild contractures. In those patients with significant neuropathy physical therapy should be initiated to prevent contractures.

Treatment may be associated with neurologic side effects as well. *N*-acetyl-penicillamine has been associated with a variety of allergic reactions that include pruritis and swelling. More chronic toxicity associated specifically with penicillamine includes hematopoetic suppression, alteration in cognitive formation, alteration in renal function, a myasthenia gravis picture and even hepatitis. (See Chapter 17.)

Long-term recovery was studied in the Iraq epidemic. The most severe cases

METALS

died within a few weeks of onset of symptoms or survived with major neurologic disability. In those with mild or moderate neurologic disability, marked improvement occurred within the first six months, especially in children and young adults. Those who had been bedridden because of ataxia regained the ability to walk and some children who were totally blind regained vision. In some of these patients, no medical or physical therapy was received and the patients were simply removed from the toxin. The question of long-term chronic forms of mercury toxicity in relation to cerebrovascular disease and other systemic vasculopathies is not resolved.

▪ STUDY QUESTIONS

Match the diagnostic "line" with the toxin:

1. Brown line that is visible along the margin of the teeth   A. Lead
2. White lines in the fingernails   B. Arsenic
3. Lines in the growing margin of the bone seen on X-ray.   C. Mercury
4. Gingival lines at border of teeth.

Answers: 1-C; 2-B; 3-A; 4-A

This question focuses on visible systemic clues for various metal toxins. Dark linear mouth lesions suggest mercury toxicity and often accompany a fetid metallic breath. Mees lines in the nails are seen in chronic, but not acute, arsenic intoxication. The lines of plumbism include X-ray findings in long bones and the gingival deposits of blue/black lead sulfide.

Mercury is toxic because:

1. It blocks sodium pumps.
2. It complexes with sulfhydryl groups of protein and enzymes.
3. It inhibits dopamine beta hydroxylase.
4. It acts as a detergent on cell walls.

Answer: 2

Inorganic mercury alters membranes by combining with sulfhydryl groups, and inhibiting glucose oxidation and enzymatic activity. The mercury-induced complexing with amino groups on proteins is not typical of lead..Sodium pump blockade is seen with tetrodotoxin, discussed in the section on biological toxins. Metals do not appear to affect dopamine beta hydroxylase, the synthesizing enzyme specific for norepinephrine, and they are not detergents.

Mercury toxicity should be a serious consideration in which of the following clinical situations?

1. A New Mexican farmer with diffuse fasciculations and hyperreflexia.

MERCURY

2. A baby who is found in the bathroom surrounded by the fragments of a broken thermometer.
3. A child with painful pink or red extremities, profuse sweating, neuropathy, and bizarre behavior.
4. A depressed 30-year-old woman who volitionally ingested a bottle of skin antiseptic prescribed for her mother's scaly dermatitis.
5. A dentist with progressive neuropathy.

Answers: 1, 3, 4, 5

The clinical picture of amyotrophic lateral sclerosis with combined findings of upper and lower motor neuron disease has been described as a form of organic mercury toxicity. Large populations of intoxicated individuals from organic mercury have been seen in the Orient, specifically in the Minamata Bay region of Japan. Grain contaminated with mercury products is a source of toxic exposure in the United States.

Metallic mercury found in thermometers is not significantly toxic unless large quantities (more than available in a thermometer) are consumed. The major danger of a broken thermometer is the glass. Acrodynia is seen in children exposed to inorganic mercury and involves autonomic dysfunction and neuropathy. The sweating and discoloration of the extremities are manifestations of autonomic dysfunction. Mercuric compounds are still available in various dermatologic antiseptics and acute mercury toxicity, often with a lethal outcome, should be a consideration in the fourth patient. Finally, dentists are exposed to substantial mercury vapor and particulate in the preparation of amalgams, and nationally, it is estimated that at least 10% of dental offices have mercury concentrations above the threshold safety limit of 0.05 mg/m^3.

Match the form of mercury toxicity with the clinical picture:

1. Childhood inorganic mercury toxicity.
2. Adult inorganic mercury toxicity.
3. Organic mercury toxicity.

A. Tremors and personality changes
B. Acrodynia
C. Neuropathy, cortical blindness and ataxia

Answers: 1-B; 2-A, 3-C

As described in the previous question, acrodynia is seen in children with inorganic mercury toxicity. Adults exposed to inorganic mercury demonstrate the characteristic tremor and often show bizarre behavior and gradual personality changes. Erethism is the psychiatric term used to describe the excessive irritability and sensitivity to environmental stimuli. Such patients are often unable to tolerate either criticism or correction and therefore are unable to maintain their jobs or stable family situations. Organic mercury toxicity is associated with the triad of neuropathy, cortical blindness and ataxia, although other clinical syndromes such as the motor neuron syndrome and early cerebrovascular atherosclerosis have been suggested as additional presentations of toxicity.

The most effective therapy for chronic mercurialism is:

A. BAL and EDTA in combination.

B. EDTA alone.
C. Dialysis.
D. Penicillamine.

Answer: D

EDTA is contraindicated in the treatment of mercury toxicity since it is associated with renal tubular damage and is not an effective in vivo chelator of mercury. Dialysis has been used in the management of patients with renal failure after acute mercury toxicity, but is only advocated to manage the renal failure and not the metal toxicity, since dialysis does not clear chelated products well. Penicillamine is an effective antidote for mercury toxicity and mercury levels in the blood can be expected to rapidly and dramatically decrease in those patients treated with this drug.

REFERENCES

1. Bates LW: Mercury Poisoning in the Industries of New York City Vicinity. National Civic Federation, New York, 1912.
2. Bakir F, Damlugi SF, Amin-Zaki L, Murtadha M: Methyl mercury toxicity in Iraq. Science 181:230-241, 1973.
3. Chang LW: Mercury, In PS Spencer and HH Schaumburg, eds., Experimental and Clinical Neurotoxicology, Williams and Wilkins, Baltimore, pp. 508-526, 1980.
4. Cohen MM: Neural toxins. In MD Cohen, ed., Biochemistry of Neural Disease, pp. 200-220. Harper and Row, Hagerstown, MD, 1975.
5. Goetz CG, Klawans HL, Cohen MM: Neurotoxic agents. In AB Baker and LH Baker, eds., Clinical Neurology. Harper and Row, Philadelphia, 1981.
5a. Gotelli, CA, Astolfi E, Cox C, Cernichiari E, Clarkson TW: Early biochemical effects of an organic mercury fungicide on Infants: "Dose makes the poison." Science 227:638-40, 1985.
6. Hamilton A: Industrial Poisons in the United States. Macmillan, New York, 1925.
7. Hryhorczuk OD, Meyers, L, Chen C: Treatment of mercury intoxication in a dentist with N-acetyl DL penicillamine. J. Toxicol. Clin. Toxicol. 19:401-408, 1982.
8. Hunter D: The Diseases of Occupations. Hodder and Stoughton, London, 1978.
9. Kantarjiam AD: A syndrome clinically resembling amyotrophic lateral sclerosis following chronic mercurialism. Neurology 11: 639-644, 1961.
10. Kark RAP: Clinical and neurochemical aspects of inorganic mercury intoxication. In PJ Vinken and GW Bruyn, eds., Handbook of Clinical Neurology, Vol. 36, pp. 147-198. North-Holland Publishing Co., Amsterdam, 1979.
11. Kazantzis G: Mercury. In HA Waldron, ed., Metals in the Environment, pp. 221-260. Academic Press, London, 1978.
12. Mantyla DG, Wright OD: Mercury toxicity in the dental office. J. Amer. Dental Assoc. 92:1189-1192, 1979.

13. Marsh DG: Organic mercury. In PJ Vinken and GW Bruyn, eds., Handbook of Clinical Neurology, Vol. 36, pp. 73-82. North-Holland Publishing Co., Amsterdam, 1979.
14. Shiraki H: Neuropathological aspects of organic mercury intoxication. In PJ Vinken and GW Bruyn, eds., Handbook of Clinical Neurology, Vol. 36, pp. 83-146. North-Holland Publishing Co., Amsterdam, 1979.
15. Takeuchi T, Matsumoto H, Saski M, Kambara T, Shiraishi Y, Hirata Y, Nobuhiro M, Ito H: Pathology of Minamata disease. Kumamoto Med J. 34:521-531, 1968.
16. Tokuomi H, Okajima T, Kanai J, Tosunda M, Ichiyasu Y, Misumi H, Shimomura K, Takaba M: Minamata disease. World Neurol. 2:536-548, 1961.
17. Warkany J: Acrodynia. Amer. J. Dis. Child 112:147-156, 1966.
18. World Health Organization: Environmental Health Criteria I: Mercury. Geneva, World Health Organization Publication, 1976.
19. Yoshino Y, Mozai T, Nakao K: Biochemical changes in the brain of rats poisoned with an alkyl mercuric compound. J. Neurochem. 13:1223-1226, 1966.

CHAPTER 3

Arsenic

DESPITE its known toxic properties, arsenic remains in common use (Table 3.1). Its employment in many insecticide sprays results in contamination of fruits and vegetables. It is also used as a disinfectant for skins and furs and in the manufacture of paints, prints and enamels. Occasionally arsenicals are employed in medicinal preparations, although its common utilization as an antileutic agent has been superseded by more effective treatment with penicillin. Lewisite, an arsenic gas that caused severe skin lesions, was used in chemical warfare in World War I. Arsine, hydrogen arsenide, is a gas with potent hemolytic properties and has poisoned numerous laboratory workers in the past. Significant arsenic intoxication still results from accidental and homicidal ingestion [9].

Although arsenic poisoning usually follows ingestion, toxic symptoms may result through other routes. Arsenic is rapidly absorbed from mucous membranes and parenteral sites as well as from the skin. It rapidly leaves the bloodstream and is stored in the liver and kidneys as well as the intestines, spleen, lymph nodes, and bone. It is deposited in the hair within two weeks of administration and stays fixed in this site for years. It also remains within bones for extended periods. Arsenic is slowly excreted in the urine and feces. The excretion begins two to eight hours after entry into the body and a single dose may require 10 days for excretion. With repeated arsenic administration, 70 days may be required before urinary levels return to normal.

The TLV-TWA for arsenic is 0.5 mg/m^3. In the USA, the maximal permissible concentration of arsenic in drinking water is 50 ppb or 50 µg/liter.

Biochemistry and Pathology

Once absorbed in the tissues, arsenic exerts its toxic effects through numerous mechanisms, the most clinically significant being reversible combination

TABLE 3.1. Occupations Associated with Potential Arsenic Toxicity and Job-Related Sources of Arsenic

Bookbinding	Enamels
Etching	Feathers
Gardening	Fertilizers
Painting-lithography	Insecticides
Taxidermy	Insulators
Tree and crop spraying	Lacquer
Welding	Linoleum
	Paints
Artificial flowers	Pharmaceuticals
Artificial leathers	Rubber
Brass and bronze	Soaps, detergents
Cosmetics	Storage batteries
Disinfectants	Velvet
Dyes	Wax

with sulfhydryl groups. Many enzyme systems are affected and pyruvate and succinate oxidation pathways are especially sensitive to arsenic toxicity. Dihydrolipoate, a sulfhydryl cofactor, is the principle site of inhibition. Additionally, arsenic prevents the transformation of thiamine into acetyl-CoA so that patients become clinically thiamine deficient. Patients with combined alcohol and arsenic intoxication may therefore show a lower threshold for the clinical signs of each [12]. Other enzymes, including monoamine oxidase, acid phosphatase, and adenyl cyclase are inhibited by arsenical compounds although the clinical significance of such inhibition is unknown [13].

A second major area of arsenical intoxication is arsenolysis. Arsenic anions can substitute for phosphate and thereby disrupt phosphorylation. High energy phosphate bonds are thus lost and energy wasted. The final result is that biochemically, oxidative phosphorylation can be altered by two completely different mechanisms at the cellular levels.

The amount of arsenic needed to induce toxic signs depends on the chemical form. Organic arsenicals release arsenic slowly and are hence less likely to result in acute symptoms. Arsenous acid is the final toxin, regardless of the initial chemical product ingested or inhaled.

In fatal arsenic encephalopathy, the brain is usually slightly congested. Numerous punctate extravasations of blood disseminated throughout the white matter have led to the designation of "hemorrhagic encephalitis" or "hemorrhagic purpura." There is fatty degeneration of the capillary endothelium and some hyalinization of the vessel wall. Hyaline and cellular thrombi completely fill the lumen of these vessels, resulting in surrounding areas of necrosis.

In nonhemorrhagic cases, perivascular lipid-filled phagocytes are present in disseminated foci of destruction or in areas of diffuse myelin breakdown, resulting in the term "medullary perivascular necrosis" [5]. Ganglion cell changes invariably occur. Many of the cortical neurons are shrunken, pyknotic, and exhibit chromatolysis and disintegration. Occasionally, a mild proliferation and swelling of astrocytes may occur, as well as moderate perivascular aggregation of mesodermal elements.

Peripheral nerves exhibit increased cellularity and thickening of the perineurium as well as increased connective tissue. There is a decrease in the number of myelinated fibers and those present exhibit degenerative changes consisting of swelling, granularity or a beaded, knotted, or fragmented appearance. Reduction in the number of axons is prominent [3].

Clinical Features

When arsenic is ingested, burning of the buccal mucosa and severe abdominal pain are prominent. Following inhalation, a hemolytic response with chills, fever, and hemoglobinemia occur. Acute toxicity is usually fulminating with a sudden rise of temperature accompanied by headache, vertigo, nausea and vomiting, nervousness, and apprehension. Marked excitement may develop, or the patient may pass into lethargy that terminates in coma. Convulsions are common. On examination there is evidence of widespread disturbance of the central nervous system. The reflexes are variable and are frequently exaggerated. Nystagmus, paralyses, or incontinence may occur. Kernig's sign is often positive, and the neck may be stiff. The cerebrospinal fluid frequently is under increased pressure. The pulse and respirations gradually increase, breathing becomes difficult and labored, and death may ensue within a few days after onset of the initial symptoms [3].

The terminal delirium of acute arsenic encephalopathy was dramatically described by Flaubert in *Madame Bovary,* where the desperate heroine, Emma, commits suicide:

> "Blind man," she screamed. And Emma began to laugh with an atrocious frenetic and desperate howl, believing she saw the hideous face of an old man, standing in the shadows like a deadly terror. A convulsion threw her against the mattress. They all approached. She was dead.

In the subacute or chronic form of arsenic encephalitis, the onset is more subtle and the course prolonged, varying from 16 days to many years. Patients frequently complain of continuous progressive headaches and marked physical and mental fatigue, resembling neurasthenia. Vertigo, restlessness, mild somnolence, and focal paresis may be present. The neurologic examination often reveals evidence of diffuse cerebral damage. The patient becomes progressively weaker, passes into coma, and dies.

Spinal cord involvement has been noted [1], consisting primarily of weakness, sphincter disturbances, motor and sensory impairment, and trophic changes. Polyneuritis is a frequent concomitant of subacute or chronic intoxication. Optic neuritis manifested by cloudy vision and field changes may also be observed. In severe cases there may be optic nerve atrophy.

Evidence of involvement of the peripheral nerves may be noted as early as two hours after exposure or symptoms can be delayed as long as two years. Most commonly, neuropathy is evident within 7 to 14 days after ingestion of arsenic in toxic amounts.

When symptoms of neuropathy occur they most commonly are mixed sensory and motor phenomena. On occasion, purely sensory involvement has been reported but only rarely has a pure motor form been noted. The neuropathy is usually symmetrical and begins with numbness and tingling in the lower extremities. With severe involvement, upper extremity symptoms subsequently appear but are not usually as severe as those in the lower extremities. Hyperalgesia and spontaneous pain are common. The patient usually notes severe burning in the soles. Touch, or any pressure, such as the weight of bedclothes, may cause extreme exacerbation of the pain, and interfere with sleep. Occasionally, paresthesias may be noted in the face. Muscle tenderness, particularly on calf pressure, and cramps are common, and increased sweating is a frequent concomitant sign of arsenic intoxication. In objective testing, decrease in the vibratory and position sense is almost uniform and up to half the patients will lose these modalities completely. Decreased touch and pinprick sensation occurs often with some areas of complete loss. Motor phenomena are manifested by weakness which often progresses to wrist or foot drop and in severe cases may continue to atrophy. Fasciculations may be present [6].

Dermatitis and dessication occur with arsenic exposure. In areas where there are folds, as around the nose and mouth, lesions may be prominent and in moist regions, axillae and scrotum especially, the dermatitis may become severe. Even after recovery extensive scarring often remains. Hyperkeratosis of the soles and palms is seen after chronic exposure. Hepatic, renal, and hemotopoietic involvements are common in subacute and chronic arsenic intoxication. Transverse white striae (Mees lines) above the lunula of the nails occur 30 to 40 days after the intoxication commences in chronic cases. Inhalation of arsine gas (AsH_3) induces massive acute hemolysis, leading to hemoglobinuria, with port wine or black urine, progressive jaundice, and renal failure.

There are numerous reports of occupational cancer associated with arsenic. These cancers focus on the respiratory system and skin. Because smelter workers are also simultaneously exposed to sulfur dioxide, silica and lead fumes, a direct extrapolation to arsenic toxicity cannot necessarily be confirmed. However, the figures suggest that caution should be exercised in all arsenic-exposing occupations. No animal model exists for the study of carcinogenic properties of arsenic.

Diagnosis

The clinical features of severe abdominal pain, dermatitis, painful peripheral neuropathy, and seizures suggest the possibility of arsenic intoxication. The conclusive diagnosis requires the history of arsenic exposure and the confirmation of toxic levels in blood, hair, urine, or nails. It is important to consider other causes of painful neuropathy whenever arsenic intoxication is considered. Alcoholic neuropathy may present with hyperalgesia and hyperpathia. Often, the patient suspected of arsenic neuropathy may also be an alcoholic. However, changes in skin pigmentation, exfoliation, and Mees lines typical of arsenical poisoning are not seen in pure alcoholic neuropathy, and the alcoholic syndromes of delirium tremens and Wernicke-Korsakoff syndrome are not typical of arsenic intoxication. Arsenic is poorly tolerated when there is concurrent use of alcoholic beverages so that a patient with alcoholic disease is at higher risk for an associated arsenic neuropathy.

Diabetic neuropathy may also appear similar to arsenical neuropathy, with pain and weakness. However, the more proximal distribution of the acute diabetic neuropathy and the mononeuritis multiplex of diabetic neuropathy are exquisitely unusual in arsenic toxicity. Nutritional neuropathies associated with beri-beri or pellagra can be difficult to differentiate from arsenic neuropathy since skin lesions are typical. Guillain-Barré syndrome should not be difficult to differentiate since high CSF protein values are atypical for arsenic neuropathy as are cranial neuropathies. The neuropathy associated with acute intermittent porphyria is usually predominantly motor and the biochemical changes in the two conditions are quite distinct [2].

Hair and nails, because of their richness in disulfide, have a high binding capacity for arsenic. The normal arsenic content in hair and nails is 0.5-1 ppm or 0.05-0.1 mg arsenic/100 g hair. In a patient with acute intoxication, hair growth may be temporarily slowed and an higher level may be detected.

The major excretion route for arsenic is the urinary tract and the measurement of urinary arsenic concentration is the more usual method chosen for biological monitoring. Importantly, high urinary arsenic levels may be seen after the consumption of seafood. Therefore, a dietary history is important before an arsenic level is interpreted to be in the absolute toxic range. Most laboratories report normal urinary arsenic values as 0.010-0.100 mg/liter. Values in excess of this or a total 24 hour excretion of 0.15 mg arsenic are indicative of arsenic poisoning [11].

ARSENIC

When concentrations of arsenic are not sufficiently elevated to allow a diagnosis, mobilization of tissue arsenic by a therapeutic regimen may increase the urine concentrations to diagnostic levels. Arsenical toxicity may occur even when blood and urine concentrations are normal. Polyneuropathy may follow a single ingestion of arsenic, but symptoms may not appear for up to two weeks, after the toxic dose has been excreted.

In intoxication of longer standing, examination of the hair may be helpful. The growing ends of the hair are the most reliable for this purpose. Concentrations exceeding 0.1 mg/100 g of hair indicate excessive ingestion or contamination. Arsenic is radiopaque, and the diagnosis has been made when ingested toxic material was visualized in the gastrointestinal tract during radiologic examination [11]. Electroencephalographic studies during intoxication may reveal a slow high-voltage activity which becomes less conspicuous as recovery occurs. The cerebrospinal fluid constituents may be within normal limits, but approximately 40 percent of patients with arsenic intoxication exhibit protein concentrations between 45 and 90 mg/100 ml of fluid. When the central nervous system involvement is hemorrhagic, red blood cells are present in the fluid. Electrocardiographic changes have also been noted [8].

Practical Management

If intoxication follows oral ingestion, gastric lavage with two to three liters of water is indicated, followed by instillation of milk or 1% sodium thiosulfate. BAL (2,3-dimercapto-1-propanol) is given parenterally in a 10% solution. In severe cases, doses of 3 mg/kg of body weight are employed six times daily for two days, followed by a similar dosage four times daily for the next three days and then by two injections each day for 10 or more days. In less severe cases, 2.5 mg/kg body weight is given 4 times daily for 10 days [7]. Intravenous fluids are essential to combat dehydration, and morphine may be necessary for the severe abdominal pain. When shock occurs, treatment with blood transfusion is indicated, and oxygen administration is utilized for the resultant hypoxia.

D-Penicillamine has also been advocated in a daily dosage of 250 mg four times daily. This drug has the advantages of oral administration and fewer side effects.

Alcoholics and opium addicts who develop arsenical neuropathy because of the adulteration of these substances with arsenic almost invariably suffer from nutritional deficiencies and these patients require a highly nourishing diet and vitamin supplements. Pain and paresthesias in the extremities can usually be managed with simple analgesics, although in resistant patients carbamazepine (Tegretol) in a dosage of 400-600 mg/day may be remarkably beneficial.

Additional systemic complications that should be anticipated after acute poisoning include hematuria and proteinuria, jaundice after 3-5 days, and unstable blood pressure. After a single dose of arsenic, excretion is complete within 14 days, except that toxin will continue to be detected in nails and hair, where the keratin has very high concentrations of sulhydryl groups.

The prognosis in severe arsenic encephalitis is poor; 50 to 75 percent of cases are fatal, usually within 48 hours [8]. When intoxication occurs during pregnancy, the outlook is particularly poor.

Once neuropathy occurs BAL treatment has been considered ineffective. However, Chhuttani et al. felt that administration of BAL decreased the duration of illness without significantly affecting the recovery rate [3].

■ STUDY QUESTIONS

Match the side effect with the drug:

1. Optic atrophy.
2. Hypokalcemic tetany after rapid infusion.
3. Seizures.
4. Hypotension.

A. BAL
B. Calcium disodium EDTA
C. Penicillamine
D. None

Answers: 1-C; 2-D; 3-A & C; 4-A

BAL is associated with hypotension that can be severe, as well as headaches, flushing, and a strange burning sensation in the genitals. Occasionally generalized weakness and restless anxiety have been described. Seizures have also occurred and are most prominent in animals treated with BAL. Convulsions appear to be due to brain capillary injury and not to hypoglycemia. While sodium-EDTA is associated with a hypokalcemic tetany after rapid infusion, calcium sodium EDTA is not. Side effects anticipated with this drug include a flulike febrile state, including chills, malaise, and myalgias after the EDTA injection and prolongation of the prothrombin time. More serious is renal damage to the proximal tubular epithelium. Penicillamine is associated with bone marrow depression, proteinuria and hematuria, and occasionally a myasthenia gravis picture. Optic neuritis and other neuropathies have been described and may relate to pyridoxine deficiency. Similarly, seizures associated with penicillamine may relate to pyridoxine alterations or GABA production.

Which occupations should raise the question of arsenic intoxication in a patient with neurologic complaints?

1. Farmer.
2. Taxidermist.
3. House exterminator.
4. Floor polisher.
5. Glass producer.
6. Automobile mechanic.
7. Nurse.
8. Worker in a paint factory.

Answers: 1, 2, 8

Arsenic is still found in insecticides used in farming and is important for its disinfectant properties in the preparation of skins and furs. Taxidermists and dry clearners specializing in the cleaning of leathers, furs, and feathers are hence definite candidates for arsenic

ARSENIC

poisoning. Exterminators are more likely candidates for methylbromide, triorthocresyl phosphate, and various other organophosphate and organochloride products. Floor polishers are exposed primarily to organic solvents like benzene, toluene, hexane and MBK. Glass producers are exposed to lead and manganese, auto mechanics to lead, methyl alcohol and gasoline. Nurses, as health professionals, have primary access to drugs and are likely to be exposed to the potential toxicity of these agents when taken illicitly. Although arsenic was formerly in some medicinal preparations, these products are now rare. Finally, the paint industry uses arsenic and workers should be considered for arsenic, lead and mercury intoxication, as well as organic solvent poisoning.

A depressed college chemistry major ingested arsenic trioxide from the laboratory and was found by his roommate on the floor of the dormitory, vomiting, delirious, and clutching his abdomen. Which is/are true?

1. Arsenic trioxide is not the likely cause since it is insoluble and not associated with toxicity except at exorbitant concentrations.
2. Probably more than just arsenic was ingested because mental changes are strikingly rare with arsenic intoxication.
3. Garlic breath would be a typical sign of arsenic intoxication.
4. Prompt lavage with water or saline should be initiated as soon as possible.

Answers: 3, 4

Arsenic trioxide is generally not well absorbed but in liquid or pulverized form it is highly toxic and even in low doses can be lethal. The clinical picture is highly typical of arsenic intoxication, and, while multiple drugs/poisons must always be considered in suicide attempts, the picture here does not suggest more than arsenic. Garlic breath is quite typical but can be obscured by the vomitus. Prompt lavage with water or saline is appropriate. If ferric chloride 30 cc or sodium carbonate 30 grams is administered subsequently, the resulting precipitant must be removed by continued lavage.

Neurologic syndromes with primary motor rather than sensory signs include:

(1) Guillain-Barré   (3) lead neuropathy
(2) poliomyelitis   (4) arsenical neuropathy

Answers: 1, 2, 3

Guillain-Barré syndrome or acute inflammatory demyelinating polyneuropathy may begin with sensory abnormalities distally, but quickly becomes a predominant motor abnormality characterized by ascending weakness, loss of reflexes and maintained bladder control. Poliomyelitis causes motor syndromes where anterior horn cells degenerate, and flaccid weakness, usually asymmetric, is characteristic. Paresthesia may occur but is not a major hallmark. Lead neuropathy classically affects adults chronically exposed to the metal and wrist drop or other motor neuropathy is characteristic. Other predominant motor neuropathies are: porphyria, diphtheria. (These five motor neuropathies are material for classical exam questions.)

In contrast, arsenic neuropathy has prominent sensory involvement and may even present as a pure sensory neuropathy. Other diseases where prominent peripheral sensory abnormalities are detected include: syringomyelia, hereditary sensory neuropathy, leprosy; diabetes, B_{12} deficiency, and amyloidosis.

■ REFERENCES

1. Blackenhorn D, Wolff HG: Myelitis following the administration of neoarsphenamine. J. Lab. Clin. Med. 33:1165, 1948.
2. Chhuttani PN, Chawla LS, Sharma TD: Arsenical neuropathy. Neurology 17:269, 1967.
3. Chhuttani PN, Chopra JS: Arsenic poisoning. In PJ Vinken and GW Bruyn, eds., Handbook of Clinical Neurology, Vol. 36, pp. 199-216, North-Holland Publishing Co., Amsterdam, 1979.
4. Dickerson OB: Arsenic. In HA Waldron, ed., Metals in the Environment, pp. 1-24. Academic Press, London, 1980.
5. Ecker AD, Kernohan JW: Arsenic as a possible cause of subacute encephalomyelitis. Arch. Neurol. Psychiatry 45:24-28, 1941.
6. Feldman RG, Niles CA, Kelly-Hayes, M, et al.: Peripheral neuropathy in arsenic smelter workers. Neurology 29:939-944, 1979.
7. Glasgow JFT: A neurological disorder associated with chlordiazepoxide therapy. Clin. Toxicol. 2:5, 1969.
8. Glatzel J, Runin H: Klinisch-elektroencephalographische verlaufs-untersuchung einer psychose nach 1 roch dosierter ACTH. Arch. Psychiatr. Nervenkr. 209:365-368, 1967.
9. Goetz CG, Klawans HL, Cohen MM: Neurotoxic agents. In AB Baker and CH Baker, eds., Clinical Neurology, pp. 1-84. Harper and Row, Philadelphia, 1981.
10. Goldstein NP, McCall JT, Dyck PJ: Metal neuropathy. In PJ Dyck, PK Thomas, EH Lambert, eds., Peripheral Neuropathy, pp. 1227-1240. WB Saunders, Philadelphia, 1975.
11. Heydlauf H: Ferric cyanoferrate 2. Europ. J. Pharmacol. 6:340, 1969.
12. Massey EW: Arsenic neuropathy. Neurology 31:1057-1058, 1981.
13. Sexton, GB, Gowdey CW: Relation between thiamine and arsenic toxicity. Arch. Dermatol. Syph. 56:634-647, 1963.

CHAPTER 4

Other Metals

IN addition to lead, mercury, and arsenic, a variety of other metals can induce neurotoxic signs. These are usually occupational or medicinally related cases, but occasional homicidal or suicidal instances exist. The ten metals in this chapter are arranged alphabetically. Table 4.1 offers a reference for occupations associated with toxic exposure. In general, chelation as outlined in the preceding chapters is advocated, along with the withdrawal of the toxic source. Where applicable, other treatments are indicated. Table 4.2 summarizes the neurologic syndromes associated with acute and chronic exposure to these naturally occurring metals. Although not technically a metal, silicon has been the source of recent research in dementia and is discussed briefly at the end of the chapter.

ALUMINUM

Aluminum is an abundant constituent of the earth's crust and is used in the construction of aircrafts and other large metal structures where light weight and corrosion resistance are required. Industrial and household utensils, electrical equipment, explosives, paints and deodorants are further sources of aluminum exposure. Medically, aluminum is available in the form of oral antacids and antidiarrheal agents and protective dermatologic pastes. It is also present in renal dialysis fluids and in commercially available albumin solutions. Patients with renal failure, and especially those on dialysis, are at greatest risk of aluminum intoxication [16a].

Aluminum toxicity has been implicated in the pathogenesis of dementias and the specific dialysis encephalopathy seen in patients with renal failure. Brains from demented patients studied at autopsy or cerebral biopsy have shown neurofibrillary changes that correlate regionally with high aluminum levels [6]. Animals exposed to aluminum show progressive deficits in short-term atten-

TABLE 4.1. Sources of Occupational Exposure to Various Metals[a]

	Aircraft manufacture and maintenance	Brass and bronze	Brick making	Cosmetics/deodorants	Disinfectants	Dyes	Enamels	Explosives	Fertilizers	Fire extinguishers	Furniture polish	Glass manufacture	Lacquer	Leather-tannery goods	Linoleum	Longshoring	Mining	Paints	Pharmaceuticals	Photography equipment	Pottery/ceramics	Rubber	Soaps, detergents	Welding
Manganese		×	×						×			×			×	×	×	×	×		×		×	×
Barium			×			×	×					×	×	×	×		×	×		×	×	×		
Bromide					×	×		×		×									×	×				
Aluminum	×			×				×		×	×							×						
Bismuth						×					×								×		×	×		
Selenium									×			×						×		×	×	×		

[a]Please see Chapters 1–3 for a discussion of occupational sources of lead, mercury, and arsenic.

Other Metals

TABLE 4.2. Neurologic Syndromes Associated with Various Metals

	Acute intoxication	Chronic exposure
Aluminum		
Dementia, encephalopathy	(subacute)	x
Seizures		x
Antimony		
Agitated delirium with seizures	x	
Barium		
Flaccid transient paralysis	x	
Bismuth		
Confusion, dysarthria, tremors	(subacute)	
Myelopathy	x	
Bromides		
Confusion, hallucination		x
Tremor and cerebellar dysfunction		x
Ocular abnormalities		x
Autonomic dysfunction		x
Gold		
Neuropathy	x	x
Manganese		
Parkinsonism and cerebellar signs		x
Emotional changes and hallucination		x
Selenium		
Motor neuron disease		x?
Thallium		
Neuropathy	x	x
Seizures	x	x
Chorea	x	x
Cranial and optic neuropathies	x	x
Zinc		
Ataxia, dysarthria, tremors		x
Anencephaly, spina bifida		x

tion, and at autopsy show neurofibrillary changes in the brain, as well as elevated aluminum brain levels [31]. For these reasons, aluminum toxicity has been proposed as a working model of Alzheimer-type dementia.

Trivalent ions, including aluminum, have been reported to be strong inhibitors of ferroxidase. In the specific case of aluminum, the inhibition is mixed competitive and noncompetitive with respect to iron (Fe^{++}). Another enzyme inhibited by aluminum is dihydropteridine reductase; reduction of brain tetrahydrobiopterin and tyrosine could thereby result.

The subacute encephalopathic syndrome of "dialysis dementia" is seen in patients with renal failure on hemodialysis. These patients receive high doses of aluminum-based phosphate-binding antacids and may be exposed to high aluminum concentrations in the dialysis fluid. The syndrome is characterized by mixed dysarthria-aphasia, significant myoclonus, gait difficulty, focal seizures and a progressive dementia. An abnormal EEG pattern showing generalized slowing and multifocal spikes and delta bursts is characteristic. Other metabolic tests, including cerebral spinal fluid studies, are not diagnostic. The encephalopathy is generally progressive and often fatal, although neuropathologic changes are nonspecific and mild. Cortical gray matter aluminum levels have been reported to be elevated, and in some cases neurologic improvement follows cessation of aluminum-based antacids [2]. Other therapies aimed at treating individual signs included anticonvulsants and levodopa, both without improvement. Treatment in England of aluminum dialysis encephalopathy has focused on the use of the chelator desferroxamine, usually 6 gr. in saline. The agent is infused in the arterial hemodialysis line with estimated aluminum removal of 3-7 mg at each dialysis; over a 10-month cycle, 500-600 mg aluminum can be removed. This agent in the United States is approved for iron intoxication [16a].

Other encephalopathies must be distinguished from this specific entity; the failure of more dialysis to improve the patient suggests that the encephalopathy is distinct from that associated with uremia. The temporal pattern of the chronic progression distinguishes dialysis dementia from the dysequilibrium syndrome where patients are encephalopathic with headaches and even seizures after the first or second hemodialysis.

The question has been raised whether the aluminum-associated encephalopathy relates to the aluminum per se or to an associated hypophosphatemic state. Aluminum antacids are known to chelate dietary phosphate and this hypophosphatemia can be corrected with phosphorus supplementation [10]. Suggestions that this metabolic arrangement in fact relates to secondary hyperparathyroidism has led to parathyroidectomies in some patients.

If aluminum toxicity is related to aluminum-containing antacids, it is reasonable to question why this dementia is not more widespread and seen in patients with ulcers or other gastrointestinal disorders who ingest these medicines. It is possible that the condition does in fact exist more generally, but is not accurately identified. Alternatively, the uremic state may itself potentiate gastrointestinal or brain absorption of the aluminum ion.

In summary, there is good, but not conclusive evidence that dialysis dementia relates to aluminum toxicity. It is a sweeping step to extrapolate aluminum's role in dialysis dementia to a pathogenic role in the more widespread phenomenon of primary dementia. The problem is further complicated by the observation that metals can accumulate secondarily in the brain after injury, so that the identification of aluminum in demented patients does not establish the metal as the pathogenic agent.

ANTIMONY

Antimony is a crystalline powder with a metallic taste. In action, it resembles arsenic, but is absorbed more slowly. Intoxication has resulted from the use of tartar emetic to provoke vomiting or with homicidal or suicidal intent. Poisoning has also resulted during the use of antimony in the treatment of bilharziasis, filariasis, and trypanosomiasis.

The acute intoxication manifests itself in abdominal pain, profuse vomiting, and diarrhea. The patient soon becomes weak, drowsy, and finally comatose. Occasionally, fainting spells or spasmodic contractions of the limbs may be present. After a period of apparent improvement, there may be suppression of urine, the temperature drops to subnormal, and delirium, convulsions, and coma may be present for hours or days before death. In less severe cases drowsiness and weakness persist for days, often accompanied by tetanic spasms of the limbs. The symptoms gradually subside, leaving only a persistent enteritis and loss of hair [13].

BARIUM

Barium is found industrially in automotive parts, in paint pigments, and in ceramics and glass. Historically, barium was used extensively in medicine, but because of its severe neurotoxicity, its use has been curtailed. Multiple cases of mass poisoning by food adulteration continue to occur, the most recent in 1964. A profound, often transient, flaccid paralysis develops with respiratory compromise, but sphincter and sensory functions unaffected [19]. The clinical similarity between this presentation and familial periodic paralysis suggests that the pathophysiologies of the two conditions may be related. Low serum potassium has been documented in the patients exposed to barium and resolution of the paralysis follows restitution of normal potassium levels. It is felt that barium acts to enhance intracellular uptake of potassium by red blood cells and hence extracellular depletion of the necessary ion [17].

BISMUTH

Although bismuth is a moderately common metal and frequently obtained as a byproduct of ore processing, neurologic toxicity has only been reported after its use in medicinal compounds. At present, bismuth drugs are used most commonly for gastrointestinal disorders, since the insoluble salts aid in decreasing odor and increasing bulk of bowel movements. Bismuth salts are especially used in patients with colostomies after surgery for colonic carcinoma.

The major neurologic syndrome associated with probable bismuth toxicity is a subacute encephalopathy characterized by confusion, tremulousness, myoclonic jerks and marked dysarthria. Most patients reported have undergone bowel resection and colostomy formation for colonic carcinoma. The encephalopathy is reversible after cessation of bismuth compounds and has been reproduced when bismuth was again administered [3]. The pathophysiology of the syndrome is unclear, but the toxic element appears to be the bismuth itself rather than the accompanying moiety since multiple bismuth compounds have been associated with the syndrome.

In Australia, where highly lipophilic forms of bismuth salts are used, the encephalopathy appears to relate directly to the dose and regularity of bismuth exposure. In France, where less lipophilic salts are used, a direct dose-effect is not clear and secondary changes such as altered gastrointestinal or dietary patterns may play ancillary roles [19]. Biochemical changes studied in experimental animals exposed to bismuth include increases in whole brain dopamine and decreases in hypothalamic noradrenaline [23].

A second neurologic syndrome reported after bismuth therapy has been described only after intramuscular use for systemic disease, usually syphilis. After multiple injections of bismuth compounds, an acute myelopathy has been reported with flaccid paraplegia and loss of bladder control [27]. Animal studies suggest that bismuth may exert a vasoconstrictive effect and the apparent myelopathy may be a vascular ischemic event. No human autopsy material has been studied.

BROMIDES

Medicinal bromides, available as inorganic salts or organic compounds, have been used historically in the treatment of epilepsy and various psychoneuroses. The mechanism of action of bromides remains unknown, but may well relate to a general effect on neuronal membranes rather than a selective alteration of enzyme systems. Abuse or inadvertent intoxication has become less common in the United States since proprietary bromide was removed from the market in 1971. Currently, triple bromide, containing potassium, sodium and chloride salts, is available in the U.S. by prescription.

Following ingestion, bromides are rapidly absorbed into the bloodstream and are distributed to all body organs with only minimal amounts reaching the brain. Bromides appear in all secretions and are present in breast milk in sufficient amounts to affect a nursing infant. Acute poisoning is distinctly uncommon, since doses sufficient to cause acute toxicity induce nausea and vomiting with expulsion of the irritant. Chronic intoxication with bromides, however, is frequently observed and the clinical manifestations of poisoning may be divided into: (1) excessive sedation, 30%, (2) delirium, 65%, and (3) hallucinosis, 5%. Excessive sedation begins at blood bromide levels above 150 mg/dl, and is an accentuation of the medicinal effect. A mild drowsiness develops, associated with loss of concentration and occasional insomnia. In bromide delirium, the patient becomes disoriented, with mood disturbances, delusions and possibly hallucinations. The hallucinatory type of toxicity differs from the delirium in that the hallucinations are experienced in an otherwise lucid setting [13].

Neurologic findings are present in approximately 60% of intoxicated patients and are commonly fluctuating. Tremor, ataxia, autonomic disturbances and eye abnormalities appear as the most frequent abnormalities. The tremor is a fine postural one and is frequently most pronounced in the tongue on extension. As intoxication progresses, speech becomes slurred and gait ataxic, although unlike barbiturate intoxication, limb and trunkal coordination are less compromised. Autonomic disturbances with unexplained fever and cardiac arrhythmias are also common, and eye signs have been a frequent source of diagnostic error. Anisocoria, extraocular palsies and dilated pupils with light/near association are reported and, on occasion, small irregular pupils suggest neurosyphilis. Furred tongue, headache, constipation, digestive disturbances, palpitations, fatigue, masked facies and insomnia have also been attributed to bromide toxicity; however, they cannot be reproduced by experimental intoxication [13].

Two nonneurologic characteristics seem common in patients with bromide toxicity and may help to suggest the diagnosis in confusing cases. The first is a state of general cachexia suggesting some form of chronic disease, neoplasm or vitamin deficiency. The physiologic basis of this picture is unclear, but when evaluation does not reveal an explainable cause for the cachexia, bromide toxicity should be considered. Secondly, skin involvement is present in approximately one-third of cases, usually manifested as an acneiform eruption over the face, arms and upper trunk. Folliculitis or pemphigoid blisters may also appear. Treatment involves the removal of all bromide substances, and the institution of hydration to promote diuresis. One liter of sodium chloride solution may need to be given intravenously every four hours. Diuretics like furosemide (1 mg/kg) will also enhance the excretion of bromide. For chronic intoxication, 2–3 grams of sodium chloride three or four times daily may be given by mouth with at least 4 liters of fluids daily. Ammonium chloride in a dose of 2–3 grams four times daily may be substituted for the sodium chloride if high sodium concentrations are felt undesirable in the patient. Severe psychosis has been managed with 300–500 mg of chlorpromazine daily. Patients with chronic exposure to bromide should be observed for three weeks.

GOLD

Gold is widely distributed in nature and detectable in small quantities in may ores and metals. Medicinal gold products are used in the treatment of arthritis, lupus erythematosis and (rarely) other inflammatory conditions. These salts characteristically have gold attached to a sulfur moiety. Water soluble gold salts are rapidly absorbed after intramuscular injection with therapeutic blood levels occurring within six hours, although there is only erratic gastrointestinal absorption [12]. The general toxicity of the metal includes fever, nausea, vomiting, diarrhea, proteinuria and hematuria, skin rash and blood dyscrasias.

The primary neurologic problem associated with gold is a neuropathy, usually presenting as a symmetric, sensory or sensory-motor distal neuropathy which may be acute or subacute in onset. Alternatively the neuropathy may be characterized by a burning stabbing pain that is transient but of great severity with cutaneous hyperasthesia not confined to any one nerve distribution (*grippe aurique*). Neuropathic changes include both loss of myelin as well as active axonal degeneration. The diagnosis of gold neuropathy may be particularly difficult in patients with rheumatoid arthritis because the disease itself is associated with a well-described neuropathy that may share characteristics similar to those of gold neuropathy [10,14].

Guillain-Barré syndrome and radiculopathies have also been reported in association with gold therapy. Additionally, myokymia has been reported. Most cases involve the extremities (fibrillary chorea of Morvan), but in fact cases involving the face and tongue do occur. The characteristic undulating involuntary movements with discomfort may respond to carbamazepine [21]. In general, myokymia is self-limited to three months after gold therapy is discontinued. It has been suggested that gold may damage terminal motor axons and result in terminal motor neuropathy [21].

MANGANESE

Manganese poisoning results primarily from inhalation of manganese dust in mining and in industry. Exposure occurs in the United States from mills separating manganese from other ore and through its use as an antiknock additive in gasoline. In Chile and India, intoxication occurs chiefly among manganese miners. Manganese is widely used in industry in the manufacture of chlorine gas, storage batteries, paints, varnish, enamel, and linoleum; in glass works for cleaning and coloring molten glass; and for coloring and graining soaps. Workers exposed to the manganese dust both inhale and swallow particles, which are absorbed from the lungs and the gastrointesintal tract.

Toxic symptoms occur in approximately 15 percent of exposed miners and are mostly referable to the extrapyramidal system. They may appear as early as 1½ months after exposure to manganese dust, although there is usually a delay of six to nine months. The onset is usually gradual, with weakness and fatigability increasing until the patient is unable to work. The gait becomes awkward with retropulsion on rising and propulsion on walking. The upper limbs show a similar awkwardness, often associated with a fine tremor of the hands and a gross rhythmic movement of trunk and head. The facial expression becomes fixed and masklike, and the speech faint, monotonous, disjointed, and occasionally unintelligible. Manganese intoxication is part of the differential diagnosis of Parkinson's disease, and if a patient has the exposure history and Parkinsonian signs, a thorough evaluation of metal levels is essential.

Almost all patients show some personality change, consisting of irritability, lack of sociability, uncontrollable laughter, tearfulness, mild euphoria and suspiciousness. Brief emotional explosions may occur during which patients become abusive or even assaultive [7]. If the exposure to manganese continues, mental languor and extreme lack of energy and muscular weakness may occur, and patients frequently fall asleep the minute they sit down, even while at work. Paresthesias have been reported, but no other sensory disturbances occur. Other symptoms and signs include sialorrhea, profuse sweating, impotence, insomnia, hallucinations, terrifying dreams and muscle cramps.

The cerebrospinal fluid may show a mild pleocytosis (up to 15 cells per cubic millimeter). Other laboratory studies are usually within normal limits. The symptoms progress as long as exposure continues, and recovery is rare once a far advanced syndrome develops. The signs and symptoms remain at their maximum for many months after exposure is stopped; however, some improvement may occur. Cotzias and his associates demonstrated that clearance of tissue concentration of manganese did not alleviate neural symptoms [5].

The diagnosis is aided by urinalysis for manganese. Mena and his associates demonstrated that total body loss of injected radioactive manganese was more rapid in healthy miners than in those with manganese poisoning [20]. They interpreted these data to indicate that tissue burdens are larger among healthy miners than among either normal individuals or manganese intoxicated miners.

Because patients with manganese intoxication are usually hypokinetic and rigid, levodopa has been used to help alleviate these symptoms. Patients studied by Mena responded to levodopa doses greater than 3 grams/day with a marked reduction in rigidity, postural reflexes and gait abnormalities as well as bradykinesia. However, no improvement of speech was noted. While on placebo, there was a rapid reappearance of rigidity. The behavioral alteration associated with levodopa therapy included marked mental improvement, and disappearance of fogginess without appearance of euphoria. In those patients with dystonic manifestations of manganese toxicity, levodopa in doses of 4-5 grams/day improved the dystonia and was associated with improvement in daily functional tasks, such as shaving or eating [20].

In the rare hypotonic manganese-intoxicated patient, 5-hydroxytryptophan, the immediate amino acid precursor of serotonin, has been used with success. Doses range from 2.6 to 4.2 grams/day and side effects included somnolence. Traditional chelation therapy has also been attempted in manganese toxic patients without marked success.

Histologic examination of tissues from manganese-intoxicated subjects demonstrates diffuse injury to the ganglion cells involving chiefly the larger cells of the pallidum. Midbrain involvement may also be severe, and damage to the substantia nigra has also been observed. Less severe nerve cell alterations have been described within the rest of the basal nuclei, frontal and parietal cortex, cerebellum, and hypothalamus. Cellular damage and glial proliferation within the corpus striatum and cerebral cortex occurred in rabbits intoxicated experimentally with manganese [22]. Vascular changes were often marked and consisted of vascular thrombi and, frequently, capillary proliferation.

SELENIUM

This unusual metal has been associated with headache, vertigo, convulsions and dermatitis, as well as a chronic motor neuron syndrome similar to amyotrophic lateral sclerosis. This latter syndrome has been reported in 4 ranchers who lived in the United States in an area of high selenium content in the soil. It was suggested that selenium entered the food chain via grasses eaten by grazing animals and eventually meat provoked the motor neuron disease. The causative role of selenium to motor neuron disease is not at all established and is the subject of prospective studies [4]. Selenium levels alter lead absorption so that low dietary selenium enhances lead absorption in animals. Motor neuron disease has also been associated with lead intoxication. As discussed in the chapter on mercury intoxication, selenium also interacts with mercury and can be effectively used to antagonize the acute inorganic mercury intoxication as well as the effects of chronic methyl mercury poisoning. The protective level of selenium is 0.5 ppm; when higher levels are in use, the protective effect of selenium against mercury intoxication is lost, possibly due to the direct toxic effects of selenium itself. These experimental studies from the laboratory have not been directly applied to human toxic situations.

THALLIUM

Poisoning due to thallium is now uncommon. Munch reviewed the literature in 1934 and found records of 778 human poisonings with 46 deaths [354]. Thallitoxicosis has resulted from industrial use, clinical use, from homicidal and suicidal attempts, and through inadvertent use in foods. Industrially, thallium occurs as a waste product in manufacture of sulfuric acid. Thallium acetate has been used clinically in the treatment of dysentery and ringworm, and as a depilatory. Thallium acetate creams have accounted for many cases of thallitoxicosis, since thallium is readily absorbed through the skin. The chief source of thallium in cases of homicide or suicide has been Zelipaste, or "Zelio," a rodent and ant poison containing 2.5 percent thallium sulfate. A few cases have been reported in which thallium sulfate had been accidentally mixed with food and eaten. The lethal dose of thallium in adults is approximately 1.7 g [22].

Recently, thallium poisoning has been implicated as the cause of numerous political poisonings. A 1980 news release by Amnesty International reported political suspects in Iraq poisoned while in custody. Some of these patients, examined and treated in the United Kingdom later, had varied thallium poisoning. It was suspected that thallium was added to the prisoner's food [29].

Like other heavy metals and metalloids, thallium ions have a particular affinity for SH groups, and are capable of binding these groups in many sulfhydryl enzymes and certain proteins. Additionally thallium ions have the capacity to replace potassium ions and may affect systems such as the Na+/K+ ATP-ase. Porphyrin metabolism is also affected as evidenced by the appearance of porphyrins in the urine [28].

Characteristically, thallium toxicity focuses on combined neurologic, gastrointestinal and hair abnormalities. Severe abdominal cramps are often the earliest sign. Alopecia usually is not seen for 2–4 weeks after the acute exposure. This triad of system involvement should suggest thallium poisoning, although additional hepatic and renal disorders can also be seen [29].

Neurologically, the onset of symptoms may be explosive or gradual, depending on the amount of thallium ingested. The earliest symptoms consist of neuritic pains in the extremities, followed by progressive, widespread flaccid paresis or paralysis and even generalized convulsive seizures. The patient may become restless, irritable, mildly confused, and sometimes severely depressed. Often, as the illness progresses, the restlessness is replaced by lethargy and coma. In many cases of chronic or subacute thallotoxicosis, the patients will manifest choreiform movements or myoclonic movements of the extremities and head. A sensory neuropathy similar to that seen with arsenic toxicity may occur, or an ascending weakness that resembles Guillain-Barré syndrome or even polio.

Involvement of the cranial nerves result in ptosis, strabismus, dilated pupils, facial palsies, vocal cord involvement, and optic neuritis with resulting optic atrophy and possible blindness. Vision may fail rapidly and often does not improve much after withdrawal of the thallium. Large scotomas usually remain in recovered cases and are often associated with irregular field defects. The deep reflexes are irregular, and the extensor toe signs may be present. In a few cases, intention tremors develop.

Recovery is uncommon, and prolonged when it does occur. Patients continue to be weak and tired and seem unable to return to a normal state. Striking residuals persist in the form of scattered pareses, visual disturbances, or severe emotional instability.

METALS

Prick described the following common major neuropathologic central nervous sytem findings in thallium toxicity [28]:

1. Ganglion cell changes in the cortex, which are marked in chronic cases, but usually less severe in the more acute than might have been expected with the intensity of the clinical symptoms;
2. Degenerative changes in the ganglion cells throughout the brain stem, and particularly severe alterations in the hypothalamus. In the latter structure, the neurons exhibited granular cytoplasm with numerous large and small vacuoles. The Nissl substance was diminished in quantity and displaced toward the periphery of the cell.
3. White matter lesions consisting, most prominently, of edema and to a lesser degree, demyelination, and axonal degeneration.
4. Mild glial alterations and rather minor involvement of the spinal cord. On light microscopic examination of involved peripheral nerves, some fibers exhibit segmental myelin degeneration.

Electron microscopy of rats experimentally poisoned with thallium revealed many nerve fibers with primary neuroaxonal degeneration accompanied by mitochondrial swelling and prominent phagocytosis.

The diagnosis of thallium intoxication is based on history and urinary excretion levels. Excretion of greater than 10 mg thallium sulfate/24 hours in the urine indicates severe intoxication [25]. Minimal amounts are excreted in the stool so that this latter assay is not of practical use.

Chelating agents such as BAL and diethyl-dithiocarbonate have been employed in the past. The latter agent has been controversial since animal studies demonstrate redistribution of chelated thallium from tissues into the central nervous system with sharp increases in brain concentrations of unbound thallium. Hence, dithiocarbonate is no longer used in acute thallotoxicosis. Prussian blue (potassium ferri-hexacyanoferrate) administered via duodenal tube has been used with success. This agent is a crystal lattic that absorbs thallium ions and is not absorbed gastrointestinally so that thallium is prevented from entering the circulation. It appears to be useful in both acute and chronic toxicity. The colloidal form is most efficacious. A dose of 250 mg/kg/day divided into four doses dissolved in 50 ml of mannitol 15 percent has been used with success, especially in acute intoxication.

Potassium appears to increase the urinary excretion of thallium, either by an inhibitory effect of the ion on the reabsorption of renal tubular thallium or by a potassium-induced displacement of intracellular thallium. However, since Papp et al. [24] noted an increase in the severity of symptoms in thallium-intoxicated patients after potassium administration, this agent must be used extremely cautiously, especially in patients with chronic poisoning. Forced diuresis and hemodialysis have been tried, but are not associated with significant efficacy [30]. Combined hemoperfusion-hemodialysis has also been used with success [9].

ZINC

Zinc is present in sheet metals, dry cell batteries and automotive equipment as well as various alloys like bronze, brass, and German silver. Although zinc is considered a relatively harmless element when compared to other metals, two neurologic syndromes are seen after toxic exposure, one following oral ingestion of zinc sulfate or chloride, the other after inhalation of zinc fumes (Brazier's disease).

Zinc compounds are used medicinally as emetics and astringents. Accidental poisoning of large populations also has occurred after ingestion of acid foods stored in galvanized containers. The syndrome of oral zinc intoxication includes nausea, vomiting, bloody diarrhea, coma and often death, with muscle spasms, weakness and residual dyspnea or lethargy in those surviving [1]. Toxicity has also been reported after an incorrect hyperalimentation formula containing 7.4 g zinc sulfate was infused parenterally.

Zinc inhalation toxicity causes a systemic disease characterized by cough, anorexia, and increasing apathy. Chills and headache develop within hours, accompanied by severe muscle cramps and pains. The victims are often unable to speak and it is unknown whether this disability relates to generalized weakness or specifically to laryngeal dysfunction. These attacks last 10-20 hours and are followed by deep sleep, from which the patient usually awakens with good recovery. While some authors describe a developing immunity to the syndrome after several attacks, others report a chronic irritability, upper extremity coarse intention tremor, incoordination and ataxia that develop after multiple attacks of "zinc fever." Cortical steroids have been recommended in an attempt to reduce the associated inflammatory pulmonary reaction [11].

Hyperzincemia has recently been suggested to play a role in the pathogenesis of anencephaly and spina bifida. Compared to 258 controls, Zimmerman found increasing content in umbilical cord in 8 of 9 newborn anencephalics and 3 infants with spina bifida. Zimmerman suggested that the fetus with neurotube defects receives but does not use zinc normally. These data have led to new caution regarding the use of high vitamin and mineral supplementation in well-nourished pregnant women [32].

SILICON

Although not strictly a metal, this environmental trace element has been the source of recent controversy regarding dementia. Hershey et al. reported

METALS

high CSF levels of the element in patients with clinical Alzheimer-type dementia (ATD), and the same finding in 71% of autopsy-proven Alzheimer's disease cases studied [16]. In a more recent prospective study using both ATD and other dementias, they found elevated silicon in approximately 30% of both groups, but in less than 5% of aged-matched nondemented controls [15]. Whether silicon relates pathogenically to dementia or is only a secondary reflection of neuronal dysfunction is undetermined. Senile plaques of Alzheimer's disease brains contain high concentrations of silicon, but histologically unaffected neurons also appear to accumulate the molecule. Silicon is known to be an essential trace element in many higher species and is required for collagen and glycosaminoglycan formation. Its role in man is unknown.

■ STUDY QUESTIONS

Match the toxin with its clinical presentation:
1. 58-year-old black woman with chronic renal failure on dialysis who develops progressive dementia, myoclonus, and gait disturbance.
2. A patient from Europe with a colostomy who develops tremor, confusion and dysarthria.
3. A thirty-year-old American Indian with rheumatoid arthritis and a new burning dysesthesia that comes and goes in the left leg, associated with hyperesthesias in that area.
4. A South American immigrant with parkinsonism.
5. Myokymia

A. Manganese
B. Bismuth
C. Gold
D. Aluminum
E. None

Answers: 1-D; 2-B; 3-C; 4-A; 5-C

Dialysis dementia has been suggested to relate to aluminum toxicity. The syndrome as described above includes progressive decline in mental function, walking difficulties, and myoclonic jerks. Bismuth encephalopathy is seen predominantly in Australia, Oceania, and Europe, where bismuth is used after colostomies and to treat gastrointestinal disorders. Patients with rheumatoid arthritis are often exposed to gold and may develop a neuropathy associated with this treatment. The fact that the patient in this case is an American Indian has no bearing on the toxicity. The patient from South America with parkinsonism may well have been exposed to manganese from Chilean or Peruvian mining industries. Myokymia has classically been associated with gold toxicity and is not seen with the other metals in the list.

Other Metals

True statements regarding manganese toxicity include:

1. Mental changes are not typical
2. Abnormal involuntary movements without weakness are characteristic
3. Manganese toxicity clinically resembles multiple sclerosis
4. Treatment with levodopa has been useful

Answers: 2 & 4

Almost all patients with established manganese toxicity show some personality change, consisting of irritability, suspiciousness, or emotional explosions. Extrapyramidal signs in the form of parkinsonism or sometimes chorea are typical and patients usually are not weak. There are rare instances of patients with an amyotrophic lateral sclerosis syndrome presenting with upper motor neuron signs that may relate to manganese exposure. These cases, however, would never be considered typical. As such, manganese toxicity clinically resembles Parkinson's disease, but does not resemble multiple sclerosis where weakness and prominent sensory abnormalities and often visual disturbances are common. Levodopa is useful in managing patients with chronic manganese toxicity and may significantly alter the patient's ability to function and his level of independence.

Which statements are true in regard to factors that might help separate a case of thallium poisoning from arsenic intoxication?

1. Only arsenic is associated with seizures
2. Only thallium has significant gastrointestinal disturbances
3. Only thallium is associated with alopecia
4. With thallium, a sensory neuropathy is typical and with arsenic a motor neuropathy is common

Answer: 3

Both arsenic and thallium may be associated with seizures. Similarly, both demonstrate dramatic gastrointestinal disturbances with explosive vomiting and severe abdominal pain. Hair is important to the accurate diagnosis of both toxins, but in completely different manners; with arsenic, analysis of the hair will document the deposition of the metal, while with thallium, clinical loss of hair, or alopecia, is the typical sign. In both arsenic and thallium intoxication, a sensory neuropathy or motor-sensory is typical. A pure motor neuropathy with arsenic would be most unlikely.

A patient with rheumatoid arthritis treated with gold and penicillamine developed a progressive glove-and-stocking sensory motor neuropathy over six months. Her specific complaints are numbness and tingling of the hands and feet and the neurologic examination demonstrates diffusely decreased reflexes. Which of the following could explain her neuropathy?

1. Rheumatoid arthritis
2. Gold therapy
3. Penicillamine therapy

4. The precipitant that results when gold and penicillamine are combined together

Answers: 1, 2, 3

Rheumatoid arthritis is associated with a symmetric sensory or sensory-motor distal neuropathy that may be acute or subacute in onset. Similarly, gold therapy can provoke a polyneuropathy. Penicillamine, when not administered with pyridoxine, has in some instances been associated with a sensory motor distal neuropathy. No precipitants have been described with the combination of gold and penicillamine, so that the final answer (4) is not correct.

A 60-year-old cachetic woman is brought for evaluation by her family for progressive mental alterations over six months. She is irritable, poorly cooperative, and the family says she sometimes hallucinates and sleeps for long periods of time. She has a fine postural tremor, has occasional myoclonic jerks, and slurred speech with ataxia. A marked acneiform rash is seen across her face.

An evaluation of progressive dementia is initiated that includes a lumbar puncture, a computerized tomography scan of the brain, thyroid test, electrolytes and blood counts, and a drug screen. Which of the following would be reasonable conclusions in this patient?

1. Bromide toxicity should be considered here in light of the acneiform rash and curious mental alterations with tremor and ataxia.
2. Gold intoxication is reasonable here because of the prominent sedation.
3. Bismuth intoxication is reasonable here, especially in light of the myoclonus.
4. Thallium toxicity is suggested by the skin rash and tremor.

Answers: 1, 3

Elderly patients often still are able to obtain bromide products as general tonics. The acneiform skin rash is a clue to the possibility of bromide intoxication, and the clinical picture certainly fits this cause. However, of course there are other possible etiologies to this patient's progressive mental alteration, and a full evaluation is in order. Gold intoxication is not reasonable, since it does not provoke a marked encephalopathy, but instead a significant peripheral neuropathy. Bismuth intoxication causes confusion and myoclonic encephalopathy, so it is reasonable if the patient has gastrointestinal disease and received bismuth salts. Arsenic poisoning presents with prominent gastrointestinal problems and peripheral neuropathy; acute intoxication without vomiting would not suggest arsenic intoxication.

■ REFERENCES

1. Brown MA, Thom JV, Orth GH, Cova P, Juarez J.: Food poisoning involving zinc contamination. Eur. Health 8:657–62, 1964.
2. Buge A, Poisson M, Masson S, Bleibel JM, Lafforgue B, Raymond P, Jaudon

MC: Encéphalopathie prolongée et réversible chez un dialysé chronique. Nouv. Presse Med. 7:2053, 1978.
3. Burns R, Thomas DW, Barron VJ: Reversible encephalopathy possibly associated with bismuth subgallate ingestion. Br. Med. J. 1:220-223, 1974.
4. Cotzias GC, Horiuchi K, Fuenzalida S, Mena I: Chronic manganese poisoning. Neurology 18:376-382, 1968.
5. Crapper DR, Krishnan SS, Quittkat S: Aluminum, neurofibrillary degeneration and Alzheimer's disease. Brain 99:67-81, 1976.
6. Davies TA, Harding HE: Manganese pneumonitis. Brit. J. Ind. Med. 6:82, 1949.
7. Day AT, Godking JR, Penicillamine in rheumatoid arthritis. Br. Med. J. 3:593-4, 1973.
8. Demarcy JM: Reflexions á propos d'une encéphalopathie myoclonique des dialysées. Nour. Presse Med. 11:456, 1982.
9. Dreisbach RH: Handbook of Poisoning, 6th Ed. Los Altos, Lange, 1969.
10. Freyberg RH: Gold therapy for rheumatoid arthritis. In, JL Hollander, ed., Arthritis and Allied Concitions, 7th ed. Philadelphia, Lea and Febiger, 1966.
11. Goetz CG, Klawans HL, Cohen MM: Neurotoxic Agents. In, AB Baker and CH Baker, Clinical Neurology, Harper and Row, Philadelphia, 1-84, 1981.
12. Hart FD, Golding JR: Rheumatoid neuropathy. Br. Med. J. 1:1594, 1960.
13. Josse M, Cerf JA, Hulin G: Effects of barium ions on the resting membrane potential of frog striated muscle fibers. Life Sci. 4:77-81, 1965.
14. Lagier G: Encephalopathies bismuthiques. Therapie 35:315-317, 1980.
15. Lewi Z, Bar-Khayim Y: Food poisoning from barium carbonate. Lancet 2: 342-343, 1964.
16. Mena I, Horiuchi K, Burke K, Cotzias GC: Chronic manganese poisoning. Neurology 19:1000-1002, 1969.
16a. Milliner DS, Shinaberger JH, Shuman P, Caburn JW: Inadvertent aluminum administration during plasma exchange due to aluminum contamination of albumin replacement solution. N. Engl. J. Med. 312, 165-167, 1985.
17. Mitsumoto H, Wilbourn AJ, Subramony SH: Generalized myokymia and gold therapy. Arch. Neurol. 39:449-450, 1982.
18. Munch JC: Human thallotoxicosis. JAMA 102:1929, 1934.
19. Olive G: Recherches menées par l'INSERM sur les encephalopathies myocloniques provoquées par les sels insolubles de bismuth. Therapie 35:305-306, 1980.
20. Papp JP, Gay PC, Dodson VN: Potassium chloride treatment in thallotoxicosis. Am. Intern. Med. 71:119-120, 1969.
21. Paulson G, Vergara G, Young J: Thallium intoxication treated with dithizon and hemodialysis. Arch. Intern. Med. 129:100-103, 1972.
22. Penalver R: Manganese poisoning. Ind. Med. Surg. 24:1-17, 1955.
23. Poilpre E, Morin P, Turpin J: Paraplegie provoquee par une injection intramusculaire de bismuth. Presse Med. 76:2013-2018, 1968.
24. Prick JJG: Thallium poisoning. In, PJ Vinken and GW Bruyn, eds., Hand-

book of Clinical Neurology, Vol. 36, North-Holland Publishing Co., Amsterdam, pp. 239–278, 1979.
25. Rasmussen OV: Thallium poisoning: an aspect of human cruelty. Lancet 1: 1164–1165, 1981.
26. Thompson DFL: Management of thallium poisoning. Clin. Toxicol. 18:979–990, 1981.
27. Troncoso JC, Price DL, Griffin JW, Parhad IM: Neurofibrillary axonal pathology in aluminum intoxication. Ann. Neurol. 12:278–283, 1982.
28. DeBacker W, Zachee P, Verpooten GA: Thallium Intoxication treated with combined hemoperfusion-hemodialysis. J. Toxicol. Clin. Toxicol. 19:259–64, 1982.
29. Zimmerman AW: Hyperzincemia and anencephaly and spina bifida: a clue to the pathogenesis of neurotube defects? Neurology (1984) 34:443–50.
30. Conradi S, Ronnevi LO, Norris FH: Motor neuron disease and toxic metals. In, Rolland LP, editor, Human Motor Neuron Diseases, Raven Press, New York, 1982. Advances in Neurology Vol. 36. 201–232.

II.
Industrial Toxins

CHAPTER 5

Organic Solvents

With the development of the plastic and chemical industries, organic solvents have exposed large segments of the population to potential toxic compounds. These products are easily available, and can lead to significant neurotoxicity when used in the improper setting. Inadvertent exposure occurs as well as volitional abuse of solvents primarily by inhalation.

Two properties are characteristic of all neurotoxic organic solvents, their liposolubility and their high volatility. The first influences not only the anatomic distribution of the toxins to organs rich in lipids (brain and adrenals), but also metabolism. In general, these lipid-soluble products are eliminated through the kidneys after several breakdown reactions to render them more water soluble. These reactions may give rise to additional compounds sometimes more toxic than the parent chemical. Volatility influences the quantity of solvents in the air and dictates the respiratory system as the primary means of initial absorption.

In spite of their wide diversity, solvents as a group precipitate a constellation of clinical abnormalities that usually help to identify the patient as a likely victim of organic solvent toxicity. Often the implicated substance (e.g., paint thinner) is in fact a mixture of several organic solvents and thus no single chemical can be definitively implicated. Hence, the first section of this chapter focuses on problems seen in patients exposed to nonspecified or mixed organic solvents: their clinical presentation, treatment and long-term prognosis. Separate discussions follow that focus on individual toxic products. Because the number of such products is growing rapidly and their control is not significantly regulated by government, industry, or the community, the discussion of these various toxins is representative, but not exhaustive. In Table 5.1 the occupations at high risk for organic solvent intoxication are listed. In Table 5.2, the threshold limit values for airborne concentrations of organic solvent neurotoxins are given.

INDUSTRIAL TOXINS

TABLE 5.1. Occupations and Job-Related Sources of Organic Solvent Intoxication

	Methyl alcohol	Ethylene glycol	Formaldehyde	Amyl alcohol	Isopropyl alcohol	Acetone	Benzene	Toluene	N-Hexane	MBK	Gasoline	Turpentine	TCE	Tetrachloroethane	Carbon tetrachloride
Airplane hangars	X						X				X				X
Alcohol distillation (brewing)	X		X	X			X								
Antifreeze	X	X													
Artificial flowers	X						X								
Artificial leathers	X					X									
Artificial pearls	X					X									
Automobile painting	X						X								
Automobile manufacturers and repair							X				X				
Bookbinding	X														
Brass and bronze	X														
Cement-plastic mixing						X	X				X				
Can sealing							X								
Cosmetics				X	X										
Degreasing and scouring						X	X	X			X		X	X	X
Dry cleaning	X						X		X	X		X	X	X	X
Disinfectants			X			X	X						X		
Dyes	X		X			X	X					X	X		X

66

Organic Solvents

Industry																						
Enamels	x																x	x		x		
Etching	x	x															x	x	x				
Explosives	x	x	x															x					
Feathers	x																x						
Fertilizers					x																		
Fire extinguishers	x							x									x	x	x	x	x	x	
Furniture polish			x					x		x							x	x	x	x	x	x	
Fuel (airplane, auto)									x										x				
Glass	x																x	x	x				
Glue					x			x		x							x	x	x	x			
Insecticides								x										x	x				
Insulators			x	x	x			x		x							x	x	x	x	x	x	x
Lacquer	x	x	x	x	x			x		x								x	x	x	x	x	x
Leather-tannery goods	x		x		x			x														x	
Linoleum	x			x				x									x	x	x		x	x	
Millinery (hats)	x			x				x		x							x	x	x				
Metal cleaners, polishers	x					x		x										x			x	x	
Paints	x			x				x		x							x	x	x	x	x	x	x
Paper workers	x				x			x															
Perfumes			x		x			x											x	x	x	x	
Pharmaceuticals					x			x									x	x	x	x	x	x	x
Painting-lithography	x			x				x									x		x				
Plastics	x		x		x			x									x	x	x	x	x	x	x
Rayon	x				x			x											x		x	x	
Refineries (petroleum)					x	x		x									x	x	x	x			

(continued)

INDUSTRIAL TOXINS

TABLE 5.1 (Continued)

	Methyl alcohol	Ethylene glycol	Formaldehyde	Amyl alcohol	Isopropyl alcohol	Acetone	Benzene	Toluene	N-Hexane	MBK	Gasoline	Turpentine	TCE	Tetrachloroethane	Carbon Tetrachloride
Rubber	×		×			×	×	×	×	×		×	×	×	×
Shoe manufacture and repair	×			×		×	×					×	×	×	×
Soaps, detergents	×		×				×						×	×	
Tobacco		×					×						×		
Vegetable oil extraction									×	×			×		
Waterproofing			×				×								
Wax							×					×	×	×	×
Welding							×								

68

Organic Solvents

TABLE 5.2. Safety Threshold Limit Values of Airborne Concentrations for Various Organic Solvent Neurotoxins

	Time-weighted average		Short-term exposure limit	
	ppm	mg/m^3	ppm	mg/m^3
Methyl Alcohol	200	260	250	310
Ethylene Glycol Vapor	100	250	125	325
Amyl Alcohol	—	—	—	—
Isopropyl Alcohol	400	980	500	1,225
Ethylene Oxide	50	90	75	135
Acetone	1,000	2,400	1,250	3,000
Benzene	10	30	—	—
Toluene	100	375	150	560
N-Hexane	100	360	125	450
MBK	25	100	40	165
Gasoline*				
Turpentine	100	560	150	840
TCE	100	535	150	800
Tetrachlorethane	100	670	150	1,000
Carbon Tetrachloride	10	65	20	130

Threshold limit values for chemical substances in workroom airs adopted by ACGIH for 1978.
*The composition of gasoline varies so greatly that a single threshold limit value cannot be determined.

■ SOLVENT MIXTURES

Table 5.3 lists various common solvent mixtures involved in solvent abuse and their constituents. Exposure to these agents can be occupational and related directly to the work area, or volitional. Volitional practices include placing a solvent in a plastic bag and inhaling the fumes, soaking a rag or handkerchief with the solvent and sniffing the rag (huffing), sniffing the solvent directly from the container, or more inventive practices, such as using perfume sprayers, filling bathtubs with solvents and locking the bathroom door, or heating the product to enhance vapor concentrations [2]. Organs in addition to the nervous system that are affected by organic solvents include the skin and mucous membranes, as well as the digestive, hepatic, and renal systems.

Below, two major neurotoxic syndromes are described in patients exposed to organic solvents, a peripheral neuropathy and an encephalopathy. The former usually occurs after chronic exposure; encephalopathic symptoms may occur acutely or after chronic use. Myopathy and cerebellar symptoms, also described in patients exposed to organic solvents, are less common than the other two syndromes; they are also described below.

TABLE 5.3. Products Involved in Solvent Abuse and Principal Constituents

Products	Main solvents
Aerosols	Dichlorodifluoromethane (Propellant 12), trifluoromethane, isobutane
Fingernail polish	Acetone, aliphatic acetates, benzene, alcohol
Gasoline	Mixture of petroleum hydrocarbons, paraffins, olefins, naphthenes, and aromatics (chiefly benzene, toluene, and xylenes) and tetra-ethyl lead.
Household cements	Toluene, acetone, isopropanol, methyl ethyl ketone, methyl isobutyl ketone
Lacquer thinners	Toluene, aliphatic acetates, methyl, ethyl, or propyl alcohol
Lighter fluid and cleaning fluid	Naphtha, perchlorethylene, carbon tetrachloride, trichlorethane
Model cements	Acetone, toluene, naphtha
Plastic cements	Toluene, acetone, aliphatic acetates (ethyl acetate, methyl-cellosolve acetate, etc.)
Typewriter correction fluid	Trichlorethane, trichlorethylene
Paint strippers	Methylene chloride

Clinical Features

Neuropathy

A progressive and often insidious symmetric neuropathy, involving both sensory and motor systems, occurs in patients exposed to mixed organic solvents. Prior to the development of clinical neuropathy or subjective complaints, objective evidence of neuropathy may often be detected. In one Scandinavian study, asymptomatic car-garage workers and painters were exposed over prolonged periods to low levels of solvent fumes. In these subjects, who did not have specific neurologic complaints, nerve condition velocities were prolonged and clinical evidence of neuropathy could be detected. These findings suggest that even at low levels, organic solvents may compromise peripheral nervous system function [33].

Huffer's neuropathy was described in patients who soaked rags with solvents, sniffed the rags, and developed a severe and predominantly motor neuropathy after several months or years of exposure. Weakness involved both proximal and distal muscles, the muscles of respiration and even facial expression. Some patients required respiratory support. Areflexia was the general rule, although sensory loss was mild. Most patients showed improvement in motor function after exposure ceased, but many showed persisting deficits.

Electromyographic studies demonstrated severely slowed conduction velocities and signs of acute denervation. Pathologic examination of sural nerves in patients with Huffer's neuropathy demonstrated depletion of myelinated axons and thinning of the myelin sheaths [25]. The single or multiple synergistic agents responsible for Huffer's neuropathy remain undetermined; analysis of the original implicated laquer thinner included xylene, 2-heptanone, acetone, isobutyl acetate and toluene [30].

Encephalopathy

Reversible mental changes are seen in subjects who volitionally inhale organic solvents and in workers who are exposed during the day and develop symptoms, but who recover when they return home. Wyse has described four stages in the development of acute mental symptoms associated with the inhalation of hydrocarbon mixtures [41]. Initially, there is euphoria, excitation, and a pleasant exhilaration. Dizziness and mild nausea may occur and occasionally hallucinations and bizarre behavior. This is the desired level of intoxication in those who volitionally inhale, although further intoxication may lead to more significant and dangerous encephalopathy. The second stage is early central nervous system depression with symptoms of confusion, loss of self-control, cramps and headache. Later, further CNS depression causes ataxia, slurred speech, and somnolence. In the fourth stage of late CNS depression the patient sleeps most of the time and may lapse into a coma. In addition, inhaling organic solvents can be fatal; over 110 sudden sniffing deaths occurred during the period of 1960–1970 that were not attributed to suffocation [4].

Chronic encephalopathic symptoms are predominantly exceptional fatigue, concentrational difficulties, impaired memory, and sleep disruption [15]. In multiple studies, these features have consistently been reported. In specific psychological tasks, impairment of verbal memory and visual intelligence has been reported, along with slowed emotional reactivity. The long-term prognosis of such mental changes in solvent-exposed subjects has been studied in two detailed studies. In 80 patients, followed for a mean of 5.8 years after initial chronic solvent encephalopathy was diagnosed, subjective symptoms of headache, tiredness and memory disturbances tended to wane, although objective clinical signs of CNS dysfunction in fact progressed [16].

In addition to these psychometric alterations, personality changes have also been described in patients exposed chronically to organic solvents [23]. In another long-term follow up of 26 encephalopathic house painters, patients demonstrated little change in neurological examinations, neuropsychological or neuroradiological alterations 2 years after solvent encephalopathy was diagnosed. Symptoms of headache and dizziness, however, were generally reported to be improved. These studies together suggest that long-term exposure to organic solvents may lead to a chronic irreversible encephalopathy where intellectual impairment remains. The progression of neurologic signs seen in the first studies cited was not seen in the latter group [7]. This difference may relate to the fact that in the first study, some patients continued to work in the solvent environment but in the second study all patients were removed from the implicated environment at the time of original diagnosis. The CT scan in patients with chronic solvent encephalopathy revealed diffuse cerebral atrophy.

Autopsy material from patients exposed to mixed organic solvents is rare. A recent detailed study of a single patient addicted to glue sniffing and thinner inhalation disclosed diffuse cerebral and cerebellar cortex atrophy and giant axonopathy centrally and peripherally. The corpus callosum was also atrophic secondary to neuronal loss in the neocortex [9].

Myopathy and Cerebellar Signs

Myopathy, characterized by an increase in creatinine kinase activity, may underlie some of the fatigue symptoms so characteristic of patients exposed to mixed organic solvents. Such patients often complain of exercise intolerance, arthralgias and muscle tenderness [28]. In animals exposed to solvents, CK elevations are induced and muscle necrosis occurs. Cerebellar dysfunction manifested as a fine action tremor, slurred speech and ataxia, may also be long-term sequelae of patients exposed to organic solvents. These symptoms may improve after the patient has left the exposed environment, although in the Scandinavian follow-up study reported above, disturbances of gait and station progressed over time. Some of this progression may relate to the natural aging of the population studied [16].

Practical Management

The only treatment for those patients chronically exposed to organic solvents is to remove them from the environment. In those patients suffering with acute oral poisoning by organic solvents, treatment with activated charcoal in combination with laxatives has been recommended.

Additional Components in Mixed Solvents

Of the many solvent mixtures associated with neurotoxic syndromes, special mention must be made of gasoline, since victims of gasoline exposure are subject to organic solvent neurotoxicity, as well as tetraethyl lead. The composition of gasoline (benzine, petrol) is extremely varied. Originally it was composed largely of butanes, hexanes and pentanes, but various other hydrocarbons have since been added. Tetraethyl lead is present in most gasolines because of its anti-knock

Organic Solvents

qualities and triorthocresyl phosphate has occasionally been used as an additive. Gasoline is extensively employed in industry as a motor fuel, solvent, and cleaning agent. Intoxication has resulted from inhalation of the vapor in industry, from the use of gasoline to wash hair, from aspiration during siphoning, and from sniffing this substance by abusers. Poisoning also follows the use of gasoline to remove plastics from the skin.

With the inhalation of toxic qualities, symptoms appear rapidly and are often accentuated by exposure to the open air. Milder intoxications produce the typical "naphtha jag," with lack of self-control, inebriation, blurred vision, incoordination, confusion, excitement and, occasionally, delirium with visual hallucinations. These symptoms are followed by depression, headache, lethargy, roaring in the ears, trembling, staggering, a sensation of heaviness, nausea, burning in the chest and a feeling of irritation and constriction in the throat. In severe cases, the symptoms progress to dyspnea, cyanosis, convulsions and, in some instances, death within 10 minutes to four hours. In the less serious cases, recovery is followed by an alcohollike "hangover." A number of symptoms may persist following recovery, including irritability, headache, speech disturbances, dyspnea, gastrointestinal disturbances, chest pain, syncope, peripheral neuritis and, in some instances, seizures, ataxia and dementia [39]. With oral ingestion of gasoline, the symptoms of local irritation of the intestinal tract are added to the systemic effects.

With prolonged exposure, inattention, irritability, and change in personality may develop. Hallucinations, myoclonus and dysmetria with poor coordination and ataxia may also occur [13]. Pallor, weight loss and insomnia may also follow. The diagnosis of gasoline/tetraethyl lead toxicity depends on an exposure history. Biochemical measurements are helpful but not always diagnostic. Laboratory values, including urinary delta amino levulinic acid, coproporphyrin, and erythrocyte protoporphyrin, may vary. These findings contrast with inorganic lead poisoning, where these values are consistently increased. No close correlation exists between blood lead levels and the severity of intoxication, making it always difficult to ascertain whether it is the organic solvent or the lead that is provoking the toxic syndrome. In children with inorganic lead toxicity, and the presentation of an encephalopathy, ataxia and myoclonus are not typical problems.

Autopsy findings in one patient with a progressive chronic encephalopathy related to gasoline-sniffing showed cerebellar cortex atrophy and gliosis in subcortical structures; the cerebral cortex was normal. The central nervous system damage in this case was attributed to the toxic effects of organic lead.

The treatment of gasoline encephalopathy is removal of the patient from the source of poisoning. Chelation has been used successfully, and is associated with clinical improvement and lower serum lead concentrations [13,39]. If the gasoline has been swallowed, the stomach should be lavaged with olive oil or mineral oil. Treatment of lead toxicity is discussed in detail in Chapter 1.

INDUSTRIAL TOXINS

Metal impurities are also present in many aerosols, and pulmonary dysfunction related to non-solvent contamination may underlie other medical complications seen in these toxin-exposed patients.

▪ SPECIFIC ORGANIC SOLVENTS

METHYL ALCOHOL

Methyl alcohol (methanol, wood alcohol) is used as a solvent, a combusible, a component of antifreeze, and as an adulterant of alcoholic beverages. Although the compound itself is only mildly toxic, its oxidation products, formaldehyde and formic acid, induce a severe acidosis and account for the signs related to methanol abuse [31].

No specific pathologic changes have been reported with acute fatal intoxication. The most constant findings include brain edema with prominent meningeal and subarachnoid petichiae. Severe degenerative changes occur within the ganglion cells of the retina [14].

The amount of methyl alcohol causing serious effects varies with the individual. Some of this variation is attributed to a protecting effect that ethyl alcohol may exert when consumed together with methanol. The two compounds share the same degrading enzyme, alcohol dehydrogenase, so that this competition by ethanol tends to diminish the rapid production of toxic formaldehyde and formic acid. In general, the oxidation and excretion of methyl alcohol is so slow that toxic symptoms do not develop for 12-48 hours and may last for several days. When toxic symptoms and signs do appear, they involve the visual apparatus, the central nervous system and the gastrointestinal and respiratory tracts. Clinical toxicity relates to metabolic acidosis as well as to the direct effects of accumulation of toxic products. Early there is nausea, vomiting, generalized weakness, severe abdominal pain, vertigo, and headache. Symptoms similar to ethyl alcoholism appear, with restlessness, incoordination, and, at times, delirium, and hallucinations. Confusion and memory defects are common.

With increasing severity of poisoning, stupor, coma, tonic muscle contractions, hyperactive reflexes, opisthotonos, and generalized convulsions may occur. Uncommon symptoms, such as hyposmia, dysdiadochokinesia, unilateral deviation of the tongue, involvement of the sixth, seventh, and eighth cranial nerves, and apoplexy have been reported. In the more severe cases, death occurs from respiratory failure.

Visual disturbance and ocular manifestations are frequent with methanol poisoning. Visual loss may commence a few hours after consumption of the alcohol or be delayed several days. Amblyopia, scotomas, or total blindness occurs in most cases and may be the first disturbance noted. The pupils may be dilated and nonreactive to light. Ocular pain is common. Ophthalmoscopic examination may reveal injection of the disks with blurring of the margins and pericapillary and macular edema. After three to six weeks, pallor of the optic disks may be noted. The vision may improve with recovery from the acute intoxication, but permanent central scotomas or total blindness often result. Profound nuchal rigidity may be present along with coma, resembling an acute meningitis. The prognosis in these cases is extremely unfavorable. The electrocardiogram may show evidence of ischemic change or arrhythmia.

In animals with methanol toxicity, leakage of fluorescein from retinal blood vessels occurs similarly to patients with raised intracranial pressure. In monkey studies, when formic acid is given to the animals, the same gross and light-microscope changes in the visual system are seen as when methanol is administered. At least for the visual system, the toxicity of methanol appears to relate directly to formic acid [14]. The acid decreases cytochrome oxidase activity and causes a reduction in adenosine triphosphate (ATP) levels. Three major effects then follow: swelling of oligodendrocytes with axonal compression, stasis of transport (and optic disc edema clinically), and a decrease in Na, K-ATPase with a resultant decrease in electrical activity and visual function.

In addition to blindness, another sequela is parkinsonlike extrapyramidal syndrome characterized by bradykinesia, low voice volume, masked facies, mild tremor and rigidity. Dementia and additional motor signs, which may include increased reflexes (upper motor neuron disease) or decreased reflexes (lower motor neuron disease), may occur. In two patients with a parkinsonlike syndrome, computerized tomographic scans showed bilateral symmetric infarctions of the frontal, central white matter and putamen. One of these brains was examined at autopsy and cystic degeneration of the putamen and subcortical white matter were seen in addition to widespread neuronal damage in the brainstem and spinal cord. The prominent putaminal necrosis seen in these patients may relate to decreased venous outflow through the veins of Rosenthal, or relate to a possible accumulation of formic acid and formaldehyde preferentially within the putamen. Levodopa when given to the more severely affected of these two patients had no effect on the parkinsonian features [24].

A three-part approach to treatment has been developed and involves the use of ethanol, bicarbonate and, in severe cases, dialysis. Frequent measurements of methanol, CO_2, bicarbonate and pH levels in the blood are essential. Ethyl alcohol administration saturates the alcohol dehydrogenase enzyme and thereby retards the conversion of methanol into its toxic byproducts (formaldehyde and formic acid). Massive and rapid alkalinization (approximately 3mEq bicarbonate/kg body weight) may be necessary to correct severe acidosis. Since methanol metabolism is slow, alkalinization must be carried out for several days to avoid relapses. Attention must be paid to the level of serum potassium, which tends to drop with bicarbonate therapy. Finally, dialysis has been advocated when the methanol blood concentration is over 50 mg%. Both peritoneal and hemodialysis have been successful, the latter being more rapid [21].

ETHYLENE GLYCOL

Ethylene glycol is commonly used as an antifreeze for automobile and airplane motors. It is also employed as a tobacco moistener, a softener for lacquers, a solvent for fruit essences, and as a constituent in the manufacture of explosives. Numerous instances of toxicity, some fatal, have resulted from drinking ethylene glycol as an inebriant.

The toxic dose approximates 100 cc and ingestion of larger doses has been associated with death usually on a renal or cardiopulmonary basis. Ingestion of this solvent results in 40 to 60 deaths per year [38].

Symptoms of toxicity may appear early or may be delayed for hours. Initially, the patient becomes restless and agitated. This is soon followed by somnolence, stupor, coma and even convulsions [29]. Death results from respiratory or cardiac failure. The patient is usually cyanotic, the pupils fail to react to light, and the corneal reflexes may be absent. Aducens and soft palate paralysis, aphasia, nystagmus, and fecal and urinary incontinence have been observed [5].

In patients who have died within 72 hours of ingestion of ethylene glycol, there is cerebral edema, vascular engorgement and hemorrhage and evidence of chemical meningoencephalitis.

Ethylene glycol poisoning should be strongly suspected when an apparently inebriated patient has no alcohol on the breath, where coma is associated with a metabolic acidosis and a large anion gap, and prominent calcium oxylate crystals are found in the urinalysis. Laboratory confirmation with ethylene glycol and oxylate acid levels may follow. Other laboratory abnormalities include an elevated white blood cell count, elevated serum potassium, and a cerebral spinal fluid demonstrating increased white blood cells, elevated protein, and usually a normal glucose level.

Ethylene glycol itself appears to be nontoxic. It does not affect respiration, the citric acid cycle, or other biochemical pathways until it is metabolized. The intermediate compounds that result from hepatic and renal metabolism include aldehydes and oxalate, which account for most of the toxicity. Aldehydes inhibit oxidative phosphorylation, respiration and glucose metabolism, as well as protein synthesis and DNA replication. These compounds reach their maximum concentration at the time of cerebral symptoms, 6–12 hours after the ingestion of the ethylene glycol. Oxalate damages renal tissue, which may induce acidosis. The product chelates calcium ions producing hypocalcemia, and the resultant calcium oxalate may further obstruct renal tubules. Calcium oxalate crystals may also be deposited in the brain and meninges, inducing cellular reaction, although in animals given small doses of ethylene glycol, no CNS symptoms develop in spite of the dense cerebral oxalate deposition. Such studies suggest that oxalate crystals are not of great significance to central toxic symptoms. Lactic acid is also formed during the breakdown of ethylene glycol.

Treatment consists chiefly of symptomatic measures, respiratory support and careful monitoring of the cardiovascular status. Metabolic acidosis must be corrected. Animal work has shown that correction of acidosis with sodium bicarbonate increases survival. Parry and Wallach [27] confirmed that the correction of acidosis in humans improves survival, although the depth of coma in individual patients may not immediately change. Hypocalcemia must be corrected. As in methyl alcohol toxicity, ethyl alcohol infusion reaching 5-10 grams per hour may be useful, since the two substances compete for the same enzyme, alcohol dehydrogenase [27]. If this infusion is to be effective, it should be initiated as soon as possible, since the half-life of ethylene glycol is only about three hours in humans. The desired blood alcohol level is between 100 and 200 mg/dl. Early dialysis will remove the ethylene glycol and at the same time treat the uremia that often accompanies toxic ingestion. Oxalate is dialyzable and aldehyde derivatives may also be removed in this way. Peterson et al. used hemodialysis and nasogastric ethanol infusion (20%) keeping the ethanol infusion rate at 237 mg/kg/hr during dialysis, and thereafter adjusted to maintain the above-noted levels [29].

Hypocalcemia may produce mild tetanic spasms. These must be differentiated from seizure activity, which may be focal or generalized. If the treating physician encounters the patient within minutes or an hour, lavage is reasonable, but since the glycol is readily and rapidly absorbed from the stomach, lavage is useless afterwards.

FORMALDEHYDE (See Methyl Alcohol)

AMYL ALCOHOL

Amyl alcohol is utilized in lacquers, solvents and ore flotation reagents, in the manufacture of amyl acetate and smokeless powder, and in the preparation of certain drugs and pharmaceuticals. It is also known as fusel oil, grain oil, potato spirits, and amyl hydroxide.

Acute intoxication occasionally results from the consumption of amyl alcohol. Initially, there is headache, dizziness, nausea, vomiting and diarrhea, followed by delirium, coma and even death. Sleeplessness, psychomotor overactivity, and changing chromatopsia have been observed following inhalation of the fumes. Chronic exposure to this solvent may produce giddiness, disturbances of smell and taste, diplopia, trembling, insomnia, delirium, and other psychic manifestations. Somnolence progression to stupor and death may develop in the more severe cases. Treatment for acute or chronic intoxication is symptomatic. The stomach should be lavaged if amyl alcohol has been ingested.

ISOPROPYL ALCOHOL

This alcohol is a solvent for certain resins and is used in the manufacture of perfumes, cosmetics, safety glass, varnishes, and lacquers. In home and hospital medical care, it is commonly used as a rubbing alcohol and in tepid sponges to reduce elevated body temperatures. The toxicity and narcotic effect is about twice that of ethyl alcohol. Acute intoxication may follow oral ingestion or the inhalation of vapors. In children, toxicity has been reported following alcohol sponge baths. With acute isopropyl alcohol intoxication, dizziness and headache occur, followed by ataxia, depression, and narcosis. In severe cases, there may be paralysis, dyspnea, coma, and death. Treatment is supportive and hemodialysis has been used with good results following ingestion of large amounts [12].

Isopropyl alcohol has a longer duration of action than ethanol, since it is metabolized more slowly and its major metabolite, acetone, is also a central nervous system depressant. With hemodialysis, one can expect to remove approximately 19 grams of isopropyl alcohol and 7 grams of acetone per hour using a 1.0 M^2 standard dialyzer. On arrival in the hospital, the blood level of isopropyl alcohol should be determined prior to dialysis. Deep coma is usually associated with a level of 150 mg/dl [32].

ACETONE

Acetone is used in the preparation of coated fabrics and rayon, as an organic solvent, and in the manufacture of chemicals, explosives, plastics and certain drugs and pharmaceuticals. Intoxication has occurred following application of casts containing certain plaster substitutes.

The toxic effects of acetone are similar to those of ethyl alcohol but may be more severe, particularly with the inhalation of heavy concentrations. Headache, a sensation of heaviness in the head, bad dreams, a feeling of oppression and, in some instance, nausea and vomiting develop. Ketosis and a diabeticlike coma may occur. Mydriasis has also been noted. Chronic exposure to acetone vapor causes symptoms similar to those of amyl acetate poisoning; vertigo and attacks of coughing predominate. Treatment consists of symptomatic measures after removal of the patient from the intoxicating fumes.

Because acetone, like toluene, is a component of many mixed solvent products, its specific toxic properties are difficult to study in man. In animals, however, acute inhalation of acetone induces sedation that clears only after 9 hours in fresh air. This prolonged activity contrasts with the intense but short-lived depressant effect of toluene. In animals exposed chronically to acetone for up to 10 weeks, no microscopic changes are seen in brain.

Organic Solvents

BENZENE

This hydrocarbon is one of the most important of the industrial poisons, ranking second only to tetrachlorethane in the production of serious intoxications. Benzene is still widely employed in industry, although its use has been curtailed because of the toxic reactions. It is utilized in the processing of rubber, motor fuel, munitions, dyes, leather, celluloid, and electric fittings. Workers in chemical laboratories and in coal tar distilleries are also subject to exposure to this toxin. Benzene has been used to a limited extent in the treatment of polycythemia vera and leukemia, but has been discarded because of the frequency of toxic reactions.

Acute benzene intoxication occasionally results from oral ingestion in suicidal attempts. More commonly, acute intoxication occurs in workmen who have been cleaning or repairing leaks in benzene tanks or have been exposed to toxic concentrations of this susbstance in the air.

Biochemical studies in experimental animals demonstrate that acute and chronic benzene intoxications alter the GABA system. GABA levels rise to 5-6 times normal in cerebellum and pons, although with very prolonged exposure levels they eventually return toward normal. Enzymatic levels of glutamic acid decarboxylase (GAD) are correspondingly increased [17].

Excessive inhalation of benzene vapor produces euphoria and an alcohol-like inebriation associated with giddiness, tinnitus, headache, drowsiness, sensations of tightness in the chest, nausea and vomiting. The gait is ataxic. Muscular twitching appears with more severe intoxication, followed by convulsive seizures passing into paralysis and unconsciousness. In very severe intoxications, there may be an almost immediate loss of consciousness and a terminal failure of respiration. In individuals who survive the acute effects, recovery is usually complete, although headache, chest pain, shortness of breath, anorexia, nausea and vomiting may be present for a brief period.

Chronic benzene intoxication has been observed during benzene therapy for leukemia. If aplastic anemia occurs as a result of the benzene, hemorrhage may result and precipitate neurologic problems. These are not considered direct results of the toxin. However, central nervous system and peripheral nervous system damage does occur additionally in patients, and may relate directly to benzene. Pyramidal tract involvement, hypesthesias, ataxia, paresthesias, paraplegia, retrobulbar neuritis, median nerve lesions and convulsive disorders have all been observed. Recovery is gradual in nonfatal cases, and pancytopenia is the characteristic feature rather than aplastic anemia in those patients with neurologic complications.

The best studied of the neurologic complications related to benzene is peripheral neuropathy. However, since toluene is often mixed with benzene, the role of benzene specifically is not fully established. Six Turkish shoemakers or leather workers who were studied neurologically and electrophysiologically, demonstrated slowed conduction velocities and often signs of denervation and clinical atrophy [3]. In rabbits, chronic benzene intoxication has effects on porphyrin metabolism and a porphyrinic-related polyneuropathy may be the foundation of benzene-induced peripheral nerve damage [18].

When acute intoxication results from oral ingestion of benzene, the stomach should be emptied and symptomatic treatment instituted with stimulants, artificial respiration, and carbon dioxide and oxygen inhalations. Lecithin, 5 to 10 ml given intravenously, has been reported to be effective. Vitamin C has also been employed. With chronic intoxication the therapy is directed principally against the hematopoietic changes. Pentanucleotide, folic acid, and pyridoxine have been recommended. Transfusions of whole blood may be essential and antibiotics may prevent fatal intercurrent infections.

TOLUENE (METHYL BENZENE)

Toluene is one of the most widely used solvents, employed as a paint and lacquer thinner, as a cleaning and dying agent and as a constituent of motor and aviation fuels. It is commonly used in histology laboratories. The toxic effects are similar to those of benzene, although toluene induces more mental changes and less bone marrow depression [2]. The important exposure entry route is respiratory and tissue concentration is highest in lipid-rich organs, adrenals, CNS, and bone marrow. After exposure, 80% is eliminated as hippuric acid and 20% is excreted unchanged in the lungs.

Neurologic signs occur after exposure to as little as 200 ppm; with concentrations of 800 ppm, signs may persist for several days. After acute exposure, there is an early exhilaration, followed by fatigue, mild confusion, ataxia, and dizziness. As a constituent of many solid mixtures, especially glue, toluene has been implicated as the cause of the neurotoxic syndrome seen in glue-sniffers. With intentional exposure by glue sniffing with the head in a plastic bag, blood levels of 6.5 mg percent may be observed. Psychotic behavior, unconsciousness, and death have been reported following such exposure [40].

Reports of neurologic changes associated with chronic pure toluene abuse are uncommon, but habituation is seen and probably relates to the euphoric effect of the solvent. Tremulousness, unsteadiness, emotional lability and insomnia are prominent features, and jaw jerk, snout and other primitive reflexes have been reported in chronically exposed patients. Intolerance to alcohol has been considered a valuable diagnostic clue, although the biochemical explanation for this observation is not clear. Cerebellar ataxia with and without severe optic nerve dysfunction has also been reported [19,36]. In chronic users, the presence of tremor and ataxia is seen, as well as memory impairment correlated with duration of abuse. CT scans revealed significant cortical and cerebellar atrophy.

Additionally, polyneuropathy has been reported to follow chronic toluene exposure. However, in such cases, patients were exposed to N-hexane, as well as toluene, the former inducing a definite peripheral neuropathy. In a well studied case of a youth who inhaled a toluene solvent without N-hexane, a severe and irreversible cerebellar syndrome developed, but there was no sign of a peripheral neuropathy. As a general rule, one can think of toluene as a central nervous system intoxicant and N-hexane as more peripheral [6].

Although many signs of toluene toxicity to the central nervous system are reversible when toluene is removed from the environment, long-term disability may be still seen. Cerebellar ataxia and blindness may be the long-term residua of abuse or inadvertent exposure to this solvent. No distinct drug withdrawal syndrome is seen with toluene and no specific therapy or antidote is known.

N-HEXANE

N-Hexane, formerly considered innocuous, has been recently identified as a significant neurotoxin. The compound is used in the printing of laminated products and in the extraction of vegetable oils, but most importantly, it is a component of numerous glues and has become a source of inhalant abuse. N-hexane causes a euphoric effect in patients with acute exposure, and a pronounced peripheral neuropathy after chronic intoxication. Although most glues contain N-hexane and toluene, the specific role of N-hexane has been established by cases in which neuropathy did not develop until the glue-sniffer changed to a glue that only contained N-hexane [37]. Enormous quantities may be inhaled in cans or plastic bags, ranging from 20-100 grams of glue per day to as much as one-third liter in an hour. Recently, a major glue manufacturer, Testor Corporation, has added a mucous membrane irritant, oil of mustard, to its glues, in an attempt to discourage volitional glue-sniffing.

N-Hexane, like methyl N-butyl ketone (MBK) [see below], is metabolized to 2, 5-hexanedione (2,5-HD), a toxin responsible for much of the neurotoxicity related to this compound. Human neurologic disease has been associated with repeated and prolonged exposure to levels of N-hexane in excess of 20-240 ppm. In the United States, the threshold limit air value (TLV) for N-hexane in workroom air is 100 ppm.

In contrast to toluene, N-hexane does not usually induce significant signs of encephalopathy. Lightheadedness and mild euphoria and narcosis, as well as occasional hallucinations, may occur acutely, but such central nervous system signs as seizures and significant delirium do not regularly occur [34].

The most pronounced nervous system disease associated with N-hexane is peripheral neuropathy. In a patient who has solvent exposure, weight loss, a gradual onset of distal paresthesias and weakness with or without ataxia should suggest N-hexane toxicity. Spasticity, a sign of upper motor neuron damage, may occur in such patients, although the predominant disease is in the peripheral nerve. Symmetric sensory dysfunction in the hands and feet is the usual presenting complaint and on examination pin, vibratory, and thermal sensation are prominently underactive. Loss of distal reflexes in the ankles also occurs, but early in the disease, no weakness is apparent. As the neuropathy progresses, however, atrophy and weakness may extend from the distal areas proximally. Volitional abusers of N-hexane (glue sniffers) may show a more rapid course and develop proximal weakness within weeks. Only rarely do cranial neuropathies occur, although abnormal color vision associated with macula damage has been reported [30].

Motor nerve conduction studies are of particular interest with N-hexane neuropathy. Although the neuropathy is predominantly axonal, there is marked slowing of velocity due to the demyelination that accompanies the early swelling of the affected axons. Motor nerve conduction slowing increases in proportion to the intensity of the clinical disease, and in the most extreme cases, no conduction can be detected. Symmetric distal fibrillation potentials and positive waves with reduced amplitude of muscle action potentials may also be seen. Sural nerve biopsies demonstrate focally swollen axons and demyelination. In animal studies, the long ascending and descending spinal cord tracts also show such findings.

2,5,Hexanedione appears to bind to glycolytic enzymes in the nerve fiber, causing a dose dependent inhibition of enzymatic activity along the length of the axon. The most distal regions of the axons would become enzyme deficient earliest, resulting in distal axonal transport malfunction and nerve fiber degeneration. Another untested hypothesis is that the energy disruption occurs by inactivation of thiamine, a required cofactor for pyruvate decarboxylase [35].

There is no specific treatment for N-hexane neuropathy other than removal from the source of exposure. Steroids and large doses of vitamin B complex have been tried, but without significant effect. After the patient is removed from the N-hexane source, recovery occurs over a period of weeks, although there may be a transient exacerbation of symptoms.

METHYL-N-BUTYL KETONE (MBK)

Until the early 1970s, this solvent was not widely used and no major instances of chronic human toxicity were reported. With wider utilization of MBK, however, as a paint thinner, cleaning agent and solvent for dye printing, numerous outbreaks of polyneuropathy have appeared. The means of exposure is usually inhalation, but oral exposure has occurred by ingesting contaminated food in work areas and cutaneous contact has also occurred.

Clinically, the sensorimotor polyneuropathy is insidious and painless in onset, beginning several months after continued chronic exposure. Weight loss may occur although autonomic involvement and cranial nerve dysfunction are not apparent. Interestingly, there is a reported dissociation of the compromised sensory modalities; light touch, pin prick and temperature discrimination are impaired, but vibratory and position senses as well as C-fiber deep pain appreciation are intact [35]. Pathologically, there is early multifocal axonal degeneration involving swelling and neurofilamentous accumulations at paranodal areas. Overlying the axonal swelling, severe myelin thinning occurs. Later, axonal degeneration occurs distally and takes on the appearance of a traditional "dying back" or terminal axonal neuropathy. It has been hypothesized that the primary effect of MBK is the paranodal induction of neurofilamentous accumulations with these accumulations secondarily blocking axonal transport leading to eventual distal axonal degeneration [26].

Since MBK is metabolized to the same gamma-diketone metabolite as N-hexane, 2,5-HD, the mechanism of action of the two toxins may well be the same (see above). The present threshold limit air value (TLV) is 25 ppm and the limit of 1 ppm is recommended by the United States National Institute for Occupational Safety and Health. These lower values reflect the concern for greater neurotoxic potential by MBK than N-hexane.

As with N-hexane, no specific therapy is available for the treatment of neurotoxic signs. Removal of the exposure source and good nutrition are the pillars of therapy.

Endogenous MBK toxicity may occur in two genetically determined amino acid disorders. MBK and methyl ketone have been identified in the urine of children with ketotic hyperglycinemia and methylmalonic aciduria [26]. However, these disorders are not associated with peripheral neuropathy.

ANILINE

Human exposure to this volatile solvent in concentrations of 7-53 ppm can cause mild symptoms of lightheadedness and confusion. Aniline causes hypoxia due to formation of methemoglobin. Cyanosis appears when the methemoglobin concentration reaches 15% or more. As the level rises to 40%, global weakness and dizziness predominate and at 70%, there is accompanying ataxia. The lethal level of methemoglobin is 85-90%. In general, high ambient temperatures will increase an individual's susceptibility to methemoglobin-forming compounds.

To diagnose aniline toxicity, methemoglobin levels can be assayed. To treat the intoxicated subject, all contaminated clothing should be promptly removed and the patient bathed, first to remove the aniline and second to cool the patient. Hair, scalp, nails and mucous membranes should be washed carefully. In general, after acute intoxication, methemoglobin concentration should return to normal within 48 hours. Bed rest and oxygen will symptomatically abate the headache and weakness. In cases of coma, with methemoglobin levels above 60%, methylene blue intravenous infusion 1-2 mg/kg over 5-minutes in a 1% solution can be used.

Chronic aniline toxicity has been suggested to play a role in the neurotoxic syndrome reported in Spain associated with rape seed oil ingestion (see botanical toxins, chapter 10).

TRICHLORETHYLENE (TCE)

This compound is an important organic solvent used occasionally in medicine as an anesthetic, but more extensively used in dry cleaning, degreasing metal parts, extracting oils and fats from vegetable products and as an adhesive in the leather industry. Deliberate inhalation of TCE induces a rapid state of euphoria and many workmen have become addicted to the fumes. Sudden death associated with bronchial constriction, pulmonary edema and myocardial irritability has been reported [22].

Neurologically, cranial and peripheral neuropathies are the most striking features of TCE toxicity. There is a propensity for trigeminal involvement, both sensory and motor, with facial nerve involvement also being characteristic [10]. Neuro-ophthalmologic complications including retrobulbar neuropathy, optic atrophy and oculomotor disturbances are associated with industrial exposure to TCE. Peripheral neuropathy is common and is usually mixed and predominantly distal. Tremor, ataxia, cerebellar and extrapyramidal dysfunction have occasionally been encountered, as well as dysphagia and other bulbar symptoms [22].

Examination of nerves from TCE victims shows extensive myelin and axon degeneration. It has been proposed that TCE acts as a demyelinating agent because of its lipid solvent qualities. Animals studies show that the agent also interferes with miniature end plate potential generation at the neuromuscular junction [20].

There is a potentiation of the effects of trichloroethylene by alcohol. A three-fold increase in serum trichloroethylene concentration is seen when there is concurrent ethanol administration in humans. Eighty-percent of trichlorethylene is exhaled unchanged by the respiratory system. The substance is highly fat soluble and may not be metabolized immediately. The remaining nonexhaled trichloroethylene is excreted in the form of trichloroethanol and trichloroacetic acid.

In any patient with a trigeminal neuralgia or trigeminal dysfunction, a history of possible trichloroethylene should be sought. Feldman has described the pattern of resolution after exposure to trichloroethylene. Twenty-four hours after significant exposure, the entire face may be anesthetic, four to eight weeks later, the far peripheral face generally has returned to normal, but the central regions of the face remain anesthetic. 20-33 weeks later, there is again retraction of the anesthetic area with the eyes, nose, and mouth regions now the only significantly affected area. By 79 weeks, only spotty hypalgesia is usually seen. This onion peel pattern has been described in other types of 5th nerve dysfunction and may relate to the known laminations of fibers in the 5th nerve bundle.

Although 5th nerve and 7th nerve dysfunction are typical of trichloroethylene exposure, electromyographic evidence of other nerve injury can often be detected. Additionally, when exposure of 100 ppm or greater over 7.5 hours occurred in six patients, visual evoked changes were detected in four. Long-term exposure or acute high level exposure caused disturbance in memory. When a human volunteer was exposed to 200, 300, and 500 ppm for over two hours, his only complaint was drowsiness. At 500 ppm, however, there was a pronounced decrease in concentration and neuropsychological tasks. The current threshold limit value of trichloroethylene is 100 ppm [10].

CARBON TETRACHLORIDE (TETRACHLORMETHANE)

Carbon tetrachloride is widely used in industry in the manufacture of refrigerants and aerosols, as a dry-cleaning fluid, as a fat solvent, and as a component in fire extinguishers, insecticides and "dry" shampoo. It has also been employed as an antihelminthic against Ascaris and tapeworm but has been discarded because of its toxicity. Acute intoxication has resulted from swallowing carbon tetrachloride and following inhalation, particularly when this solvent has been employed as a dry shampoo for hair or wig cleaning. The ingestion of alcohol concomitant with or preceding exposure to this toxin increases the susceptibility to poisoning. Pretreatment of rats with phenobarbital has also been reported to increase susceptibility to carbon tetrachloride poisoning. Obesity, diabetes and liver or kidney disease appear additionally to lower the threshold to the toxic effects of carbon tetrachloride.

Postmortem examination in fatal cases has demonstrated chromatolysis and vacuolization of the cortical ganglion cells and some hypertrophy of the neuroglia. Pontine necrosis and demyelination, Purkinje cell damage, cerebellar venous thromboses and hemorrhagic infarcts have been reported [8]. Edema and hemorrhage of the brain have also been noted. Degenerative changes in the kidney and liver are common with subacute or chronic intoxication.

Central nervous system symptoms are predominant in the acute intoxication. Following oral ingestion, headaches and drowsiness develop, often associated with abdominal pain, nausea, vomiting, diarrhea and hiccups. The acute symptoms are usually more severe following inhalation and may consist of feeling a fullness in the head, vertigo, a staggering gait, confusion, lethargy and unconsciousness. Optic atrophy with amblyopia or constriction of the visual fields occasionally occurs. Generalized convulsions and delirium terminate in death.

The most prominent and serious effects with subacute or chronic intoxication are on the liver and kidneys. Instances of toxic amblyopia, mental confusion and polyneuritis have been observed as well as parkinsonism after chronic carbon tetrachloride exposure. In specific reference to the latter clinical syndrome, chronic administration of the neurotoxin to experimental animals is associated with neuronal loss and astrocytosis in the corpus striatum.

If the solvent has been ingested orally, gastric lavage should be performed and saline cathartics administered. Oils should be avoided, as should epinephrine, which has been observed to cause syncope when administered during carbon tetrachloride intoxication. Calcium gluconate has been recommended and hemodialysis has been used with success [11]. Parenteral nutrition also may be helpful in preventing protein catabolism and promoting hepatic regeneration in poisoned patients.

■ STUDY QUESTIONS

Which statements are true regarding methanol intoxication?

A. Patients are usually severely acidotic due to the production of numerous organic acid metabolites of methanol.
B. Liver ethanol catalase is the main enzyme inactivated by methanol.
C. Ocular injury usually occurs two weeks to one month after the acute ingestion of methanol.
D. Parkinsonism may be a sequela of methanol intoxication.

Answers: A, D

Methyl alcohol, or methanol, is primarily oxidized to formaldehyde and formic acid resulting in a severe metabolic acidosis which contributes to CNS depression. Lactic acid also accumulates. Since methanol is metabolized very slowly, toxic metabolites may accumulate over days. The major enzyme that metabolizes methanol is alcohol dehydrogenase. This enzyme also metabolizes ethanol, and this shared metabolic pathway is the basis for the infusion of ethanol into patients with methanol toxicity. Because of competition with the ethanol, methanol will be slowly metabolized and toxic accumulation will be decreased. Ocular damage is seen usually in the first week after acute methanol ingestion. Sequelae related to methanol ingestion include visual compromise with optic atrophy and motoric dysfunction which may include parkinsonian signs.

Match the organic solvent with the characteristic presentation.

A. Trichloroethylene
B. Ethylene glycol

1. Severe chorea
2. Calcium oxalate crystals in the urine of an encephalopathic patient

Organic Solvents

C. Hexane
D. Methanol

3. Trigeminal nerve dysfunction
4. Prominent peripheral neuropathy in a glue sniffer
5. None of the above

Answers: A-3; B-2; C-4; D-none of the above

Trichloroethylene is an anesthetic agent that is associated with a typical 5th nerve neuropathy when it is abused. Facial nerve neuropathy is also seen and other mononeuropathies may occur. Ethylene glycol causes prominent renal dysfunction because of the toxic effect to renal tubules, as well as the precipitation of calcium oxalate crystals. The neurologic signs often include an encephalopathy. Hexane is a component of many glues and causes an euphoria acutely, but with chronic use can precipitate a prominent peripheral neuropathy. Methanol is described in question one and is not associated with any of the possible choices.

A patient has inadvertently swallowed antifreeze. Which of the following statements is true?

A. The likely toxin is ethyl alcohol and calcium lactate infusion may be useful acutely.
B. Ethylene glycol is the likely toxin and hypocalcemia is a significant danger in the patient.
C. Toluene is the likely toxin and infusion of alcohol will help to compete for the metabolizing enzyme.
D. Tetraethyl lead is the major toxic product here and an irreversible encephalopathy is the major risk in the patient.

Answer: B

The major toxic component in antifreeze is ethylene glycol. Several intermediates, including glycoaldehyde, glycolic acid and glyoxylic acid are produced and later metabolized to oxalic acid. The precipitation of calcium oxalate crystals can lead to significant hypocalcemia with tetany and carpopedal spasms. Sodium bicarbonate increases the amount of sodium and citrate excreted in the urine. In the alkalinized urine, calcium citrate is formed in preference to calcium oxalate and the former product is not toxic. Ethyl alcohol should be infused, since the metabolic enzyme, alcohol dehydrogenase, is shared by ethylene glycol and ethyl alcohol.

Match the toxin with its common and non-neurologic complication.

A. Benzene
B. Carbon tetrachloride

1. Pancreatic islet cell necrosis
2. Myocardial ischemia
3. Bone marrow suppression
4. Hepatic and renal necrosis

Answers: A-3; B-4

INDUSTRIAL TOXINS

Benzene provokes bone marrow depression and in fact has been used to treat leukemic states. Aplastic anemia and pancytopenia are medical complications of benzene exposure. Carbon tetrachloride, while it produces significant neurotoxicity, is predominantly a renal and hepatic toxin. Fulminant renal and hepatic damage may occur after both chronic or acute exposure.

■ REFERENCES

1. Allen N: Solvents and other industrial organic compounds. In PJ Vinken, G Bruyn, eds., Handbook of Clinical Neurology, Vol. 36, pp. 361-390. North-Holland Publishing Co., Amsterdam, 1979.
2. Barnes GE: Solvent abuse; A review. Int J. Addict 14:1-26, 1979.
3. Baslo A, Aksoy M: Neurologic abnormalities in chronic benzene poisoning. Environ. Res. 27:457-465, 1982.
4. Bass M: Sudden sniffing death. JAMA 212: 2075-2079, 1970.
5. Berger JR, Ayyar OR: Neurological complication of ethylene glycol intoxication. Arch. Neurol. 38:714-716, 1981.
6. Boor JW, Hurtig HI: Persistent cerebellar ataxia after exposure to toluene. Ann. Neurol. 2:440-442, 1977.
7. Bruhn P: Prognosis in chronic toxic encephalopathy. Acta Neurol. Scan. 64:259-272, 1981.
8. Cohen MM: Central nervous system in carbon tetrachloride intoxication. Neurology 1:238-246, 1957.
9. Escobar A, Aruffo C: Chronic thinner intoxication: clinical pathologic report. JNNP 43:986-994, 1980.
10. Feldman RG: Trichlorethylene. In PJ Vinken, and GW Bruyn, eds., Handbook of Clinical Neurology, Vol. 36, pp. 457-464. North-Holland Publishing Co., Amsterdam, 1979.
11. Fogel RP: Carbon tetrachloride poisoning treated with hemodialysis and total parenteral nutrition. Can. Med. Assoc. J. 114:560-561, 1983.
12. Freireich AW, Cinque TJ, Xanthaky G, Landau D: Hemodialysis for isopropanol poisoning. New Engl. J. Med. 277:699, 1967.
13. Hansen KS, Sharp FR: Gasoline sniffing, lead poisoning and myoclonus. JAMA 240:1375-1376, 1978.
14. Hayreh MS, Hayreh SS, Baumbach GL, Cancilla P, Martin-Amat, G. Tephly TR, Martin KE, Makar AB: Methyl alcohol poisoning. III. Ocular toxicity. Arch. Ophthalmol. 95:1851-1858, 1977.
15. Hernberg S: Neurotoxic effects of long-term exposure to organic hydrocarbon solvents. Epidemiologic aspects. In B. Holmstedt and R. Lauwerys eds., Mechanisms of Toxicity and Hazard Evaluation, pp. 307-317. Elsevier/North-Holland, Amsterdam, 1980.
16. Juntvnen J, Antti-Poika M, Tola S, Partgnen T: Clinical prognosis of patients with diagnosed chronic solvent intoxication. Acta Neurol. Scand. 65: 488-503, 1982.

17. Kadyrov GK, Saforov MI, Sytinsky IA: Effects of benzene vapour on the GABA system in rat brain. Biochem. Pharmacol. 24:2083-2087, 1975.
18. Kahn H, Muzyka V: Chronic effect of benzene on porphyrin metabolism. Work Environ. Health. 10:140-143, 1970.
19. Keane JR: Toluene optic neuropathy. Ann. Neurol. 3:390, 1978.
20. Kennedy RD, Galindo AD: Comparative site of action of various anaesthetic agents at the mammalian myoneural junction. Br. J. Anaesth. 47: 533-540, 1975.
21. Keyvan-Larijami H, Tannenberg AM: Methanol intoxication. Comparison of peritoneal dialysis and hemodialysis treatment. Arch. Intern. Med. 134: 293-296, 1974.
22. Lawrence WH, Partyka ER: Trigeminal anesthesia after trichlorethylene exposure. Ann. Intern. Med. 49:205-209, 1981.
23. Lindstrom K, Marbelin T: Personality and long term exposure to organic solvents. Neurobehav. Toxicol. 2:89-100, 1982.
24. McLean DR, Jacobs H, Mielke BW: Methanol poisoning. Ann. Neurol. 8: 161-167, 1980.
25. Means ED, Procktop LD, Hooper GS: Pathology of lacquer thinner induced neuropathy. Ann. Clin. Lab. Sci. 6:240-250, 1976.
26. Mendell JR, Sahenk Z, Saida K, Weiss HS, Savage R, Couri D: Alterations of fast axoplasmic transport in experimental methyl n-butyl ketone neuropathy. Brain Res. 133:107-118, 1977.
27. Parry MF, Wallach R: Ethylene glycol poisoning. Am. J. Med. 57:143-145, 1974.
28. Pedersen W, Nygaard E, Nielsen O: Solvent induced occupational myopathy. Occ. Med. 22:603-607, 1980.
29. Peterson CD, Collins AJ, Himes JM, Bullock ML, Keane WF: Ethylene glycol poisoning. N. Engl. J. Med. 304:21-23, 1981.
30. Prockop, LD, Alt M, Tison J: Huffer's neuropathy. JAMA 229:1083-1084, 1974.
31. Roe O: Past, present and future fight against methanol blindness and death. Trans. Ophthalmol. Soc. U.K. 89:235-242, 1969.
32. Rosansky SJ: Isopropyl alcohol poisoning treated with hemodialysis. J. Toxicol. Clin. Toxicol. 19:265-271, 1982.
33. Seppalainen AM, Husman K, Martenson C: Neurophysiological effects of long term exposure to a mixture of organic solvents. Scand. J. Work. Environ. and Health 4:304-314, 1978.
34. Spencer PS, Couri D, Schaumburg HH: n-Hexane and methyl n-butyl kettone. In PS Spencer and HH Schaumburg, eds., Experimental and Clinical Neurotoxicology, pp. 456-475. Williams and Wilkins, Baltimore, 1980.
35. Spencer PS, Schaumberg HH, Sabri MI, Veronesi B: The enlarging view of hexacarbon neurotoxicity. CRC Crit. Rev. Toxicol. 1980:279-356.
36. Takeuchi Y, Hisanaga N: Cerebellar dysfunction caused by sniffing of toluene-containing thinner. Ind. Health 19:163-169, 1981.
37. Towfighi J, Gonatas NK, Pleasure D, Cooper HS, McCree L: Glue sniffer's neuropathy. Neurology 26:238-243, 1976.

38. Vale JA, Widdop B, Bluett NH: Ethylene glycol poisoning. Postgrad. Med. J. 52:598-602, 1976.
39. Valpey R, Sumi SM, Compass MK, Goble GJ: Acute and chronic progressive encephalopathy due to gasoline sniffing. Neurology 28:507-510, 1978.
40. Winek CL, Wecht CH, Collom WD: Toluene fatality from glue sniffing. Penn. Med. 71:81-86, 1968.
41. Wyse G: Deliberate inhalation of volatile hydrocarbons. A review. Can. Med. Assoc. J. 108:71-74, 1973.

CHAPTER 6

Gases

NERVE gases gained chilling notoriety first in World War I and later in Viet Nam, where they were used as vaporous war weapons. Gases may affect man as industrial or medicinal fumes, as naturally occurring or volitionally inhaled substances. Nitrogen mustard, the original "nerve gas," significantly inhibits cell growth, particularly myeloid and lymphoid tissues, and as a result, this agent is used in the treatment of various carcinomas (see Chapter 16). The large variety of neurotoxic organic solvents are discussed in Chapter 5; although highly volatile and absorbed by the pulmonary route, they are naturally liquids.

CARBON MONOXIDE

Carbon monoxide, an odorless and nonirritating gas, is the most abundant air pollutant in the lower atmosphere. Acute poisoning accounts for over 3,000 accidental or suicidal deaths each year in the United States. The effects of chronic exposure to carbon monoxide, due to inhalation of polluted air, are of increasing concern to scientists and clinicians.

Carbon monoxide is produced both by exogenous sources and by natural production of the chemical in the body. Natural sources include volcanoes, forest fires, and photochemical degradation of organic compounds. Industrial sources include hotwater heaters, furnaces, and at-home fireplaces that are inadequately ventilated. Automobile exhaust is, however, the major source of carbon monoxide production with concentrations of approximately 50,000 ppm. Cigarette smoking may be one of the major sources associated with chronic carbon monoxide toxicity, although it probably plays an insignificant role compared to acute intoxication. Although cigarette smoke contains approximately 40,000 ppm of carbon monoxide, the toxin is diluted with air to an average of

INDUSTRIAL TOXINS

200-400 ppm. Importantly, paint stripper compounds containing methylene chloride are also dangerous sources of carbon monoxide, since the methylene chloride is absorbed and metabolized specifically to carbon monoxide. A three hour exposure to paint stripper vapors can result in the accumulation of toxic concentrations of carboxyhemoglobin. Medications including barbiturates and phenytoin induce an increased production of carbon monoxide, and the natural catabolism of hemoglobin produces the gas as well [10,28].

The threshold limit value of carbon monoxide has been set at 50 ppm, causing a carboxyhemoglobin saturation level of 8-10% after an 8 hour exposure. Levels of carboxyhemoglobin which exceed 50% saturation are considered life threatening and levels of 70-75% are usually fatal. Such saturation levels may occur either by exposure to very high acute concentrations or by exposure to relatively lower concentrations for a chronic period. The threshold limit value assumes that the carbon monoxide comes from a single source and does not take into account endogenous factors or smoking which can also increase the victim's baseline saturation.

Biochemistry

As carbon monoxide enters the bloodstream by pulmonary absorption, it reversibly binds to hemoglobin. Hemoglobin's affinity for carbon monoxide is approximately 225 times greater than that for oxygen. The resultant carboxyhemoglobin causes a decrease in the amount of oxygen carried by the red blood cells and an alteration of the oxyhemoglobin dissociation curve. Tissue oxygen tensions fall, and whatever oxygen is on blood cells is bound tighter. The net result is more pronounced tissue oxygen deprivation than would be produced by either an equivalent reduction in environmental oxygen concentration (pure hypoxia) or an equivalent reduction in hemoglobin (pure anemia) [7].

Other biochemical functions are also compromised. Carbon monoxide binds to intracellular proteins and inhibits their function. Myoglobin function and the cytochrome oxidase system may be affected.

Clinical Features

Acute carbon monoxide toxicity may cause signs of global dysfunction or signs related directly to focal lesions. In Table 6.1, several signs of carbon monoxide toxicity are listed. They of course are not pathognomonic but their presence along with the history of exposure to carbon monoxide will establish the diagnosis. Importantly, the conditions under which the poisoning took place may alter the order of appearance of these signs and symptoms. For example, if a patient is suddenly exposed to concentrations of carbon monoxide in excess of 50,000 ppm, fatal cardiac arrhythmias and death may occur before the

TABLE 6.1. Neurologic Manifestations of CO Poisoning [17]

Mild:	Dizziness
	Headache
	Increase of visual threshold
Severe:	Severe throbbing headache
	Convulsive disorders
	Coma
Persistent/Chronic:	Blindness
	Deafness
	Pyramidal signs
	Extrapyramidal signs
	Convulsive disorders
Miscellaneous:	Dysphagia, anisocoria, palsies, neuritis, tremors, ataxia, agraphia, visual-perceptual problems, akinetic mutism

carboxyhemoglobin concentration has been elevated significantly. In infants, hypotonia and convulsions may occur along with severe metabolic acidosis [34].

Neurologic damage associated with carbon monoxide poisoning primarily focuses in the globus pallidus, Ammon's Horn, and the white matter. The mechanism of such damage probably is indirect through circulatory mechanisms in the globus pallidum and Ammon's Horn, and through edema and functional disturbances in capillary permeability for the demyelination that occurs in the white matter. Mild neurologic effects include headache, dizziness and visual disturbances; more severe toxic reactions include convulsive disorder, pyramidal and extrapyramidal signs, cerebral blindness and deafness. Such symptoms may be transient to persistent appearing immediately or days or weeks after the intoxication. Myositis and calcification in the muscles with mild necrosis may also occur, related to the direct effects of the toxin on myoglobin and the crushing effect of the patient's own body on muscles.

Behavioral and psychiatric alterations, including irritability and violent behavior, personality disturbances, inappropriate euphoria, confusion and impaired judgement may all occur. In a follow up study, three years after carbon monoxide poisoning, 13% of patients showed gross neuropsychiatric damage, 33% showed a deterioration of personality and 43% demonstrated impaired memory.

More recent concern over the chronic effects of carbon monoxide focus on patients with continued industrial or urban exposure to the gas. Cigarette smokers also fit into this potential category. Langsjoen et al. reported six patients with leaking exhaust systems in their automobiles who were chronically self-exposed to carbon monoxide [19]. Over weeks they developed an insidious syndrome of somnolence and mental decline with gait difficulty, incoordination and slurred speech. When the exhaust system was corrected, their carboxyhemoglobin levels reduced and their symptoms resolved. However, results from human and animal studies have not confirmed direct histotoxic effects of such carbon monoxide exposure. Suggested symptoms related to chronic low dose carbon monoxide exposure include changes in cognitive function, fatigue, headache, dizziness and disturbed sleep. Physiological studies demonstrate that oxygen deficiency due to mild carbon monoxide poisoning in the brain usually can be compensated by increasing cerebral blood flow [7]. A more focal neurologic syndrome that has been reported after acute and chronic exposure to carbon monoxide is parkinsonism [16].

Some patients show diffuse neurologic involvement associated with parkinsonian features, while others demonstrate a true parkinsonian picture. This clinical syndrome is usually associated with globus pallidus lucency on the CT scan and pallidal atrophy histologically. Patients may respond to levodopa or to anticholinergic drugs although the response is unpredictable.

The only specific laboratory test in cases of acute carbon monoxide poisoning is the direct determination of the level in the blood (expressed as percent saturation of hemoglobin by carbon monoxide). If toxic levels of carboxyhemoglobin are determined, the diagnosis of carbon monoxide poisoning is safely made. However, the level of carbon monoxide is not indicative of the severity of the poisoning since a patient removed from the intoxicated environment and allowed to breathe fresh air will show a rapid decline in the carboxyhemoglobin levels. Nevertheless, if a patient dies of carbon monoxide poisoning, the level of carboxyhemoglobin determined postmortem represents the actual levels at the moment of death since carbon monoxide cannot be excreted without active respiration and is not converted in the body to other products. This fact is of significant medical and legal importance.

Practical Management

Upon discovery of the patient with carbon monoxide poisoning, the physician should immediately remove the patient from the contaminated environment. Fresh air and inactivity are recommended to maintain the tissue demands for oxygen at an absolute minimum. Resuscitation in the contaminated environment may be dangerous to the rescuer as well as to the patient himself. If the patient cannot breathe, artificial respiration will be indicated. One hundred percent oxygen should be started as soon as possible through an oral/nasal mask. The half-life of carboxyhemoglobin is 40 minutes after the administration of 100% O_2. As a substitute for O_2, some scientists use carbogen (a mixture of 95% O_2 with 5% CO_2). This mixture eliminated carbon monoxide more rapidly than oxygen alone but the added respiratory acidosis produced by CO_2 may exacerbate the already present metabolic acidosis seen in severe CO_2 poisoning. In general, 100% oxygen is preferred to the administration of carbogen.

Hyperbaric oxygen will reduce the half-life of carboxyhemoglobin to less than 25 minutes. When it is used the following recommendations are offered: 46 minutes of 100% O_2 at 3 ATM absolute pressure, followed by 2 ATM absolute pressure for 2 hours or until the proper carboxyhemoglobin level is achieved [17,30]. Hyperbaric oxygen is considered to be the treatment of choice for carbon monoxide poisoning and if possible should be administered to every patient who presents with signs and symptoms of severe intoxication. In premature infants, the toxicity of oxygen must be considered and weighed against the likelihood of the diagnosis in questionable cases.

To decrease the tissue demand for oxygen, hypothermia has also been advocated. Patients covered in ice are maintained for 8 to 12 hours at a temperature of 30-32°C. Shivering which increases the metabolic rate is to be prevented and can often be controlled by the administration of chlorpromazine 25 mg. If seizures develop they may be treated with barbiturates. Cerebral edema associated with severe hypoxia may be treated with steroid medications such as dexamethasone 16-20 mg/day.

The prognosis for patients with significant carbon monoxide poisoning is difficult to determine immediately after the patient is discovered. Patients with carboxyhemoglobin levels as low as 20% have died after a carbon monoxide poisoning while others with much higher levels have survived. Significantly, however, long term follow-up does demonstrate that patients with intoxication often have neurologic residua. Cortical blindness, seizures, cognitive impairment with amnesia, polyneuropathy and the parkinsonian syndrome are all possible long terms effects of significant intoxication.

NITROUS OXIDE

This anesthetic, commonly used in dental practices, can be a significant source of neurotoxicity. Volitional gaseous inhalation of this neurotoxin has gained increasing popularity especially among dentists and other health workers [21]. The gas is also available commercially in various compressed dispenser cartridges and may account "for whipped cream dispenser" polyneuropathy [25]. In dentists heavily exposed to nitrous oxide in their practice, the rate of neuropathic complaints was four times greater than for nonanesthetic exposed dentists. For dental assistants heavily exposed to nitrous oxide, a three-fold increase in these same complaints was noted [3]. Nitrous oxide neuropathy may be predominantly distal or follow a radicular pattern. Most cases are mixed with both sensory and motor involvement. A peculiar "reverse l'Hermitte" sign, involving a tingling sensation passing up the toes to the neck, after neck flexion, was characteristic in one series. Often the history of a gradual progressive disorder that starts with numbness, paresthesia and clumsiness in the extremities is obtained; afterwards, weakness, gait disturbance and a loss of sphincter control may become increasingly incapacitating. Nerve conduction studies suggest an axonal neuropathy and sural nerve biopsy changes while nonspecific are characterized principally by axonal degeneration [9,21]. In one clinical study, where half of the dentists in an American city were examined, those who used nitrous oxide extensively in their practice were not different in terms of their neurologic condition, motor and sensory nerve conduction or sensory function. This latter study suggests that the usual exposure of nitrous oxide in a dental practice may not be as toxic as suggested by the four-fold increase in neuropathic symptoms described earlier [3].

In addition to a neuropathy, signs of upper motor neuron disease may also coexist, a picture resembling that of subacute combined degeneration (B_{12} deficiency). In fact, nitrous oxide has been shown to inactivate certain B_{12}-dependent enzymes in the presence of normal levels of the vitamin [5]. Whereas 3-5 years of a vitamin B_{12} deficient diet would be necessary to produce significant neurologic damage in the monkey, exposure to nitrous oxide for two months can effect the neurologic damage consistent with subacute combined degeneration [8]. Cessation of exposure to nitrous oxide is associated with gradual clinical improvement although the recovery may be prolonged for several months. No specific treatment is advocated other than good nutrition and removal of the nitrous oxide.

Methionine synthesis in the brain is profoundly affected by nitrous oxide. This may be an indirect result of nitrous oxide-induced or late deficiency, and may underlie the development of neuropathy [5]. In experimental studies, a monkey placed in a chronic oxide environment for two months became unsteady and uncoordinated with progressive ataxia. The spinal cord showed degeneration of myelin sheaths and axons in the posterior columns and lateral cortical spinal and spinal cerebellar tracts. In subsequent studies, the investigators found that such changes only occurred after 18 days' exposure to nitrous oxide and that the clinical picture began with a minor tremor of the hind limbs and progressed to ataxia. The early clinical changes were reversible by returning the animal to a normal air environment [8].

HYDROGEN SULFIDE

Hydrogen sulfide toxicity is seen in industries involving petroleum refining, tanning, the manufacture of rayon and in the handling and breakdown of protein wastes. Reactions occurring with cleaning solutions in contact with plaster sludge products have also occurred [22]. The gas is a colorless product with a noxious smell. The clinical picture of hydrogen sulfide intoxication is respiratory distress, tremors, coma, cyanosis and convulsions. The proposed safe air concentration is 10 ppm. It has been suggested that the cyanosis so characteristic of hydrogen sulfide poisoning relates to direct depression of the hypothalamic respiratory center [29].

As with cyanide poisoning, hydrogen sulfide toxicity is thought to relate primarily to the inhibition of cytochrome oxidase activity. A complex formation between the HS⁻ anion and ferric ion of cytochrome oxidase results in inactivation of the electron transport respiratory chain with resultant inhibition of aerobic metabolism [27].

In low concentrations (200 ppm), hydrogen sulfide depresses the nervous system; in higher concentration, it in fact stimulates respiration and in even greater quantities (1,000 ppm) it again paralyzes central nervous function, including respiratory systems. Additionally, the toxic effect of sulfide on the heart has been associated with arrhythmias and conduction disorders [22]. Since methemoglobin, known to bind cyanide, also inactivates sulfide, nitrite has been suggested as a possible therapy. Nitrites induce methemoglobin accumulation by competitively binding the hydrosulfide anion and then reversibly releasing the toxic product for metabolic detoxification. Recent reports indicate that amyl nitrite inhalation for 30 seconds per minute for five minutes and then 300 mg of sodium nitrite given intravenously during three minutes, as well as 12.5 grams of sodium thiosulfate intravenously, has been associated with recovery.

The role of oxygen in the treatment of hydrogen sulfide poisoning remains controversial; while oxygen promotes oxidative detoxification, work with animals has not confirmed that oxygen has a protective effect [12]. For further discussion of nitrite therapy, see Cyanides.

CARBON DISULFIDE

This compound is involved in the manufacture of viscose rayon, cellophane and adhesives and can be absorbed by inhalation or skin contact in its liquid form. Although carbon disulfide neurotoxicity was a common acute and subacute syndrome, with improved factory ventilation only intermittent and chronic insidious forms are now seen [11,32].

Historically, the acute fulminant intoxications resulted in toxic psychosis with agitated delirium and frequently a sequela of mental impairment [15]. The more important chronic syndrome involves the development of progressive mental impairment with cranial and peripheral neuropathies. Mental changes include irritability, personality changes and emotional lability. A characteristic cranial nerve dysfunction has been reported involving a selective loss of corneal reflex function without facial sensory complaints. This finding has been associated with loss of the pupillary light reflex, and various impairments of vision, ranging from scotomas to night blindness [12]. The peripheral neuropathy, relatively mild, is mixed and predominantly distal. An unusual parkinsonian presentation has been reported after carbon disulfide toxicity with characteristic tremor, rigidity and bradykinesia, but associated with peripheral neuropathy and very marked mental impairment [32].

In patients with chronic exposure to carbon disulfide, nerve conduction studies demonstrate normal motor conduction velocities and terminal latencies, but hypoexcitability of distal motor thresholds. In patients with clinical neuropathy, decreased amplitude of sensory evoked potentials after digital fiber stimulation, mild slowing of sensory conduction velocities and decreased amplitude of the evoked potentials in the distal muscles suggest that carbon disulfide polyneuropathy may relate to a primary distal axonopathy [33].

Psychologic effects have been monitored in patients exposed to carbon disulfide [15]. Three groups of patients were compared, one with clinical poisoning, one with chronic exposure from 5-20 years, but without clinical symptoms, and a control group without exposure or with only mild or intermittent exposure. Psychomotor functioning, dexterity and alertness were all compromised in those patients with clinical poisoning who also showed a decline in intellectual function requiring visual activity and speech. The chronically exposed latent group also showed motor disturbances and impaired visual function, but did not show significant speech or personality aberrations [12].

Pathologic changes have been demonstrated both centrally and peripherally, although these changes appear to be nonspecific. In the CNS, neuronal degeneration with pallor, chromatolysis and vacuolation are seen diffusely with maximal intensity in the frontal lobes, globus pallidum and putamen. Studies of peripheral nerves show myelin swelling and fragmentation. In experimental animals, multifocal axonal swelling with neurofilament accumulation can be seen.

The mechanism of action of carbon disulfide has not been clarified. Metabolites of the compound are known chelators, and it has been proposed that depletion of necessary trace metal contributes to the clinical neuropathy. For this reason, metal supplementation of copper and zinc has been advocated in the treatment of human carbon disulfide toxicity [31]. Animal data suggest the possibility of a pyridoxine metabolism disorder related to carbon disulfide and has led to the clinical use of vitamin supplementation.

ETHYLENE OXIDE

Ethylene oxide is a gas used to sterilize heat sensitive materials. It is widely used, and acute toxic effects include skin lesions, mucous irritation, pulmonary edema and neurologic symptoms, such as headache, nausea, vomiting, and cloudy consciousness. In 1979, Gross et al. described a patient with acute encephalopathy and three patients with peripheral neuropathy after chronic exposure to ethylene oxide [14]. These patients were exposed to high levels of ethylene oxide (>700 ppm) for up to eight weeks before symptoms started. The electromyographic studies indicated decreased amplitude of muscle action potentials and decreased conduction velocities, and they suggested that the disease was predominantly an axonal neuropathy. More recent studies by Kuzuhara where nerve biopsies were performed confirmed the axonal neuropathy and showed mild changes in the myelin sheath. Unmyelinated fibers were also involved. Muscle biopsy showed typical denervation atrophy. Symptoms improved after exposure to ethylene oxide terminated [18].

In addition to the acute encephalopathy and chronic polyneuropathy, a chronic encephalopathy may be seen with gradual dementia or decline in intellectual function. Headache and the signs of peripheral neuropathy usually accompany chronic encephalopathic symptoms. In one such case there was generalized slowing on the EEG and a normal cerebrospinal fluid examination [26].

Through its alkylation of guanine and adenine as well as sulfhydryl, amino carboxyl, and hydroxyl groups of protein, ethylene oxide reacts with almost all cellular components including vitamins, cofactors and nucleic acids. The current U.S. standard for occupational exposure for ethylene oxide is 50 ppm or 90 mg/m^3 of air for an 8 hour exposure. Other countries, however, have established different standards (the USSR 0.5 ppm and Sweden 20 ppm). Reports of carcinogenic, teratogenic and mutagenic properties of ethylene oxide have prompted a current reassessment of the dangers of ethylene oxide exposure to man.

METHYL CHLORIDE

This product has been used as an anesthetic, but it is mainly a refrigerant or a volatile constituent of polystyrene foam used especially for insulation boards. It is also used as an aerosol propellant for insecticides, as a catalyst solvent, and as an intermediate in methylation reactions. The threshold limit value is 100 ppm by volume in air.

The effects of methyl chloride in the nervous system relate primarily to depression. The narcotic effects of the agent may increase up to 48 hours after removal from the methyl chloride source. In general, there is somnolence, apathy or agitation, all indicative of a generalized encephalopathy. Occasional early reports documented focal areas of brain damage, specifically frontal and parietal lobes, in addition to the generalized alterations. Long-term residua following acute intoxication include gait ataxia, emotional stability, and tremor. Only in the most severe cases of acute exposure will the patient lose consciousness, develop seizures, and proceed to respiratory collapse [14,24].

Chronic or subacute exposure to methyl chloride produces similar symptoms, but they are usually less severe and more prolonged. Findings in chronic cases include mild to moderate headache, drowsiness, vague weakness, incoordination, slurred speech and mental disturbances. Dementia and gradual ataxia occur, and since there is no single exposure accident, the history of methyl chloride exposure may be overlooked. Also reported is a residual sensitivity to methyl chloride that remains long after recovery from an earlier exposure. The development of sudden toxic symptoms even at low doses has occurred in such patients [20].

The question of long-term toxicity of methyl chloride even in dose ranges within the threshold of limit value has been studied. 122 methyl chloride workers exposed to chronic concentrations of 33.6 ppm were compared to 249 control subjects [24]. Neurologic examinations revealed no significant differences in the presence of abnormal neurologic symptoms or EEG abnormalities between the two groups. However, when patients were tested for speed and accuracy of simple tasks, there was a relationship between methyl chloride exposure and poor performance. Hence, it appears that chronic exposure to the gas even below the TLV may induce quantifiable behavioral changes [23].

Diagnosis is difficult without the knowledge of occupational exposure. The symptoms are vague and do not point to any single area of the nervous system. Interestingly, peripheral neuropathy, so common with many industrial products, is not a prominent feature with methyl chloride. No definitive clinical test is available to differentiate intoxication with this compound from others. Treatment is supportive and no specific antidote is recommended. From studies with alcohol, caffeine, and diazepam, toxic depressive effects of methyl chloride appear to be additive, but not synergistic [20].

HALOTHANE

Halothane is a gas used in clinical medicine as a general anesthetic. It is usually mixed with oxygen and nitrous oxide. Headaches, ataxia and lethargy have been associated with the use of halothane and may relate to bromide accumulation which is one of the breakdown products of the anesthetic (2-bromo-2-chloro-1,1,1-trifluoroethane). Even in subanesthetic concentrations (.001 percent), there are reports of impaired memory, bizarre psychomotor activity and altered behavior [4]. Anesthesiologists exposed chronically to low doses suffer from a high incidence of headaches. The characteristic halothane headache is frontal, above or between the eyes, and throbbing with a duration of 2-8 hours. Seizures and tetany have also been reported, but may relate to hypoxia rather than a direct toxic effect. Halothane has also been ingested, inducing coma lasting 36 hours in one patient and 72 hours in another. Both patients, however, experienced complete recovery without neurologic residua [35].

Halothane alters electron transport and decreases mitochondrial respiratory control in the liver, but not in the brain. However, cerebral oxygen consumption decreases with halothane while cerebral blood flow increases. Hence, there is enhanced oxygen delivery to the brain with a decrease in oxygen requirements. Importantly, halothane does not appear to protect the ischemic brain as do the barbiturate drugs. In a series of animal experiments with middle cerebral artery ligation, barbiturates, halothane or no anesthesia was administered. With barbiturates, there were the fewest infarctions while with halothane there was the highest incidence [6]. This effect may be related to the increased cerebral flood flow and increased cerebral pressure or may relate to a direct toxic effect of halothane on the brain. From further animal studies of rats exposed to halothane, Chang and colleagues concluded that the biological membrane system may be the primary target of halothane activity [6].

Clinical Features

Halothane and other general anesthetics may induce the catastrophic neurologic disorder, malignant hyperthermia, in susceptible individuals. This disorder is associated with a mortality rate of approximately 70 percent. The dramatic features of the disorder are fever which may reach 45°C and the profound rigidity seen in a large number of affected patients [13].

In contrast to heat stroke, malignant hyperthermia occurs in individuals with apparently normal heat dissipating mechanisms, but with a sudden increase in heat production. Accelerated cellular metabolism and sustained muscle rigidity generate the heat that characterizes the hyperthermic crisis. Experimental and *in vitro* studies have recently clarified the biochemistry of this unusual disorder and suggest that it relates to an underlying muscle membrane defect acutely exacerbated by the anesthetic agents. These studies offer a foundation for rational therapy and preventive planning. Retrospective analyses of patients who develop malignant hyperthermia demonstrate that 20-30 percent of patients have preexistent congenital muscle or muscular skeletal abnormalities [2]. Such defects include kyphoscoliosis, strabismus, ptosis, hernias and spontaneous joint dislocations. No single myopathy appears to encompass cases of malignant hyperthermia, but the remarkable frequency of mild underlying muscle disease in patients with hyperthermic crises suggest that the two conditions may pathogenically or pathophysiologically be related.

It appears that the basic underlying mechanism of malignant hyperthermia relates to intracellular calcium metabolism. General anesthetics, including halothane, release calcium from the probable defective calcium storage membrane in muscle cells to both the extracellular space and the intracellular myoplasm [1]. As a result, total muscle calcium falls while serum calcium and probably myoplasmic calcium rise. The likely site of defective calcium storage is the sarcoplasmic reticulum. Modest increases in intramyoplasmic calcium activate phosphorylase kinase activity so that glycogen is broken down to pyruvate. During the often anaerobic phase of a malignant hyperthermic crisis, excess lactate may be produced which when carried to the liver is oxidized with a considerable production of heat. Another major intracellular heat producing site is the mitochondria. The eventual result of these and other heat generating mechanisms is the exhaustion of ATP content in muscle cells with continued toxic myoplasmic calcium concentration and massive heat generation. As ATP declines, muscle membrane permeability increases and ions, enzymes, and myoglobin move along their concentration gradients. As a result, the primary muscle membrane defect in calcium storage, whether genetically induced or acquired by an unknown source, could remain barely compensated until the triggering exposure to anesthesia.

Practical Management

The most reasonable approach to the management of malignant hyperthermia is to diagnose the condition before anesthesia [13]. Evidence of a prior rigid and hyperthermic episode, related anesthetic exposure or family history of such occurrence should assist in the diagnosis. However, one or even several normal anesthetic procedures in the past does not eliminate the possibility of a malignant hyperthermic crisis on the subsequent occasion. An elevated serum creatinine phosphokinase level will suggest a mild myopathy which puts the patient at a significant risk for the development of malignant hyperthermia. During the anesthetic procedure, continuous temperature monitoring, cardiographic recording, and the central venous pressure line will help to detect abnormalities at the earliest point. Prophylactic cooling blankets in the person who is suspected to suffer from this condition can be used as well as the ready availability of a method for delivering internal cooling. It has been suggested that a general anesthesia is necessary, the preferred combination is nitrous oxide, barbiturate, narcotic, diazepam or neuroleptic-analgesic agents. Large doses of procaine, approximately one gram intravenously over several minutes, have empirically proven to be of benefit. Procaine and procainamide both lower myoplasmic calcium by accelerating calcium uptake into the sarcoplasmic reticulum [1]. The lowering of myoplasmic calcium then reverses the sequence of heat generation and enhanced muscle metabolism characteristic of the malignant hyperthermic crisis. Lidocaine, which accelerates calcium release from sarcoplasmic reticulum, is to be avoided. Intravenous calcium gluconate in hypocalcemic patients is an important adjunct as it will presumably interrupt the secondary hypothalamic febrile reaction. Acidosis and electrolyte abnormalities must be corrected.

■ STUDY QUESTIONS

The toxic mechanism of action of carbon monoxide is:

A. Disruption of cytochrome oxidase

B. Inactivation of sulfhydryl groups on the heme molecule
C. Irreversible dissociation of the heme molecule and that of vitamin B_{12}
D. Production of carboxyhemoglobin

Answer: D

Hemoglobin has an affinity for carbon monoxide that is over 200 times greater than for oxygen. Hence, with carbon monoxide poisoning, the patient is deprived of the necessary oxygen. Cytochrome oxidase inhibition is seen with cyanides, and sulfhydryl attachment is typical of heavy metals. The heme molecule itself is not altered by carbon monoxide.

In addition to the removal of the patient from the carbon monoxide intoxicated environment, the following is recommended:

A. Carbon dioxide by mask or nasal canula
B. Pure oxygen
C. Stimulant drugs to increase respiration
D. Nitrous oxide

Answer: B

One hundred percent oxygen is the most efficient means of correcting carbon monoxide intoxication. In ambient air, carboxyhemoglobin levels will decrease by 50% in 4 hours. When pure oxygen is inhaled, the half life is reduced to only 40 minutes. Blood transfusion will also enhance oxygen utilization.

A dentist is brought for a neurologic evaluation. From his occupational history alone, which toxins should the examiner specifically consider?

A. Mercury
B. Arsenic
C. Carbon monoxide
D. Nitrous oxide
E. Methylene chloride

Answers: A and D

The three major toxins to which dentists are exposed are lead, mercury, and nitrous oxide. Metal exposure relates to the amalgams that they prepare. A dentist presenting with mental alterations, peculiar movements, especially tremor, and global complaints of weakness would suggest chronic mercurialism. The mental picture may include marked irritability, depression, and intolerance of emotional tensions. The evaluation of a demented dentist must include careful evaluation for mercury toxicity. Nitrous oxide is an anesthetic used by many dentists in the United States and is occasionally abused by dentists volitionally. Neuropathy occasionally associated with signs of upper motor neuron disease may suggest the diagnosis of B_{12} deficiency or subacute combined degeneration. In this patient a careful history may assist in the diagnosis.

Which of the following toxins causes toxicity similar to cyanide poisoning and is similarly treated?

INDUSTRIAL TOXINS

A. Carbon dioxide
B. Carbon disulfide
C. Hydrogen sulfide
D. Methyl chloride
E. Carbon monoxide

Answer: C

Hydrogen sulfide toxicity is thought to relate primarily to the inhibition of cytochrome oxidase activity. The formation between the sulfhydryl anion and ferric ion of cytochrome oxidase inactivates the electron transport respiratory chain.

Encephalopathy with polyneuropathy would be the usual presentation for which of the following gaseous neurotoxins?

A. Ethylene oxide
B. Carbon disulfide
C. Hydrogen sulfide
D. Nitrous oxide
E. Methyl chloride

Answers: A, B, D

Hydrogen sulfide usually presents with respiratory distress, tremors, prominent cyanosis and convulsions. The pathophysiology relates to cyanide-like toxicity. Methyl chloride presents as prominent encephalopathy and mental impairment, but a significant peripheral neuropathy would be relatively unusual, although not impossible. The more likely gaseous toxins would be carbon disulfide, ethylene oxide and nitrous oxide where the combination of encephalopathy and neuropathy are expected. The mechanisms of action for the different gases may be entirely distinct from each other.

Which is true regarding anesthesia-related malignant hyperthermia?

A. The development of the disorder is a dose related toxic syndrome where children are the most susceptible
B. Halothane acts to release calcium from a defective calcium storage membrane in muscle cells
C. One means of identifying patients at higher risk of malignant hyperthermia before anesthesia is to assay their creatinine kinase activity
D. Substitution of halothane with another general anesthetic will abort the development of malignant hyperthermia

Answers: B, C

Malignant hyperthermia is a genetic disorder and patients may be entirely normal before receiving anesthesia. On the other hand, many have an underlying muscle defect that can be clinically detected or can be surmised by an elevated CK. It is wise to notify the anesthesiologist and make certain that the operating room staff is equipped with treatment for a hyperthermic crises if it develops. Although halothane is often associated with the induction of this disorder, multiple agents that enhance calcium release from the myoplasmic reticulum can induce this syndrome. The syndrome is not a dose-related toxic phenomenon and even small doses in a subject with the underlying disorder may be lethal.

■ REFERENCES

1. Bianchi CP: Cell calcium and malignant hyperthermia. In BA Britt and RA Gordon, eds., International Symposium on Malignant Hyperthermia, pp. 147-151. Springfield, Ill., Thomas, 1973.
2. Britt BA: Malignant hyperthermia and the mitochondria in human patients. IN BA Britt and RA Gordon, eds., International Symposium on Malignant Hyperthermia, pp. 387-398. Springfield, Ill., Thomas, 1973.
3. Brodsky JB, Cohen EN, Brown, BW, Wu ML, Whitcher CE: Exposure to nitrous oxide and neurologic disease among dental professionals. Anesth. and Analg. 60(5): 297-299, 1981.
4. Bruce DL: Trace anesthetic effects on perceptual and cognitive skills. Anesth. Rev. 1:24-25, 1974.
5. Chanarin I: The effects of nitrous oxide on cobalamins, folates, and other related events. CRC: Crit. Rev. Toxicol. 20:179-213, 1982.
6. Chang LW: Pathologic changes following chronic exposures to halothane: A review. Environ. Health Perspect. 21:195-210, 1977.
7. Coburn RF: Mechanisms of carbon monoxide toxicity. Prev. Med. 8:310-322, 1979.
8. Dinn J, McCann S, Wilson P, Reed B, Weir DG, Scott JM: Animal model for subacute combined degeneration. Lancet 2:1154-1155, 1978.
9. Dyck PJ, Karnes J, Lois A, Lofgren EP, Stevens JC: Pathologic alterations of the peripheral nervous system of humans. In PJ Dyck, PK Thomas, EH Lambert, R Bunge, eds., Peripheral Neuropathy, Vol. 1, pp. 760-870. WB Saunders, Philadelphia, 1984.
10. Fagin J, et al.: Carbon monoxide poisoning after accidentally inhaling paint remover. Br. Med. J. 281:1461-1462, 1980.
11. Fajen J, Albright B, Leffingwell SS: A cross-sectional medical and industrial hygiene survey of workers exposed to carbon disulfide. Scand. J. Work Environ. Health 7: (suppl. 4) 20-27, 1981.
12. Feldman RG, Ricks NL, Baker EL: Neuropsychological effects of industrial toxins: A review. Am. J. Indust. Med. 1:211-227, 1980.
13. Goetz CG, Klawans HL: Hyperthermic states: heat stroke and malignant hyperthermia. In PJ Vinken and GW Bruyn, eds., Handbook of Clinical Neurology, Vol. 38. North Holland Publishers, Amsterdam, 1980.
14. Gross JA: Ethylene oxide toxicity. Neurology 29:978-983, 1979.
15. Hanninen H: Psychological picture of manifest and latent carbon disulphide poisoning. Br. J. Ind. Med. 28:374-381, 1971.
16. Klawans HL, Stein RW, Tanner CM, Goetz CG: A pure parkinsonian syndrome following acute carbon monoxide intoxication. Arch. Neurol. 39: 302-304, 1982.

17. Koumbourlis AC, Skoutakis VA: Carbon monixide poisoning: diagnosis and treatment. Clin. Toxicol. Consult. 4:51-69, 1982.
18. Kuzuhara S, Kanazawa I, Nakanishi T, Egashira T: Ethylene oxide polyneuropathy. Neurology (Cleveland) 33:377-380, 1983.
19. Langsjven HA, Langsjven PH, Rasmussen K: Syndrome of subacute carbon monoxide poisoning. Neurology 34:9-92, 1984.
20. Lanham JM: Methyl chloride: an unusual incident of intoxication. Can. Med. Assoc. Journ. 126:593-596, 1982.
21. Layzer FB, Fishman RA, Schaefer JA: Neuropathy following abuse of nitrous oxide. Neurology 28:504-506, 1978.
22. Peters JW: Hydrogen sulfide poisoning in a hospital setting. JAMA 246:1588, 1981.
23. Putz-Anderson V, Setzer JV, Croxton JS, Phipps FC: Methyl chloride and diazepam effects on performance. Scand. J. Work Environ. Health 7:8-13, 1981.
24. Rapkero JD, Lasley SM: Behavioral neurological toxic effects of methyl chloride: A review of the literature. CRC Crit. Rev. Toxicol. 6:283-302, 1979.
25. Sahenk Z, Mendell JR, Couri D, Nachman J: Generalized polyneuropathy: Inhalation of N_2O cartridges through a whipped cream dispenser. Neurology 28:485-488, 1978.
26. Salinas E, Sasich L, Hall DH, Kennedy RM, Morriss H: Acute ethylene oxide intoxication. Drug Intell. Clin. Pharm. 15:385-388, 1981.
27. Smith RP, Kruszyna R, Kruszyna H: Management of acute sulfide poisoning. Effects of oxygen thiosulfate, and nitrite. Arch. Environ. Health 31:166-169, 1976.
28. Stern FB, Lemen RA, Curtis RA: Exposure of motor vehicle examiners to carbon monoxide. A historical prospective mortality study. Arch. Environ. Health 36:59-66, 1980.
29. Stine RJ, Slosberg B, Beacham BE: Hydrogen sulfide intoxication. Ann. Intern. Med. 85:756-758, 1976.
30. Strohl KP, Feldman NT, Saunders N, et al.: Carbon monoxide poisoning in fire victims: A reappraisal of their prognosis. J. Trauma 20:78-80, 1980.
31. Teisinger J: New advances in the toxicology of carbon disulfide. Am. Ind. Hyg. Assoc. J. 35:55-61, 1974.
32. Tuttle TC, Wood GD, Grether CB: Behavioral and neurological elevation of workers exposed to carbon disulfide (CS_2). Final report for National Institute for Occupational Safety and Health. Contract HSM 99-73-35, June 1976.
33. Vasilescu C, Florescu A: Clinical and electrophysiological studies of carbon disulfide polyneuropathy. J. Neurol. 224:59-70, 1980.
34. Venning H, et al.: Carbon monoxide poisoning of an infant. Br. Med. J. 284:651, 1982.
35. Wooley EJ: Neurologic complications of anesthesia. In A. Silverstein, ed., Neurological Complications of Therapy, pp. 199-268. Futura, Mount Kisco, New York, 1982.

CHAPTER 7

Pesticides and Other Environmental Toxins

BESIDES solvents and toxic gases, many other chemicals can pollute the environment, and provoke neurological syndromes of clinical significance. Often these compounds are purposely dispersed over an enormous planted area to control crop pests and enhance eventual harvests. Designed to be preferentially toxic to insects, fungi, and other vermin, these chemicals are only relatively selective and man is not spared. In other instances, toxic chemicals accumulate in the environment because they are poorly degradable wastes. Over time, the populations nearby become exposed or water-ways become polluted. With such products, cumulative doses, rarely calculated with accuracy, are probably the most important feature of chronic toxicity. The entries in this chapter are not exhaustive and new neurotoxins in the environment are reported yearly. As a group they demonstrate the significant environmental dangers of rural and urban existence and the variety of toxic mechanisms that interact to produce neurologic disability. Threshold limit values for most of the agents discussed are listed in Table 7.1.

ORGANOPHOSPHATES

Organophosphates are powerful inhibitors of acetylcholinesterase and pseudocholinesterase. In man, the former enzyme occurs in nervous tissue and erythrocytes and the latter in liver and plasma. Inhibition of these enzymes by organophosphate compounds results from binding of phosphate radicals to the active sites of the enzymes forming phosphorylated proteins. The acute toxicity of organophosphates relates primarily to the inhibition of neurologic acetyl-

INDUSTRIAL TOXINS

TABLE 7.1. Safety Threshold Limit Values for Neurotoxins

	Time weighted average (TLV-TWA) mg/m³	Short-term exposure limit (TLV-STEL) mg/m³
TOCP	0.1	0.3
DDT	1	3
Deldrin	0.25	0.75
Endrin	0.1	0.3
Toxaphene	0.5	2.0
Chlordane	0.5	2
Strychnine	0.15	0.45
Methylbromide	60	—
Phenol	19	38
Styrene	420	525
Camphor	12	18
Acrylamide	0.3	0.6

cholinesterase. This enzyme is found in the brain, spinal cord, and myoneural junction, at pre- and post-ganglionic parasympathetic synapses and at preganglionic and some post-ganglionic sympathetic nerve endings. The abundance of active acetylcholine rendered by the inhibition of its metabolic enzyme causes overstimulation and then inhibition of cholinergic synaptic transmission [34].

Biochemistry

Organophosphate insecticides have been introduced because their toxicity is high to insects and comparatively low to man and domestic mammals. Nevertheless, man is not totally resistant to the neurotoxic effects and hence is at continuing risk for the development of acute or chronic intoxication. The organophosphate insecticides have by and large replaced chlorinated hydrocarbon insecticides such as DDT because the latter compounds are so slowly hydrolized and have significant longterm cumulative effects on the environment.

The absorption of organophosphate insecticides in most instances occurs through the skin or the respiratory tract. As such, the high risk occupations for such intoxication include agricultural workers during or shortly after the spraying of crops and, less commonly, factory workers involved in the formation or transportation of the compounds. People who eat foods freshly sprayed with insecticides and who have not allowed sufficient time for organophosphate hydrolysis would also be at significant risk for acute intoxication. Organophosphate ingestion is commonly used to kill experimental animals, but has little if any significance clinically to man.

Clinical Features

Most instances of major organophosphate poisoning have been due to parathion or methylparathion. The incidence of organophosphate intoxication is relatively low in the United States, although mass epidemics have occurred in India, Egypt, and Mexico. Clinically, intoxication with organophosphate may range from latent asymptomatic poisoning to a life threatening illness. In latent poisoning, the diagnosis depends entirely on the estimation of a serum cholinesterase activity which is inhibited by 10-50 percent. In such instances, no treatment is necessary, although observation for six hours or more is recommended.

In cases of mild poisoning, the patient's complaints are usually those of vague fatigue, headache, dizziness, nausea and vomiting. There may be excessive sweating and salivation, as well as abdominal cramps. The patient may also complain of tremor, numbness and tingling of the extremities. The pupils are small. In moderate poisoning, the weakness is more marked and the patient may also have bulbar weakness with difficulty speaking or swallowing, and becoming short of breath easily. Muscular fasciculations may now be seen. In this case, serum cholinesterase activity is usually 20 percent or less of the normal value. Severe poisoning is associated with depressed levels of consciousness, marked myosis and no pupillary response to light. The patient may become cyanotic from respiratory weakness, and marked secretions in the mouth and nose cause aspiration. Muscles are flaccid with diffuse fasciculations. In such cases, the serum cholinesterase activity is lower than 10 percent of normal [6].

It is impossible to estimate with accuracy the numbers of farmers or commercial applicators dealing with organophosphates who in fact develop mild toxic syndromes. A single study of 98 persons with regular contact to organophosphates and carbamate insecticides showed significant reductions in serum cholinesterase activity in 30%. In 22% of the 98, symptoms were elicited compatible with mild organophosphate pesticide poisoning, but in all cases, these symptoms were ignored and never brought to the attention of a physician [44].

The signs and symptoms of acute organophosphate poisoning are attributable mainly to the massive accumulation of acetylcholine in the cholinergic synapse with subsequent depolarization blockade. Such accumulation occurs both at the muscarinic and nicotinic receptor sites peripherally and centrally. These signs and symptoms are listed in Table 7.2. The time interval between intoxication and symptoms may be very short after massive ingestion (within five minutes) or subacute occurring within 12-24 hours [14,34].

Neuropathy is a prominent toxic sign of organophosphate exposure. Although generally neuropathy has been reported as an effect of chronic organophosphate exposure, recent cases after acute poisoning have been described with such products as methamidophos. In 10 patients reported, all demon-

TABLE 7.2. Signs and Symptoms of Organophosphate Poisoning

Central nervous system manifestations:
    Anxiety and restlessness
    Nightmares, headaches
    Tremor
    Confusion
    Slurred speech and ataxia
    Progressive generalized weakness
    Convulsions
    Depression of respiratory and circulatory centers
Muscarinic manifestations:
    Wheezing with bronchial constriction
    Nausea and vomiting with cramps
    Excessive sweating and salivation
    Bradycardia with hypotension[a]
    Myosis and blurring of vision

Nicotinic manifestations:
    Muscular twitching, fasciculations and cramps
    Sympathetic ganglia: Pallor tachycardia, and elevation in blood pressure[a]

[a]The final heart rate and blood pressure determinations will depend on the relative activity of muscarinic and nicotinic stimulation.

strated acute and severe cholinergic symptoms and unconsciousness on admission to the hospital. After recovery from the initial cholinergic toxicity (8-14 days later), a delayed progressive neuropathy developed. The main symptoms included foot drop, weakness of intrinsic hand muscles, absent ankle jerks, and weakness of hip and knee flexors. In 6 patients who were followed for more than 2 months, pyramidal tract involvement as evidenced by spasticity also developed. This combined involvement of upper and lower motor neuron systems recalls the syndrome seen after chronic exposure to organophosphates [41].

The best studied instances of chronic exposure and delayed neuropathy involve triorthocresyl phosphate (see below), although neuropathy has been reported with tri-aryl phosphate poisoning, nipafox, and trichlorphon compounds [21]. Resolution after cessation of exposure is usually prolonged and often incomplete.

With nipafox, an organophosphate compound with a potential use for insecticide purposes, two patients developed neuropathy which was still present ten and six months after the cessation of exposure. Such case histories suggest that organophosphates as a group have the potential to induce significant neuropathic effects. Whether all products are equally dangerous or not is still undetermined. In one five-year follow-up of 398 workers who handled organophosphate insecticides, including 108 subjects who suffered from acute poisoning, no neuropathy or myopathy was detected [23].

Although parathion and its biologically active metabolite, paraoxon have been thought to be associated with minimal risk of a delayed onset polyneuropathy, such cases have in fact been well described both after chronic exposure to parathion and after a single high dose intoxication in suicide attempt [7]. As in the other cases, recovery is slow and seldom complete.

Peripheral neuropathy has been documented as a residual of organophosphate toxicity in experimental animals. In such instances, the neuropathy was of rapid onset with dioxathion and disulfoton, but delayed with such agents as triorthocresyl phosphate. Neuropathy with additional evidence of usual spinal cord involvement was detectable and the administration of atropine and pralidoxine did not prevent the development of such neuropathy. This failure of agents directly aimed at reversing cholinergic toxicity suggests that neuropathy relates to a different pathogenic mechanism. It has been suggested that phosphorylation of a neurotoxic esterase protein bound to the membrane of nervous tissue results in degeneration of axons and clinical neuropathy within 3 weeks after exposure. As such, this phosphorylated esterase would leave a negatively charged phosphate group covalently bonded to an active membrane site ("aging"). The sequence of events following the phosphorylation of the enzyme and the resulting distal axonopathy remains unknown [6]. The catalytic activity of neurotoxic esterase may be used in the future to predict the neuropathic potential of new organophosphate compounds, and its activity in lymphocytes from workers may be used in screening likely victims of intoxication [5].

Various other neurologic manifestations may range from mild giddiness and anxiety with emotional lability to progressive tremor, slurred speech, ataxia, and gradually profound weakness and bulbar dysfunction. In addition to neurologic toxicity, long term effects on liver function, blood coagulation, skin and respiratory function have also been reported.

Diagnosis

The diagnosis of organophosphate intoxication depends on a history of exposure to such compounds, the clinical picture as described above, the determination of an abnormally low cholinesterase activity in the blood, and improvement (in acute poisoning) after the administration of pralidoxine and atropine. The history of exposure is usually obtained without difficulty and in those cases where a history is unavailable, a characteristic garlic odor on the patient's breath is a sign suggestive of organophosphate intoxication. Organophosphates can be detected by gas or thin layer chromatography from gastric aspirates and urine as well. Intravenous injection of pralidoxine generally causes recovery from signs and symptoms of organophosphate intoxication. In the unconscious patient, intravenous administration of pralidoxine leads to recovery of consciousness and abatement of weakness and fasciculations within 40 minutes.

Although intramuscular or oral administration can be effective, the intravenous route is more reliable in inducing a prompt alteration in function. If the manifestations recur, treatment in the form of 2.5 percent pralidoxine at a rate of up to 0.5 grams/hour can be used. The major action of pralidoxine is to reactivate organophosphate-inhibited acetylcholinesterase activity. The compound removes the phosphate group bound to the esteratic site [36].

Although oxenes are thought to lack access to the central nervous system in humans, multiple reports of patients awakening after pralidoxine administration suggest that at least in the acute organophosphate intoxication, some oxine can cross the blood-brain barrier. This is supported by a recent description of a patient in coma whose EEG suddenly altered 2 minutes after the infusion of pralidoxine with reversal of slow wave frequency as the patient awoke [27].

Practical Management

Pralidoxine 1 gram intravenously should be administered to a patient whose clinical history and presentation suggest organophosphate intoxication. Also atropine 1 mg subcutaneously should be administered every 20-30 minutes until sweating and salivation disappear. If no improvement is seen after the administration of these doses of pralidoxine and atropine, another gram of intravenous pralidoxine should be administered. If no improvement follows, pralidoxine at a rate of 0.5 grams/hour and atropine 5 mg intravenously every 20-30 minutes may be instituted until sweating and salivation disappear. An open airway should be maintained and necessary oxygen given. Organophosphate can be washed from the skin and conjunctivae and gastric lavage can be instituted as well. If the patient has seizures that are not controlled by the administration of atropine and pralidoxine, diphenylhydantoin may be given.

The side effects related to pralidoxine administration are usually minimal. In a small number of patients, unusual excitement, confusion, tachycardia, headache and blurred vision may occur. These may relate to central and systemic anticholinergic toxicity. However, it is difficult to separate the cholinergic from anticholinergic toxic effects in all cases.

If death occurs, it is usually within the first 24 hours in untreated cases, or within two weeks in treated patients. The major fear for longterm morbidity is severe anoxia and residual brain damage. In many patients, alterations in the central nervous system and peripheral nervous system are detectable even when documented anoxic damage did not occur. Of sixteen subjects with prolonged exposure to organophosphate insecticides, eight demonstrated impaired memory, seven depression, six impaired concentration and five psychotic reactions lasting sometimes up to one year [11]. Of 114 subjects with organophosphate poisoning, ten patients complained of neurologic or behavioral alterations and nine of headache for periods of at least six months.

Pesticides and Other Environmental Toxins

TRIORTHOCRESYL PHOSPHATE (TOCP)

The neurotoxicity of this compound was already recognized early in the century when peripheral neuropathy accompanied phosphocreosote therapy for tuberculosis. In the 1920s, an epidemic of Ginger paralysis in the southern United States stimulated new interest in the neurotoxicity of TOCP, since the large number of patients involved clarified the characteristic pattern of the disease. Ingestion of the toxic oily substance in amounts approximating one gram was followed twelve hours later by gastrointestinal upset. One to two weeks later, a progressive flaccid paralysis developed, beginning distally in the legs and accompanied often by aches and tingling paresthesias. With larger doses, the paresis spread to involve the intrinsic hand muscles, the pelvic girdle and thighs. Cranial nerves remained spared and sensory involvement was markedly less than motor. With recovery of the apparent neuropathy, residual signs of central nervous system damage, including spasticity and ataxia became evident [33].

TOCP is an aryl phosphate, used primarily as a high temperature lubricant. It is chemically an organophosphate compound related to the insecticides described above, and acts as a cholinesterase and pseudocholinesterase inhibitor. While TOCP metabolites do in fact inhibit these enzymes, maximal effect in experimental animals is at 48 hours, a time that does not coincide with the clinical onset of neurologically important toxic signs in man or animals. Cholinergic overactivity may be important to the predominantly gastrointestinal prodrome, but would be unlikely to play a pathogenic role in the delayed neurotoxicity of TOCP. In experimental animals, TOCP produces a primary axonal degeneration. Disintegration of the myelin sheath occurs, but is a secondary problem. Pathologic changes in the peripheral nerve become visible around the eighth day after intoxication, and their appearance correlates well with the onset of clinical signs in the animals. At the same time that the pathologic changes occur peripherally, definite lesions are also observed in the spinal cord itself. Ultrastructural alterations include proliferation and distention of vascular elements of the endoplasmic reticulum and the disintegration of organelles. Presynaptic nerve terminals are particularly affected by TOCP intoxication, and synaptic vescicles become markedly inflated. Most authors believe than an essential early step in the neurotoxic effects of TOCP must be the inhibition of an important esterase by phosphorylation. If TOCP affects a direct alteration of the axon by altering some structural component, these changes would account for the delayed onset of neurotoxic signs [15].

PICROTOXIN AND STRYCHNINE

Picrotoxin and strychnine are two important pesticides with severe neurologic toxicity. Both are central analeptic agents and cause seizures as their major toxic manifestation.

Picrotoxin has been shown to block presynaptic inhibition in neurons, and blocks several types of inhibitory synapses in lower animals [9]. Evidence suggests that the agent is a central GABA antagonist [50]. The initial symptoms of picrotoxin intoxication consists of burning sensations in the pharynx and esophagus, abdominal pains, nausea and vomiting, salivation and diarrhea, followed by headache and giddiness. The respirations are at first short and rapid, but later become slow. The pulse rate may increase or decrease and palpitations may occur. These symptoms are rapidly followed by stupor, and at times, loss of consciousness and coma. Within 20 minutes to three hours, severe trembling and generalized seizures develop. In fatal cases, convulsions are followed by paralysis. Death usually occurs from asphyxia or gastrointestinal hemorrhage in one half to several hours.

With oral intoxication, the stomach should be immediately emptied by lavage or by emetics such as apomorphine. The convulsions should be controlled by intravenous administration of barbiturates.

Picrotoxin has been used therapeutically in the treatment of poisoning by CNS depressants, specifically barbiturates. Its narrow margin of safety, however, makes this drug the source of continued pharmacologic controversy. Doses used in treating barbiturate overdose may reach 20 mg, a dose known to induce severe toxic effects by itself.

Strychnine, in addition to its effect as a potent pesticide, is still a component of various tonics and cathartic pills. The lethal dose of strychnine seems to depend largely on absorption dynamics and individual susceptibility since as little as 20 mg has been fatal, and yet some patients have recovered after consuming as much as 249 mg. The usual lethal dose approximates 80 mg. The mechanism of action of strychnine appears to relate to an interference with central postsynaptic inhibitory mechanisms. This has been best demonstrated at the synapses between Renshaw cell and motor neuron, but is probably active at many levels throughout the brain and spinal cord. Strychnine is known to act as a competitive inhibitor of glycine at postsynaptic receptor sites [24].

If taken by mouth, symptoms appear in one half to two hours. Early there is a sense of excitement and marked irritability. Mild paresthesias appear in the face or lower limbs, associated with stiffness and fasciculations in the musculature throughout the body. The limbs, especially the lower extremities, become extended and rigid, while the arms occasionally become fixed in a flexed position. Involvement of the back muscles produces opisthotonos. Trismus and the characteristic risus sardonicus result in difficulty in speech and swallowing. This generalized muscular spasm may last from a few minutes to almost half an hour and is occasionally followed by a clonic convulsion of a generalized type. If the seizure is severe, the patient becomes comatose and cyanotic, with rapid irregular pulse and shallow respirations, often of the Cheyne-Stokes variety.

Intellect remains clear, except for the short periods of unconsciousness accompanying the more severe convulsions. Additional neurologic signs are usually minimal, and deep tendon reflexes may be exaggerated symmetrically. The course is usually rapid, and if patients die, they usually do so within the first 24 hours [1]. If the patient can be kept alive for one day, complete recovery almost invariably occurs. However, sequelae and delayed reactions may occur.

Treatment is supportive and centers on respiratory control and prevention of seizures. Short acting barbiturates and, more recently, diazepam have been successful [18]. The treatment otherwise resembles that for tetanus with complete quiet in a darkened room and freedom from external stimuli. If the patient is seen early, the stomach may be emptied by emetics or lavage and a 1:1000 solution of potassium permanganate may be instilled as a chemical antidote. It may be necessary to use a general anesthetic to control seizure activity. Morphine and apomorphine should be used with extreme caution because of the possibility of synergistic medullary depression.

HYDROCARBON AND OTHER PESTICIDES

The chlorinated hydrocarbon insecticides, with *dichlorodiphenyltrichloroethane (DDT)* as the prototype, share numerous toxicologic properties, although certain individual variations exist. They are all highly soluble in fats and oils and most are of extremely long duration in the environment, making chronic toxicity the most serious ecologic and clinical problem. As a group, these compounds are primarily toxic to the nervous system with the major manifestations being tremor and convulsions. Blood levels associated with toxicity and serum half lives of selected chemicals are listed in Table 7.3.

DDT is associated with acute and chronic neurotoxicity. With acute toxicity, the patient notices a metallic taste in the mouth, and within one hour, dryness of the mouth and extreme thirst develop. Drowsiness or extreme insomnia may develop, the eyes burn, and a gritty sensation is felt within the lid. Some degree of night blindness may be evident, concentration becomes difficult, and later aching of the limbs, muscular spasms, tremors, and stiffness and pain in the jaw may develop. After chronic low dose exposure, weakness of the upper extremities may occur and progress to a complete wrist drop. Mononeuropathy, optic neuropathy and polyneuropathy have all been described with chronic intoxication [4]. When these symptoms result from exposure of the skin to DDT, they may be limited to the limb or limbs touched by the toxin [29]. With chronic high dose exposure, generalized convulsions, coma and death may ensue [46].

The tremor described in patients with DDT toxicity may well be a combination of generalized hyperexcitability and postural tremor along with fasciculations and myoclonus. Patients who are awake may describe "shaking all

TABLE 7.3. Toxicity of Selected Insecticides [46]

Insecticide	Serum half-life	Blood level associated with toxicity	Predicted first symptom
DDT	months	1.0 ppm (μg/ml)	tremors
Hexachlorcyclohexane	several hours	0.1 ppm (μg/ml)	nonspecific
Dieldrin/aldrin	several hours to 1 month	0.1–0.2 ppm (μg/ml)	convulsions
Chlordane	21–88 days	2.7 ppm (μg/ml)	vomiting, seizures
Toxaphene	hours	unknown	convulsion
Endosulfan	probably days	unknown	? malaise
Mirex	months	unknown	hyperexcitability
Chlordecone	150 days	1.0 ppm (μg/ml)	tremor

over" and are observed to have marked twitching. With hands extended, they may have a fine postural tremor and demonstrate hyperactive reflexes, a feeling of irritability, anxiety and unexplained fear.

Exposure may be by respiratory, oral or skin routes. Patients with densely contaminated clothes have been reported to develop neurotoxic signs and patients who had contaminated hands that were scratched on bushes have developed tremors, tinnitus, and later more diffuse signs of DDT toxicity. It is generally difficult to establish a dose of exposure, although in those cases where a dose could be estimated, it appears that the symptoms are in fact dose related. A dose of 10 mg/kg orally has been associated with clinical manifestations of neurotoxicity and there is some indication that heating DDT (as with DDT mistakenly used for baking powder) markedly reduces its toxic effects. Dissolving DDT in organic solvents appears to enhance its danger, although it is unclear whether the organic solvent is causing its own additional form of toxicity or whether it enhances absorption [46].

EEG recordings of 73 workers involved in the production of DDT and other chlorinated hydrocarbon insecticides demonstrated that 21 percent had abnormal tracings. The abnormality was mainly bitemporal, sharp wave activity with shifting lateralization. In these patients there were no convulsions or history of epilepsy and the patients had no clinical neurologic manifestations or known complaints [30].

No significant pathologic lesions have been observed in fatal human cases of DDT toxicity. Central necrosis of the liver lobules, accompanied by tubular degeneration of the kidneys and pulmonary edema, has been noted on general examination. Haymaker et al., using extremely high doses in experimental animals, induced cerebellar degenerative changes [16].

There is no specific antidote for DDT and the therapeutic mainstays are supportive measures and anticonvulsants. After chronic exposure, diphenylhydantoin may be additionally effective in reducing fat sequestration of DDT. Hydantoin administration reduces DDT half-life in fat from 26 to 6.4 months [5].

The neurotoxic mode of action for DDT and the other hydrocarbon insecticides is not completely understood. It has been suggested that these agents cause excessive and spontaneous release of acetylcholine [23]. This would contrast with the proposed mechanism of action for the organophosphates which acutely block the metabolism of acetylcholine extracellularly. In both instances, however, cholinergic overactivation and depolarization blockade are the final result.

Hexachlorocyclohexane contains a number of isomers of which its gamma variety is the most active as an insecticide, generally accounting for 10-35 percent of the total product. The mean lethal dose of the total product is estimated to be 400 mg/kg in man; however, the gamma isomer is much more toxic with a lethal dose of 125 mg/kg pure. The alpha and gamma isomers appear to be central nervous system stimulants while the beta and delta portion are thought to be depressants [13]. Clinically, however, CNS stimulation and seizures are the usual clinical neurotoxic signs associated with the pesticide and hence the presentation is similar to other chlorinated hydrocarbon products. After acute exposure to this product, patients develop severe spasms of voluntary muscles. Cyanosis and seizure activity occur within hours along with severe confusion. Seizures, when they develop, are usually generalized. The gamma constituent can be analyzed in the serum. Although the level associated with neurotoxicity is not fully established, in one instance of acute intoxication (a child who ate insecticide pellets and developed seizures), the gamma fraction was 0.86 ppm (micrograms/ml) at two hours and 0.49 ppm (micrograms/ml) at four hours. The calculated dose of pure gamma toxin was 59 mg/kg. The half-life estimated from this case was in the range of a few hours as judged from the two and four hour levels. The onset of action in the acutely intoxicated patient is very rapid and recovery is complete within a matter of several days. Unlike DDT, this substance does not appear to be cumulative in the organism and either is eliminated or metabolized. Nonneurologic manifestations of hexachlorocyclohexane include bone marrow suppression [46].

Chronic poisoning may also occur with hexachlorocyclohexane, where symptoms include predominant lack of coordination and nervousness. This syndrome is not universal as 79 individuals exposed chronically to the gamma isomer either during chemical production or via a home vaporizer demonstrated no evidence of clinical disease [40]. In those cases where incoordination is prominent, there are descriptions of muscular jerking and even myoclonus. EEG's showed minor nonspecific abnormalities that were not diagnostic. Treatment of the intoxicated individual focuses on general support measures, gastric lavage in the case of an acute oral exposure and symptomatic control of seizures with standard anticonvulsants [46].

Chlordane is another chlorinated hydrocarbon insecticide. As described with other products of this class the major neurotoxicity relates seizures and tremor. Importantly, this compound can be administered along with organophosphate insecticides giving a complicated picture of mixed intoxication. Dinman reported a case where pralidoxine reversed some weakness, leaving the patient with a more classic picture of hydrocarbon intoxication [8]. Although chronic exposure to low doses of chlordane have not been reported to demonstrate significant clinical toxicity in man, spontaneous tremors in rats became evident at the end of twelve weeks of feeding. These reports suggest that chronic exposure could potentially result in significant neurotoxicity. The seizures that can occur with chlordane may appear without prior neurologic complaints. The diagnosis is based on the history, the clinical findings, and a toxic serum level of chlordane in the range of 0.2 mg%. Treatment involves general supportive care and the control of seizures. Since the half-life is long with this compound, careful observation for seizures should last several days.

Dieldrin, aldrin, endrin, and *isobenzan* give a similar toxic picture. *Toxaphene,* a chlorinated derivative of camphene, and *endosulfan* (Thiodane) are two regularly used insecticides also associated with tremor and seizure activity [46]. The toxicity of chlordane is similar except that focal seizures have been reported with unusual frequency with this toxin [35].

Tetrachlorethane is the most dangerous of all the chlorinated hydrocarbons, and use of this solvent is restricted in many countries because of its toxicity. Nevertheless, tetrachlorethane is still widely employed in some areas as an insecticide, a dry-cleaning agent and as a solvent in the leather, rubber and glass industries. It has been commercially marketed under the names of Alanol, Cellon, Emaillet, Novania, Tetralen and Westron.

This hydrocarbon exerts a prolonged narcotic effect. Unconsciousness, loss of corneal reflexes, cyanosis and death have followed within 12 hours after ingestion. More commonly, tetrachlorethane poisoning results from chronic exposure to excess concentrations of the vapor in the air. In such cases, headache, giddiness, anorexia, nausea and other nonspecific complaints may precede the appearance of more serious symptoms. The most significant damage is to the liver. Weakness of the interossei, palatal paralysis, parethesias, and disturbances of the reflexes have also been noted. During the intoxication, large mononuclear cells may constitute up to 40 percent of the circulating leukocytes. The treatment of tetrachlorethane toxicity is aimed chiefly at protection of the liver from further parenchymal damage.

Chlordecone (Kepone) is a chlorinated hydrocarbon insecticide that gained notoriety in the mid-1970's when extensive over exposure of the pesticide was found about a plant site in Virginia and later in the local environment and waterways draining the region. Fish and shell fish were discovered to contain variable quantities of chlordecone and as a consequence, the James River was completely closed to fishing in late 1975. Four years later, this ban remained in effect due to the persistence of the chemical in the sediment of the river, and continued traces of chlordecone in fish [47].

Trembling (Kepone-shakes) is the most prominent feature of this intoxicant. The tremor was usually small in amplitude and irregular in direction seen both at rest and during action, although most marked in the action or fixed posture positions. The tremor abates during sleep and increases with anxiety or fatigue. When the tremor involves the trunk or lower extremities, mild instability and gait disturbance may be seen. End point exacerbation or cerebellar incoordination is not seen. In general, the tremor begins approximately six weeks or more after exposure to the compound. With time, the tremor progresses so that subjects may no longer be able to fasten clothing, or handle small tools or eating utensils with their usual dexterity.

Irregular saccade movements were also seen in 15 patients exposed to high chlordecone levels. These aberrant movements provoked complaints of blurred vision and on examination were seen both conjugately and disconjugately. Additionally, irritability and memory loss may be present, occurring in over half of 23 patients examined in the above mentioned contamination incident. These mental changes persisted for several weeks after chlordecone exposure had halted, but were eventually reversible. With levels as high as 33 ppm, auditory and visual hallucinations have been reported, as well as incapacitating myoclonic jerks; low grade papilledema and headaches were evident with lower levels but still elevated. In three patients studied, elevated cerebrospinal fluid pressures were detected.

Muscle biopsies in six patients with chlordecone exposure demonstrated increased lipofucin and lipid-like droplets, as well as the predominance of type one fibers. Serial nerve biopsies in five patients demonstrated a diminished number of poorly myelinated fibers and an increase in endoneural collagen.

In the outbreak in Virginia, over half of the active employees of the affected plant were moderately ill. A few required hospitalization for months, but severe toxic signs generally abated when patients were removed from the toxic environment. However, four years afterwards, several workers continued to manifest a significantly incapacitating tremor.

Non-neurologic effects of chlordecone include hepatomegaly, arthralgias and pleuritic chest pain of unknown pathogenesis. The half-life of chlordecone in untreated patients averaged 165 days. Cholestyramine significantly increased fecal excretion of the pesticide so that following 16 grams per day of this product, the half-life of chlordecone in blood was reduced to a mean of 80 days. Other forms of therapy such as activated charcoal (40 grams/day) and plasmaphoresis have not been successful in lowering blood chlordecone levels. The specific treatment of the tremor has been attempted with propranolol in doses of 200 mg/day with some amelioration.

The mechanism of action of chlordecone is undetermined. Since propranolol does abate the tremor, it has been suggested that the toxin may affect beta adrenergic systems. The cholinergic system may also be affected, since a closely related compound, dieldrin, is known to cause increases in cholinergic activation. Both the Na,K-ATPase and the Mg-ATPase are inhibited by chlordecone in catfish brain [47].

Pyridylmethy-nitrophenyl urea, (PNU, VACOR) is the active ingredient used in major rodenticides aimed at controlling rats and mice. This compound is available in over-the-counter pest killers, as well as in powder available only to professional operators. It has been promoted as an "ideal rodenticide" because its LD_{50} in primates is much higher than in rodents. Furthermore, it is effective in a single dose and nicotinamide is an antidote in animals. The LD_{50} for rats is 500 times that for monkeys, but several human poisonings suggest that the LD_{50} for man may be quite close to that of rats (5 mg/kg). The minimal lethal dose observed in adult man was 390–780 mg total dose [10].

The mechanism of action of PNU toxicity appears to involve nicotinamide antagonism. Similar in structure to two known diabetogenic agents, alloxan and streptozotocin, PNU may be directly toxic to pancreatic beta cell membranes. Experimental animal studies demonstrate that nicotinamide protects pancreatic beta cells against the cytotoxic action of alloxan. PNU may act similarly and induce a depression of intracellular NAD levels. It has been suggested that PNU may produce autonomic neuropathy and diabetes by reducing nicotinamide adenine dinucleotide concentrations in the brain and pancreas, although this has not been proven [32].

The neurologic abnormality described in patients exposed to PNU includes slight dizziness and diffuse weakness within hours after ingesting the rat poison. Numbness of the hands and lower extremities follow within several hours and weakness, instability and poor coordination gradually increase. The patient may develop diabetes requiring insulin therapy and postural hypotension and gastrointestinal hypomotility may become prominent. The duration of these autonomic changes may range from eight weeks to as long as ten months and theoretically could be irreversible. In cases where there is substantial postural hypotension, mineral corticoids (fludrocortisone) may be needed. Peripheral neuropathy may be quite prominent and longstanding, manifesting in diffuse weakness, ataxia and diminished pin sensation. Some patients may demonstrate fine tremors as well. In those patients who have died from PNU toxicity, prominent ketoacidosis and cardiac arrhythmias were the major features.

Methyl bromide is widely used as an insecticide, fumigant or delousing agent and is important as a methylating agent especially in the manufacture of chemicals and dyes. Despite industrial safeguards, cases of both acute and chronic methyl bromide intoxication continue to occur. The lungs, kidneys and nervous system appear to be most profoundly affected.

The neurologic manifestations of acute methyl bromide toxicity have been divided by Wyers into three categories: a) a premonitory stage with nausea, vomiting, vertigo and headache; b) a cerebral irritative stage with tremors, convulsions, delirium or mania; and c) a recovery stage with apathy, amnesia, incoordination and often hallucinations or aphasia [52]. In children, the clinical picture closely resembles Reye's syndrome of acute encephalopathy with fatty degeneration of the liver [42].

Chronic intoxication induces visual disturbances, confusion, chronic hallucinations and speech difficulties. Progressive weakness and paresthesias occur and convulsions and coma, followed by death, have been reported.

Neuropathologic changes include small subarachnoid hemorrhages, capillary proliferation and demyelination with loss of neurons centrally. The sites of involvement are cerebral cortex, quadrigeminal bodies, red dentate, and olivary nuclei.

While the pathophysiology of methyl bromide toxicity is not understood, it is clear that neither inorganic bromide nor methyl alcohol are primarily responsible. Residual tremor, ataxia and incoordination as well as action myoclonus may follow intoxication. No specific treatment is available, although chelation has been used experimentally [19].

OTHER ENVIRONMENTAL POISONS

Tetrachlordibenzo-P-dioxin (TCDD), has been the source of an intense controversy in industrial medicine. A large scale dioxin intoxication occurred in Seveso, Italy in 1976, although prior episodes had in fact been reported. Dioxin may be associated with skin lesions, including chloracne, multiple irregularities in blood chemistries, and neurologic and psychiatric alterations [48].

Dioxin is a solid substance, insoluble to water and only slightly soluble in fats and chlorinated solvents. It is a contaminent of such herbicides as Agent Orange. It is highly heat stable and exerts its biological effects at extremely low concentrations. Its half-life in soil is estimated at approximately one year and microbial degradation only rarely occurs. Although there are significant differences in specie susceptibility to the toxin, the toxic effect occurs slowly and progresses several days or weeks after a single dose. Since the Seveso accident, long-term follow up has been conducted on intoxicated patients from this group as well as from a group of 80 patients from Czechoslovakia [37].

INDUSTRIAL TOXINS

The earliest symptoms of intoxication are the gradual formation of chloracne, a global feeling of sickness, fatigue and weakness. Usually this occurs days or weeks after the initial exposure, although in some patients these consistent findings did not occur until several months after work with dioxin was completed. In the Czechoslovakian series, 23 percent of patients exposed to chronic dioxin showed initial evidence by clinical exam or electromyographic study of polyneuropathy. In most cases, the neuropathy progressed and then stabilized after four years. In addition, four patients showed signs of facial weakness as evidence of a peripheral 7th cranial nerve lesion. Encephalopathy occurred initially in 7 percent of the patients and progressed in chronic follow up to include 9 percent of those studied. Early psychiatric signs included neurotic symptoms, neurasthenia with depression occurring in 83 percent of patients which tended to decrease in severity and was only present in 58 percent in long-term follow up.

Importantly, these symptoms did not occur initially. Polyneuropathy in some patients occurred only in the third or fourth year after exposure had ceased. The origin of this abnormality is unclear, since many of the patients had abnormal glucose tolerance tests and other metabolic abnormalities, including hypercholesterolemia, hyperlipemia and a high pre-beta fractions. In contrast, the psychiatric problems tended to be predominantly anxiety and depression that were seen early on and may well have related to exogenous influences, including fear of death, disfigurement from the cutaneous manifestations and concerns about job permanency. In a series of patients who were examined by the author and who were exposed to dioxin and other chemicals in an American worksetting, 20 of 46 (43%) had an intention tremor, most of the postural type, and over half had evidence of peripheral neuropathy (unpublished).

Polychlorinated biphenyls (PCB's) were first synthesized in Germany in the nineteenth century. In the late 1920's, American synthesis of the compounds was initiated for electrical equipment because of their highly efficient insulation properties. However, short-term exposure to PCB's can produce skin irritation, hepatic damage, myocardial and renal damage. Neurotoxicity was reported in Japan after PCB's leaked into rice oil that was used for cooking by 15,000 people. Over 1,000 people became ill with gastrointestinal or neurologic symptoms of peripheral neuropathy. The latter complication included endocrine disorders and malignant tumors. Other instances of neurologic disorders with PCB contamination are not clear, and the entire class of compounds may not be uniformly neurotoxic. Treatment of patients exposed to PCB's involves only rapid removal of the victim from the toxic environment. Of patients with liver disease related to PCB's, it is estimated that 50% will die.

Phenol is a toxic product to which workers in coal synthesis or distillation may be exposed, as well as workers with resins, disinfectants, perfumes and pharmaceuticals. Neurologic toxicity includes headaches, seizures and tinnitus.

Phenol has been injected intrathecally and epidurally, as well as directly on to peripheral nerves during neurolysis procedure for the management of pain and spasticity. Such neurolytic effects in man may be transient or permanent. The pathological consequence of phenol exposure is Wallerian degeneration and in the peripheral nervous system, both large and small fibers are affected. The nerve cell and myelin do not show distinct abnormalities. After phenol application, transient conduction blockade of nerve action potentials follows. Electron microscopy studies corroborate the axonal degeneration that occurs in fibers of all sizes, although evidence of some demyelination is apparent, especially at low phenyl doses [35,51].

Hexachlorophene used in high concentrations as an antimicrobial agent in soaps and detergents, is also a broad spectrum plant fungicide and pesticide in agriculture. It is soluble in ethanol, acetone and other organic solvents and is absorbed through skin and mucous membranes. The primary target of the toxin appears to be the cell plasma membrane, causing vacuolation and disruption of myelin. Biochemically, hexachlorophene is a potent uncoupler of oxidative phosphorylation.

Most cases of intoxication in man have resulted from skin application or ingestion of liquid detergents. In babies with diaper rash, application of detergents containing this product led to more rapid absorption than would have been anticipated in normal skin. Similarly, burn patients are subjects at high risk for extensive absorption of hexachlorophene [49].

In man, intoxication has occurred after acute or subacute exposure. With dermal or vaginal exposure, convulsions, paralysis, and behavioral changes such as withdrawal, irritability and erratic behavior predominate. Oral exposure provokes hyperthermia, hypotension and less commonly the neurologic signs discussed with dermal application. In cases with acute and fatal outcome, neuropathologic changes may be observed as early as three days after intoxication. In such instances the cerebral hemispheres are enlarged and the optic nerves show intramyelinic edema. Curiously, the brains of low birth weight, premature infants appear to be particularly susceptible to the toxic effects of hexachlorphene. In a study of 69 newborn infants bathed with the detergent, Powell and associates found no changes in full-term or premature infants, but significant vacuolation of myelin in brainstems of premature infants weighing less than 1400 grams [38]. In those patients with acute or subacute hexachlorophene intoxication who recovered, no apparent sequelae remained. Treatment focuses on withholding this chemical and prompt attention to life support measures. In animal studies, hexachlorophene also produces vacuolation of myelin in the peripheral nervous system [49]. Because of these outbreaks of problems, the United States Food and Drug Administration has withdrawn hexachlorophene from the over-the-counter availability that it once enjoyed and now the preparation is strictly controlled by prescriptions.

Styrene is used in the production of plastics and resins and is associated with widespread toxicity in workers who inhale the chemical. In addition to neurologic toxicity, hepatic, renal and pulmonary effects are also reported, as well as mutagenic actions. Older individuals may be more prone to develop styrene neurotoxicity than younger subjects. The neurologic effects are those of visual motor dysfunction, reduced short-term memory, paresthesias and weakness. In spite of the clinical problems, peripheral nerve conduction velocities may not be altered and sensory functions may be more abnormal on electromyographic studies than motor. The mechanisms of styrene-induced toxicity is not known, although it has been proposed that the chemical induces an increase in the production of intracellular free radicals [39].

Camphor is a mildly irritating and antiseptic material. Children may become poisoned by the ingestion of camphor-containing mothballs. In adults, toxic symptoms have resulted from the use of the spirits as an intoxicant, as an abortifacient and in suicide attempts. The amount of camphor that will produce toxic symptoms varies with the individual but is approximately 10 ml of camphorated oil or 15 ml of spirits of camphor.

Following ingestion of toxic amounts of camphor, the initial symptoms are irritation of the throat, thirst, nausea, and vomiting. Headache, sensations of warmth, blurring of vision, vertigo and colicky abdominal pains then appear. After a period varying from a few minutes to hours, the patient becomes confused and delirious. A twitching of the buccal and oral mucosa may develop, as well as a generalized rigidity with tetanic contraction of the masseter muscles, resulting in trismus [3]. Loss of consciousness may follow and persist for hours. Generalized convulsions appear from one to two hours after the administration of the drug and may recur for several hours. Rarely, excitement associated with anxiety, assaultiveness, and hallucinations may occur. The patient's breath and urine have a strong camphor odor. The face is initially flushed and then becomes pale, and the pupils are dilated. The temperature may rise to 101 degrees F. Difficult respiration and cyanosis occur in the more severe cases. Death is uncommon but may result from respiratory failure, asphyxia, or circulatory collapse.

When the drug has been taken orally, the material should be removed by gastric lavage. If alcoholic spirits of camphor have been ingested, olive oil should be instilled to dissolve the camphor, and the stomach contents, including the olive oil evacuated. Apomorphine in doses of 5 to 10 mg has been recommended as a substitute for the gastric lavage. If convulsions occur, they may be controlled with intravenous or intramuscular administration of barbiturates or paraldehyde. Lipid dialysis has been successfully employed in acute camphor intoxication [12].

Hydrazine is a major corrosion inhibitor in metal processing and is additionally used in the production of plasticizers and photographic developers. Recurrent exposure to as little as 0.5 ppm has resulted in fatality [43].

The route of exposure determines the prominent clinical effects; after vapor inhalation, irritation of mucous membranes and respiratory complaints develop followed by excitatory and depressive CNS effects; after oral ingestion, convulsions and coma rapidly develop.

The mechanism of action of hydrazine neurotoxicity appears to involve alterations in the GABA system. The GABA synthesizing enzyme glutamic acid decarboxylase (GAD) is inhibited by hydrazine through the depletion of the necessary co-factor pyridoxyl phosphate [31]. Treatment of hydrazine toxicity has thereby focused on replenishment of the co-factor and pyridoxine administration has been used with success. In mild cases, 200 mg intravenously and 400 mg intramuscularly have reversed symptoms within twenty minutes. After severe intoxication with seizures and coma, higher doses of 25 mg/kg, (one-third intramuscularly, two-thirds by slow intravenous infusion over three hours) has been recommended. Complete recovery can usually be anticipated [22].

Acrylamide is used as a chemical grout which is pumped into dirt, clay, and stone walls of excavations and then polymerized for a water-tight seal. In its nonpolymerized form, it appears to be neurotoxic; clinical intoxication was noted by Kuperman and confirmed experimentally in rats [25]. Acrylamide may be absorbed through skin, lungs or mucous membranes and has been implicated in numerous cases of industrial intoxication where workers were exposed in tunnels or other poorly ventilated spaces.

The neurologic features of acrylamide intoxication depend on the speed of exposure. In a Japanese family encephalopathic symptoms including confusion, disorientation, memory impairment and hallucinations developed one month after their water well became contaminated with 400 ppm acrylamide [20]. A mild peripheral neuropathy and ataxia developed subsequently. As these subjects were probably exposed to a higher dose of acrylamide than other humans, their case is exceptional, and encephalopathic symptoms of this severity are not typical of the usual intoxicated acrylamide patient.

With more mild exposure, encephalopathic symptoms may develop within a few weeks after the exposure, and include drowsiness and lack of concentration. Truncal ataxia is the most prominent feature in these patients and appears to relate to cerebellar rather than sensory dysfunction. In one series, the ataxia was already improving or had disappeared by the time symptoms of peripheral neuropathy were detectable [20]. Dysarthria is also prominent in such patients and nystagmus may be present. Gradually, a peripheral neuropathy develops and is an additional hallmark of the subacutely intoxicated patient. Such patients demonstrate both motor and sensory impairment most prominently distally in the limbs.

In those patients with a low level of chronic exposure, neurologic symptoms may not develop until several months of exposure. In such cases, a sensorimotor neuropathy is the prominent feature and neither encephalopathy nor ataxia is prominent.

The peripheral neuropathy associated with acrylamide intoxication affects both motor and sensory fibers, predominantly distally. Patients often complain of weakness and clumsiness. Wasting and fasciculations may be clinically present, as well as depressed tendon reflexes. It is of clinical interest to note that all tendon reflexes may be lost early in the course of the disease, unlike many other toxic peripheral neuropathies where only the ankle jerks are lost. Paresthesias and dysesthesias may predominate and muscle tenderness has been described as well. Autonomic dysfunction, including excessive sweating, cold and blue extremities or alternately redness and exfoliation of the hands may occur.

No specific neurologic or laboratory tests confirm the diagnosis, but a combination of truncal ataxia and prominent peripheral neuropathy should suggest acrylamide intoxication in the patient with the appropriate exposure. Electrophysiologic alterations include only mild changes in the conduction velocity of motor and sensory fibers. Sensory nerve action potentials are usually abnormal and although motor nerves may be more clinically affected, measurement of sensory nerve action potential amplitudes appears to be the most sensitive electrophysiologic test in patients with acrylamide intoxication [26]. Fullerton described the histological changes in serial nerves focusing predominantly on axonal degeneration.

The toxic mechanism of acrylamide appears to relate to the direct effects on axonal metabolism. In in vitro studies, acrylamide-treated axons demonstrate impaired regeneration in spite of continued delivery of transported organelles. It has been suggested that acrylamide combines directly with protein sulfydryl groups to impair neuronal metabolism.

A reduction of toxic signs and symptoms follows removal from the source of acrylamide. In patients with the acute encephalopathy, mild ataxia and neuropathy, complete recovery is usual. In those more severely affected patients, residual abnormalities may persist even after months of improvement. The residua include mild ataxia, distal weakness, persistent reflex loss and sensory disturbance. No treatment is available other than removal of the toxin.

▪ STUDY QUESTIONS

Organophosphates provoke acute toxicity via:

A. Increased reuptake of presynaptic acetylcholine similar to botulism.
B. Increased extracellular metabolism of acetylcholine similar to black widow spider venom.
C. Inhibition of enzymes that synthesize acetylcholine from serotonin.
D. None of the above.

Answer: D

Pesticides and Other Environmental Toxins

Acute organophosphate toxicity relates to excess cholinergic activity by means of inhibition of extracellular cholinesterase. This leads to cholinergic crisis and eventual depolarization blockade. The answers given are not only wrong but also unreasonable. Botulinum toxin blocks the release of acetylcholine. Black widow spider provokes the forced release of acetylcholine and has no effect on extracellular enzymes. Acetylcholine is synthesized from choline and acetyl-CoA and serotonin is not a precursor.

Patients with organophosphate toxicity become weak because:

A. Acetylcholine normally inhibits the neuromuscular junction.
B. Too much acetylcholine causes depolarization blockade.
C. The toxin causes enzymatic degradation of acetylcholine transferase.
D. The toxin has GABA-like activity.

Answer: B

Electrophysiologically, when excess neurotransmitter is available at the postsynaptic receptor site, these receptor sites are stimulated and increased activity is effected. When the excess is exceptional, the postsynaptic receptor function may become inactivated and the cell becomes blocked because it is continually depolarized without a chance to reestablish its baseline potentials.

Match the toxin with the prominent clinical toxic picture.

A.	Chlordecone	1.	Severe neuropathy with signs of spinal cord involvement.
B.	Triorthocresyl phosphate	2.	Risus sardonicus and trismus
C.	Strychnine	3.	kepone shakes
D.	Hexachlorophene	4.	Seizures in low birth weight babies.
E.	Dioxin	5.	Diabetes and neuropathy.

Answers: A-3, B-1, C-2, D-4, E-5

Chlordecone is a pesticide that caused an epidemic of neurotoxicity in the Virginia region. Tremor and shaking were the predominant features along with neuropathy. Triorthocresyl phosphate, an organophosphate used primarily as a lubricant rather than an insecticide, has been associated with a progressive neuropathy with signs of spinal cord disease as well. As such, patients may have neuropathy plus spasticity with the clinical picture resembling amyotrophic lateral sclerosis (ALS) when there is minimal sensory involvement. Strychnine causes general increased excitability in the nervous system and can look similar to tetanus with a classic risus sardonicus and trismus. Hexachlorophene, no longer available as an over-the-counter disinfectant, provoked seizure activity in low weight babies. Dioxin, a toxin of increasing publicity in America, has been associated with the induction of significant neuropathy and diabetes. Whether the neuropathy relates directly to the toxin or to the secondary effects of diabetes is unclear. Patients with exposure to dioxin have also been observed to suffer with memory problems and prominent postural tremors.

A patient has accidentally ingested rat poison. The likely active products are:

INDUSTRIAL TOXINS

A. Methyl bromide
B. Vacor (PNU)
C. Warfarin
D. Corticone

Answer: B and C

Vacor is a major toxin in rodenticides. Its mechanism of action is not entirely clear but it may inhibit nicotinamide and therefore may provoke autonomic nervous system as well as myoneural junction abnormalities. Warfarin affects the coagulation system and is a systemic toxin that may have neurologic consequences. Methyl bromide is used predominantly as a fumigant and chlordecone as an organophosphate pesticide.

A child presents with new onset of hyperextension of the neck, stiff arched posture and severe facial grimacing. He ingested an unknown substance within the last few hours. Which of the following can provoke this sort of clinical presentation?

A. Phenothiazine drugs
B. Strychnine
C. Vacor
D. Triorthocresyl phosphate

Answer: A and B

This patient, from the information given, could be having an acute dystonic reaction from a phenothiazine. Such patients may have opisthotonic posturing with the neck arched and the body held in a contorted position. Also, the patient could have ingested strychnine, provoking the generalized hyperexcitability state with marked painful spasms. These patients are usually very sensitive to stimulation so that loud shouts or slamming of doors can induce the spasms whereas a phenothiazine induced dystonia is not sound sensitive. The other two products (C and D) are not applicable to this presentation.

■ REFERENCES

1. Aikman J: Strychnine poisoning in children. JAMA 95:1661-1664, 1920.
2. Barnes R: Poisoning by the insecticide chlordane. Med. J. Aust. 1:972-973, 1967.
3. Benz RW: Camphorated oil poisoning with no mortality, JAMA 72:127-129, 1919.
4. Committee on pesticides: Pharmacology and toxicologic aspects of DDT (chlorophenothane, U.S.P.). JAMA 145:728-729, 1951.
5. Davies JE, Edmundson WF, Maceo A, Irvin III BL, Cassady J, and Barquet A: Reduction of pesticide residues in human adipose tissue with diphenylhydantoin. Food Chem. Toxicol 9:413–423, 1971.

6. Davis CD, Richardson RJ: Organophosphorus compounds. In PS Spencer and HH Schaumberg, eds., Experimental and Clinical Neurotoxicology, Chap. 36, pp. 527-545. Williams and Wilkins, Baltimore/London, 1980.
7. De Jager AEJ, van Weerden TW, Houthoff HJ, de Monchy JGR: Polyneuropathy after massive exposure to parathion. Neurology 31:603-605, 1981.
8. Dinman BD: Acute combined toxicity due to DDVP and chlordane. Arch. Envir. Health Vol 16:765-769, 1964.
9. Eccles JC, Schmidt R, Willis WD: Pharmacologic studies on presynaptic inhibition. J. Phys. London 168:500-506, 1963.
10. Gallanosa AG, Spyker DA, Curnow RT: Rodenticide poisoning: A review. Clin. Toxicol. 18 (4):441-449, 1981.
11. Gerson S, Shaw FH: Psychiatric sequelae of chronic exposure to organophosphorus insecticides. Lancet 1:1371-1372, 1961.
12. Ginn HE, Anderson KE, Mercier RK, Stevens TW, Matter BJ: Camphor intoxication treated by lipid dialysis. JAMA 203:230-231, 1968.
13. Gosselin E, Hodge C, Smith P, Gleason N: Clinical Toxicology of Commercial Products, 4th ed. Baltimore, Md, Williams and Wilkins, 1976.
14. Gourley DR, Haggerty JA, Spigiel RW, Holcslaw TL: Organophosphate pesticide poisoning. Clin. Toxicol. Consult. 3 (1):41-45, 1981.
15. Gross D: Clinical aspects; diagnosis and symptomatology. In AV Albertini, D Gross, WM Zinn, eds.), Triaryl-Phosphate Poisoning in Morocco, 1959, pp. 14-28. George Thieme, Stuttgart, 1968.
16. Harris S, Jr.: Jamaica ginger paralysis (peripheral polyneuritis) South. Med. J. 23:375-380, 1930.
17. Haymaker W, Ginzler AM, Ferguson RL: The toxic effects of prolonged ingestion of DDT on dogs with special reference to lesions in the brain. Am. J. Med. Sci. 212:423, 1946.
18. Herishanu Y, Landau H: Diazepam in the treatment of strychnine poisoning. Br. J. Anaesth. 44:747-748, 1972.
19. Hine CH: Methyl bromide poisoning: A review of ten cases. J. Occup. Med. 11:1-19, 1969.
20. Igisu H, Goto I, Kawamura Y, Kato M, Izumi K, Kuroiwa Y: Acrylamide encephalopathy due to well water pollution. J. Neurol., Neurosurg., Psychiatry 38:581-589, 1975.
21. Johnson MK: The delayed neuropathy caused by some organophosphorus esters: mechanism and challenge. CRC Crit. Rev. Toxicol. 3:289-292, 1975.
22. Kirklin JK, Watson M, Bondoc CC, Burke JF: Treatment of hydrazine-induced coma with pyridoxine. N. Engl. J. Med. 294:938-939, 1976.
23. Kovarik J, Sercle M: The influence of the organophosphate insectides on the nervous system. 15th International Congress on National Health. Abstract of Papers. 6 1966.
24. Kuno M, Weakly JN: Quantal components of the inhibitory synaptic potential in spinal motoneurons of the cat. J. Physiol. Lond. 287:224-226, 1972.
25. Kuperman S: Effects of acrylamide on the central nervous system of the cat. J. Pharmacol. Exp. Ther. 123:180-182, 1958.

26. Le Quesne PM: Acrylamide. In PS Spencer, HH Schaumburg, eds., Experimental and Clinical Neurotoxicology, pp. 309-313. Williams and Wilkins, Baltimore, pp. 309-313, 1980.
27. Lotti M: Pralidoxine in parathon poisoning. J. Toxicol. Clin. Toxicol. 19: 121-124, 1982.
28. Lotti M, Becker CE, Aminoff MJ: Organophosphate polyneuropathy: pathogenesis and prevention. Neurology 34 65-62, 1984.
29. Mackerras IM, West RFK: DDT poisoning in man, Med. J. Aus. 1:400, 1946.
30. Mayersdorf A, Israeli R: Toxic effects of chlorinated hydrocarbon insecticides on the human electroencephalogram. Arch. Environm. Health, 28: 159-163, 1974.
31. Meldrum BS: Epilepsy and gamma-aminobutyric acid-mediated inhibition. Int. Rev. Neurobiol. 17:1-36, 1975.
32. Miller L, Stokes JD, Silpipat C: Diabetes mellitus and autonomic dysfunction after vacor rodenticide ingestion. Diabetes Care 1:73-76, 1978.
33. Morgan JP, Penovich P: Jamaica Ginger Paralysis: 47 year followup. Arch. Neurol. 35:530-531, 1978.
34. Namba T, Nolte CT, Jackrel J, Grob D: Poisoning due to organophosphate insecticides. Ann. Intern. Med. 50:475-492, 1971.
35. National Institute for Occupational Safety and Health: Criteria for Recommended Occupational Exposure to Phenol. NIOSH, Cincinnati, 1976.
36. O'Leary JF, Harrison B, Groblewski G, Wills JH: The effect of 2-formyl-l-methylpyridinium iodide oxine (2-PAM) on reactivation of tissue cholinesterase following poisoning by a certain phosphate anticholinesterase. Fed. Proc. 18:430, 1959.
37. Pazderova-Vejlupkova J: Development and prognosis of chronic intoxication by tetrachlordibenzo-p-dioxin in men. Arch. Environ. Health 36:5-11, 1981.
38. Powell H, Swarner O, Gluck L, Lampe P: Hexachlorophene myelinopathy in premature infants. J. Pediatr. 82:976-978, 1973.
39. Rosen I, Haeger-Aronsen S, Rehnstrom S, Welinton H: Neurophysiological observation after chronic styrene exposure. Scand. J. Work Environ. Health 4:184-186, 1979.
40. Samuels AJ, Milby TH: Human exposure to lindane: clinical, hematological and biochemical effects. J. Occup. Med. 13:147-151, 1971.
41. Senanayake N, et al: Acute polyneuropathy after poisoning by a new organophosphate insecticide. N. Engl. J. Med. 306:155-157, 1982.
42. Shield LK, Coleman TL, Markesbery WR: Methyl bromide intoxication: Neurologic features including simulation of Reyes Syndrome. Neurology 27:959-960, 1977.
43. Sotaniemi E, Hirvonen J, Isomaki H, Takkunen J, Kaila J: Hydrazine toxicity in the human. Ann. Clin. Res. 3:30-33, 1971.
44. Spigiel RW, Gourley DR, Holcslaw TL, Young B, Haggerty JA: Organophosphate pesticide exposure in farmers and commercial applicators. Clin. Toxicol. Consult. 3:45-50, 1981.

45. Tabershaw IR, Cooper WC: Sequelae of acute organic phosphate poisoning. J. Occup. Med. 8:5-8, 1966.
46. Taylor JR, Calabrese VP, Blanke RV: Organochlorine and other insecticides. In PJ Vinken and GW Bruyn, eds., Handbook of Clinical Neurology, Vol. 36, pp. 391-404. Amsterdam, North-Holland Publishing, 1979.
47. Taylor JR, Selhorst JB, Calabrese VP: Chlordecone. In PS Spencer, HH Schaumburg, eds., Experimental and Clinical Neurotoxicology, pp. 407-408. Williams and Wilkins, Baltimore, 1980.
48. Tognoni G, Bonaccorsi A: Epidemiological Problems with TCDD (A Critical View). Drug Metab. Rev. 13:447-469, 1982.
49. Towieghi J: Hexachlorophene. In PS Spencer, HH Schaumburg, eds., Experimental and Clinical Neurotoxicology, p. 407, Williams and Wilkins, Baltimore, 1980.
50. Usherwood PNR, Grundjest H: Inhibitory postsynaptic potentials. Science 143:817, 1964.
51. Wood KM: The use of phenol as a neurolytic agent: a review. Pain 5:205, 1978.
52. Wyers H: Methylbromide intoxication. Br. J. Ind. Med. 2:24-29, 1945.

III.
Biological Toxins

CHAPTER 8

Bacterial Toxins

ALTHOUGH bacterial infections are often associated with acute and chronic neurologic syndromes, three major bacteria cause neurologic deficits specifically because of their potent exotoxins. Diphtheria and tetanus produce exotoxins as part of a systemic infectious process, while botulism usually results from the ingestion of exotoxin already produced anaerobically. Traditionally, these exotoxin-syndromes are felt to be unusual in the predominantly urban American society, although botulism and tetanus are not rare. The clinical history and characteristic presentations are particularly important in establishing the diagnosis of these conditions.

DIPHTHERIA

Diphtheria is acquired by droplet transmission and there are two clinical forms, oropharyngeal and cutaneous. Both manifest neurologic complications. Once infestation is established locally, the *Corynebacterium diphtheriae* gives off a powerful circulating exotoxin that preferentially affects muscle and myelin [9]. Neurologic complications may be due to either direct damage to muscle and peripheral nerve or to indirect damage from hypoxia and airway obstruction. Direct central nervous system involvement is uncommon because the exotoxin does not penetrate the blood-brain barrier appreciably [27]. Local palatal and bulbar mononeuropathies may occur within the first two weeks of the disease. Ocular involvement with paralysis of accommodation follows and has been seen in approximately half of those patients with post-diphtheritic neurologic dysfunction [23]. Further peripheral neuropathy involving somatic nerves is characteristic in the sixth and seventh weeks with a predominant sensory polyneuropathy or a proximal motor neuropathy that extends distally [20]. The picture of a Guillain-Barré syndrome with visual blurring and palatal involvement should immediately suggest diphtheria.

Pathologically, the neuropathy is a non-inflammatory demyelinating process. The ganglia of the peripheral nervous system are the most affected with adjacent segmental demyelination in peripheral nerves and roots. Cranial and somatic nerves are similarly affected. Specifically, the area of the node of Ranvier is preferentially altered, correlating experimentally with slowing of conduction. The distribution of the lesions has been explained by the existence of a "blood-nerve barrier" which prevents access to nerve parenchyma of negatively charged proteins like diphtheria toxin [27].

Muscle involvement is primarily cardiac although diphtheria toxin appears to be toxic to skeletal muscles as well. Direct injection of toxin into muscle results in necrotic lesions similar to bacterial myositis from other Clostridial infections [1].

In the rare event that central nervous extension occurs, the pathophysiology is felt to relate to focal embolization to the CNS from mural thrombi in the diseased heart or to non-specific systemic effects of a "toxic encephalopathy." The former may give signs of hemiparesis or hemichorea [7,11]. The toxic encephalopathy is characterized by alterations in mental status, drowsiness, and on occasion convulsions [14]. Diphtheritic meningitis remains a distinct rarity [18]. Diffuse cerebral damage after airway obstruction and hypoxia are not distinctive for this condition and appear microscopically the same as in other situations.

There is no specific treatment for the neurologic complications of diphtheria. It is generally agreed that antitoxin should be administered within 48 hours of the earliest signs of diphtheric infection. The incidence and severity of complications appears less when antitoxin is given within this time period. The general measures of care for diphtheria focus on rest, antitoxin, and maintenance of proper airway and cardiac function. Local therapy of the diphtheric pharyngeal lesion is useless. Once the patient's sensitivity to horse serum has been determined using a skin or eye test, antitoxin may be administered. Mildly symptomatic cases are usually treated with 10,000-20,000 units, moderate cases with a pharyngeal membrane are treated with 20,000-40,000 units, and severe diphtheria with laryngeal involvement 50,000-100,000 units. The total dose should be given at one time rather than spread over a longer period. If the skin tests to horse serum are positive, desensitization should be attempted. Since the antitoxin is only capable of binding or inactivating toxin present in the blood or extracellular fluid, the rapid administration of the antitoxin is important. In the event that airway obstruction develops, intubation and tracheostomy are indicated. If the patient becomes anxious, sedative or hypnotic agents must not be given since they may obscure progressive respiratory difficulties. The carditis that is associated with significant morbidity is poorly treated.

Quinidine and procainamide have been used with some success. Circulating exotoxin is not affected by antibiotics. Patients with diphtheria should be quarantined until two successive cultures of the nose, throat, or other infected areas taken at least 24-hours apart from one another are negative.

Diphtheria is a preventable disease, and immunization at the age of three months should be routine. Booster doses at the age of one year and again just before the child enters school are also recommended.

Treatment of unimmunized adults exposed to an active case of diphtheria is unsettled. One may receive 3,000 units of antitoxin intramuscularly or cultures may be taken and a primary series of immunizations administered. If symptoms should occur, then antitoxin would be immediately given. In those who have previously been immunized and are then exposed to active diphtheria, a booster dose of toxoid is sufficient.

TETANUS

Clostridium tetani produces a powerful exotoxin under the anaerobic conditions of wounds or soil-contaminated injuries. Less common sources of disease are vaccinations and unclean needles used by drug addicts. Although neonatal tetanus due to infection of the stump of the umbilical cord is traditionally felt to be of only historical interest, seven cases were reported for the United States in 1970 [8]. Additionally, tetanus has followed dental procedures, suggesting that unclean instruments or infection after dental trauma can lead to this potentially lethal disease.

Both the central and peripheral nervous systems as well as the muscular system are involved in tetanus toxicity. Centrally, the predominant effect is one of disinhibition related to a toxic effect on grey matter gangliosides, and a presynaptic antagonism of amino acid transmitter release by interneurons (GABA or glycine) [16]. Both the alpha and beta motor neuron systems are disinhibited by the toxin [25]. In high concentrations, tetanus toxin acts similarly to botulinum toxin to prevent the release of acetylcholine at cholinergic synapses including the neuromuscular junction [21]. Muscle fibers are grossly degenerated with high levels of creatine phosphokinase and aldolase released; whether this effect is due to direct muscle toxicity or to neurogenic muscular atrophy is unsettled, but the latter is suggested by recent studies of chronic tetanus [12,22].

Tetanus gains access to the nervous system through retrograde axonal transport from the site of inoculation. The incubation period is usually from 5 to 25 days, but may be as short as a few hours. In most cases, the clinical onset is quite characteristic, with a seemingly preferential affinity of the toxin for the facial and bulbar muscles. Premonitory signs may consist of chill, headache and restlessness, with pain and erythema at the site of injury. A sensation of tightness in the jaw and a mild stiffness and soreness in the neck are usually noticed within a few hours. Pain between the shoulder blades may also be present. These early complaints are often vague and indistinct but are followed within a day or two by the more definite symptoms that characterize this disease. The jaw becomes stiff and tight; trismus results. This muscular involvement soon spreads to the throat muscles, producing dysphagia, and when the facial muscles are involved, facial asymmetry and a fixed smile (risus sardonicus) results. As the disease progresses, muscular hypertonicity may spread and become generalized, involving the muscles of the trunk and extremities. The rigidity of the back muscles produces an arching of the spine which, together with the retraction of the head, results in opisthotonos. The abdominal muscles gradually assume a board-like rigidity; this may cause a forward arching of the back in some cases (emprosthotonos). Spasms or tonic contractions occur in any muscle group and may be spontaneous or precipitated by the slightest stimulus, such as noises, touching the patient or even touching the bed. The tetanic contractions are usually periodic and are associated with most agonizing pain. During these convulsions, the jaws are usually rigidly locked, the back arched, the limbs extended and stiff, the fingers clenched, and the abdomen boardlike. Profuse perspiration accompanies these episodes which are exhausting and often terrifying to the patient. Flaccid tetraplegias and long-lasting muscle weakness may be seen in the post-tetanic phase, and are believed to be due to the peripheral action of the toxin [19]. In some of the more severe cases, convulsions, marked dyspnea and cyanosis also occur, and may terminate in asphyxia and sudden death. Mentation usually remains unaltered throughout the illness, but the patient suffers from great anxiety and mental and physical anguish.

Localized, relatively benign forms of tetanus may rarely occur in partially immunized patients and be confined to a wounded extremity or the head (cephalic tetanus). This latter condition is characterized by a short incubation period, facial paralysis and dysphagia associated with infection of the face or head. Localized tetanus, however, is unusual and should generally be thought of as only the earliest manifestation of more extensive disease.

Another tetanus syndrome seen in partially immune patients is generalized but non-fulminant disease after a minor injury. Resembling traditional tetanus with generalized muscle stiffness, spasms and even risus sardonicus and trismus, this syndrome may be prolonged for many months. The history of a prior wound several months before the initial presentation, the high titre of serum antibody to tetanus, a history of partial immunization and the clinical signs of non-fulminant tetanus solidify the diagnosis. The major entity that must be distinguished is stiff-person syndrome or Moersch-Woltman syndrome [2,4,22]. Well established trismus is not typical of stiff-person syndrome. Chronic tetanus has been used to support the concept that muscle injury in this disease is not simply due to excessive muscle trauma. Chronic denervation with associated renervation has been seen in such cases [22].

Histopathologic changes within the central nervous system may be extensive and permanent. Usually, when death occurs before the fifth day of illness very few lesions are visible. The first elements to become involved are the nerve cells, which are irregularly damaged, with swelling and perinuclear chromatolysis. The most severe changes occur within the nerve cells of the cortex and the brainstem. If the illness lasts more than five days, many other changes appear, consisting primarily of perivascular areas of demyelination and gliosis. Hemorrhages occur in many severe toxic states, and their presence in tetanus is not surprising.

Patients must be hospitalized in an intensive care unit. Necrotic tissue and foreign bodies should be removed from an infected wound and the patient placed in the quietest room available where stimuli will not induce tetanic contractions. Aspiration should be prevented by positioning the patient carefully and frequently suctioning the nasal pharyngeal secretions. Staff members should never assume that the patient cannot understand their discussions and should be aware that the patient is awake and alert.

Antiserum does not neutralize toxin fixed in the central system, and will do little to abate symptoms already present. Human tetanus immune globulin (TIG) is available in the United States and is superior to horse antiserum. One dose of 3,000-6,000 units intramuscularly into three sites simultaneously is indicated. If human antitoxin is not available, equine antiserum can be given. Local infiltration at the site of the wound is of no value. Intrathecal injections have been performed. Since the disease does not confer natural immunity, once the patient has recovered, active immunization should be done.

Muscle relaxation is paramount and the patient must be kept away from extraneous stimuli. Barbiturates, including phenobarbitol (50-100 mg, q3 hr) may produce enough sedation to decrease stimulus-sensitive spasms. Diazepam is a relatively safe tranquilizer with muscle relaxant properties as well. It should never be administered with barbiturates, however.

Tracheostomy is an important adjunct to therapy and protects against suffocation due to laryngospasm. Most patients with mild tetanus can be managed without it, although in patients who are ventilating poorly, the need for tracheostomy should be recognized early so that it can be performed electively and not as an emergency amidst a tetanic crisis. Curarization may be needed. Tracheostomy is indicated in all heroin addicts because there exists a high incidence of cardiac arrhythmias and hyperthermia [29]. In those patients with autonomic hyperactivity, propranolol has also been helpful [26].

Antibiotics have been often used in the past to treat an infected wound, although there is no indication that they ameliorate the tetanus itself. Penicillin G is highly effective against tetanus bacillus, but of course has no effect on the actual toxin. Cultures may be taken throughout the disease to establish secondary infectious sources and those may be appropriately treated.

Tetanus is prevented by active immunization. Current recommendations are that children two months-six years of age should be immunized with diphtheria, pertussis vaccine and tetanus toxoid (DPT). The first dose should be administered within three months of birth and the second and third should follow in 4–6 week intervals. The fourth dose should be given one year after the third. A routine booster of adult type tetanus and diphtheria toxoids should be given every ten years. If a patient is a victim of a wound, a toxoid booster given less than five years previously is sufficient; if a longer period has elapsed, a booster should be readministered.

Prognosis in tetanus remains poor; over the 17-year period between 1950 and 1967, case fatality rates were unchanged at about 65%. Death occurs rapidly between the third and fifth day of illness, and is usually due to (1) exhaustion, (2) medullary failure, (3) asphyxia resulting from spasm of the glottis or spasms of the diaphragm and intercostal muscles during the convulsions, or (4) circulatory failure from the great demand upon the heart.

Occasionally, following the use of tetanus antitoxin, particularly as a prophylactic, serum reaction develops, involving primarily the peripheral nervous system but occasionally the central nervous system. In most cases there seems to be a selective action on the cervical cord and its branches, with the fifth and sixth cervical segments mainly involved. Approximately 10 days after the innoculation, severe pain develops in the shoulder girdle, radiating to the neck. This pain persists and is soon accompanied by weakness primarily in abduction of the upper extremity. Atrophy of the involved muscles, especially the supraspinati and infraspinati, the rhomboids and the deltoids, may develop. In most cases, the prognosis is good, complete recovery generally occurring within six months. About 20 percent of the patients show some residual weakness and atrophy, especially in the deltoid muscles. Although other serums and vaccines may cause this condition, most of the cases are due to tetanus antitoxin. Treatment is symptomatic.

BOTULISM

Botulinum toxin is the most potent poison known (10^{-5} micrograms in a mouse is lethal), and is produced by spores of *Clostridium botulinum*. Three varieties of the disease occur and should be distinguished, since the incubation and course may be quite distinct.

Food-borne botulism occurs primarily after the ingestion of contaminated home canned fruits and vegetables. Less commonly, outbreaks may follow the consumption of fish products or solid meats [3]. In 1974, there were 32 cases of botulism reported in America with seven deaths. In contrast to diphtheria and tetanus, as well as the other forms of botulism, food-borne botulism is caused by the preformed toxin and hence human infection by *Clostridium* is not a prerequisite for disease. Botulinum toxin may be produced by spores in the anaerobic environment of sealed cans or jars so that it is already produced at the time of ingestion. As a result, toxic signs appear rapidly and a prolonged incubation period is not expected.

Typically, neurologic signs appear within hours or at most by one week after the ingestion of contaminated food. Nausea and vomiting with abdominal pain and diarrhea are thought to be due to local effects of the ingested toxin. Later constipation may result from local paralysis of the mesenteric autonomic nervous system. The presence of early gastrointestinal symptoms helps to differentiate this form of botulism from the much rarer wound botulism where neurologic complications develop without premonitory nausea and vomiting [10].

Wound botulism is both an infection and an intoxication. The organism enters the subcutaneous tissue as a result of a laceration or compound fracture. Gas or suppuration occur in only half of the cases and the wound may be small and seemingly of little consequence. It is thought that the spores germinate locally in the tissues and produce the potent exotoxin which then produces systemic neurologic effects as with food borne botulism.

The third form of botulism, infantile botulism, occurs in the first six months of life and appears to relate to the absorption of *C. botulinum* from the gastrointestinal tract. This syndrome is clinically distinct from the neurologic complications of food borne and wound associated botulism and will be discussed separately.

After contaminated food containing exotoxin has been ingested or after the exotoxin has been produced locally in a wound, the toxin is transported by blood, lymph and possibly nerves to attach to motor nerve terminals. The basic pathophysiology of botulism neurotoxicity relates to its inhibitory effect of acetylcholine release from the junction. Individual toxin types differ in their affinity for neural tissue with type A the most potent, followed by type E and type B [13].

Cranial nerve signs appear early with eye symptoms the most common. Patients complain of eye strain and mistiness of vision, followed by blurring and diplopia. There may be both an internal and external ophthalmoplegia. Rapid involvement of other cranial nerves produces vertigo, deafness and dysphagia as the throat becomes filled with viscid mucus that obstructs the upper airway. Swallowing ultimately becomes impossible and liquids are regurgitated through the nose. The voice often has a nasal quality and may be hoarse.

Clinical presentation of ptosis, extraocular paresis and progressive weakness always suggest myasthenia gravis, and this diagnosis must be excluded in any patient presenting with the possible diagnosis of botulism. Typically, with botulism, there is pupillary dilatation which is not seen with myasthenia. A Tensilon test cannot be used to definitely distinguish the two, since the test may be positive in up to 26% of botulism cases [17].

Muscular weakness is usually characteristic of botulism and is commonly generalized, appearing on the second to fourth day of the illness. A first the limbs may feel tired, and the patient is unable to climb stairs. This weakness may become so severe that moving about or even turning in bed is impossible. Often this muscular involvement is limited to the neck muscles, so that the patient is unable to raise his head. The head usually falls forward and the hands must be used to turn the head in any direction. The muscular weakness may occasionally be the presenting symptom; the patient suddenly falls down and is unable to raise himself [3].

The weakness is often descending so that proximal muscles are affected before distal extremities. This pattern is extremely rare for Guillain-Barré syndrome (1-4 percent of such cases begin proximally) and this feature helps in differentiating the two conditions.

While there is no objective sensory involvement in botulism, paresthesias may occur in as high as 14 percent of cases [17]. Consciousness is maintained, although restlessness and agitation are prominent. Throughout the illness autonomic dysfunction is manifested by an obstinate constipation and a reduced urinary output.

Because cholinergic function is felt to be important to memory, patients have been tested during their intoxicated state with type A botulism to assess this function. Botulism severe enough to block peripheral cholinergic transmission did not alter formal memory testing, suggesting that in fact this toxin does not penetrate the central nervous system, nor affect central cholinergic synapses [15].

In severe cases the course is rapidly downhill, and terminally, the illness is characterized by labored respirations intermixed with prolonged periods of apnea and a gradual change from restlessness to somnolence. If the patient survives, recovery begins within a few weeks, with the first improvement usually occurring in the eyes. Swallowing improves, so that at the end of two to three weeks the patient is able to take soft foods. Strength returns slowly, and muscular fatigability often persists long after many of the cranial nerve palsies have disappeared.

Many cases of botulism are mild and present only transient disturbances of vision or swallowing. These patients may complain of extreme fatigue and inability to walk fast or chew adequately. Such mild cases may be overlooked except in the event of an outbreak.

The differential diagnosis of botulism includes such entities as myasthenia gravis, Guillain-Barré syndrome, tick paralysis, chemical intoxication (e.g., carbon monoxide, belladonna, barium carbonate, methyl chloride, methyl alcohol, organic phorphorus compounds and atropine), trichinosis, diphtheritic polyneuritis, psychiatric syndromes and the Eaton-Lambert syndrome, usually associated with bronchogenic carcinoma. While similar to atropine toxicity, the absence of hallucinosis in botulism is striking and helpful in distinguishing the two entities. Mushroom and various marine toxins are also often anticholinergic, but sensory complaints and violent vomiting and diarrhea are also present. The absence of fever in botulism helps to exclude poliomyelitis.

Toxin-induced paralysis of cholinergic nerves involves three basic steps:

1. The binding of exotoxin to external receptors at ganglionic synapses, postganglionic parasympathetic synapses and neuromuscular junction.
2. A translocated step during which the toxin molecule or some portion of it passes through the nerve or muscle membrane.
3. The paralytic step during which the release of acetylcholine is usually blocked.

Two mechanisms have thus far been proposed to explain the latter final step. One proposal suggests that the toxin impairs the ability of vesicles to become loaded with acetylcholine so that the diminished quantity of acetylcholine is released as depolarization. A second more widely held belief is that the toxin acts on the nerve or muscle membrane that regulates the release of transmitter with impaired calcium-induced exocytosis [24].

Confirmation of the diagnosis depends on detection of the toxin in the patient or in implicated food. The patient himself and all exposed subjects should be hospitalized for antitoxin therapy and observation. Respiratory monitoring is crucial, and intensive care facilities are usually required. Trivalent ABE antitoxin has been recommended, one vial intravenously and one intramuscularly, to be repeated once in two to four hours if symptoms persist. Guanidine, which enhances acetylcholine release from presynaptic terminals, has been used with experimental success but remains controversial in humans [10]. Because there is a small possibility that spores may still be releasing toxin within the gastrointestinal tract, penicillin has been advocated, although definite penicillin efficacy has only been established for wound related botulism.

Quite a different clinical syndrome occurs in infants as a result of *Clostridium botulinum*. In this instance, the spores actually germinate in the infant's intestine and hence produce botulinum toxin in vivo. As with most other infectious diseases, infant botulism has a spectrum of clinical severity and may range from a mild out-patient illness to fulminant sudden death. This is a disease described only within the last decade and hence most cases reported have been recognized in infants so weak and hypotonic that they required hospitalization. Infantile botulism is part of the differential diagnosis for infants with flaccid paralysis (hypotonic or floppy infant syndrome) in the first six months of life. The early manifestations are usually constipation and an inability to suck or swallow with a weak cry. As such, the clinical syndrome is not unlike that seen with the food borne and wound related botulism, but the age group is so different that it requires separate mention. In these babies, serum assays for toxin are usually negative, but both toxin and spores can be found in the stool. If proper life support measures are administered, the disease appears to be self-limited even without the administration of antibiotics or antitoxin. It is possible that focal systemic immunity occurs in the gastrointestinal tract or that there is a reduced absorption of toxin eventually since spontaneous recovery is frequently observed in such cases. Botulinum toxicity has been offered as a possible explanation for the sudden infant death syndrome (SIDS, crib death). The curious age distribution of the SIDS with peak incidence between two and four months is remarkably similar to that seen in the identified infantile botulism. Ten cases identified in California in 1977 with SIDS had evidence of intestinal infection of *C. botulinum* [6]. It has been suggested that botulism causes sudden death in infants as a result of flaccidity of the upper airway or tongue muscles leading to airway obstruction during sleep [5].

Respiratory care is the most important in patients with botulism and assisted ventilation should be available for rapid use. If respiratory difficulties are suggested, an elective tracheostomy should be performed before the onset of significant respiratory failure. If no ileus is present, lavage and enemas may help to remove unabsorbed toxin from the intestine. Magnesium citrate and magnesium sulfate should never be given as magnesium ion will potentiate neuromuscular block produced by the botulinum toxin.

The patient should be rapidly tested for hypersensitivity to horse serum and treated with trivalent ABE antitoxin. If sensitization is present, desensitization measures must be performed prior to further treatment. In infants, where multiplication of ingested organisms may be an important factor to the botulinum syndrome, antibiotics may be justified. In adults, where clostridial multiplications are not important, antibiotics are not of definite benefit either for food or wound botulism.

▪ STUDY QUESTIONS

Botulism induces:

(1) circulating antibodies to the post-synaptic acetylcholine receptor
(2) decreased responsiveness of the post-synaptic membrane to acetylcholine
(3) increased deep tendon reflexes and weakness
(4) impaired release of acetylcholine from the presynaptic nerve terminal.

Answer: 4

Botulinum toxin blocks the presynaptic release of acetylcholine. Circulating antibodies to the acetylcholine receptor are seen in myasthenia gravis. Curare and similar drugs bind at the post-synaptic membrane to acetylcholine and provoke decreased responsiveness.

Bacterial Toxins

Weakness and increased reflexes are seen in upper motor neuron diseases, such as cerebrovascular accidents, multiple sclerosis, or lateral sclerosis.

Which actions are associated with diphtheria toxin?

1. Binds to Schwann cells.
2. Arrests protein synthesis.
3. Provokes demyelination.
4. Impairs conduction of electrical information down the axon.

Answer: All of the above

Schwann cells make myelin and these cells are attacked by diphtheria toxin. Protein synthesis and effective myelination are inhibited. Myelin coats axons to increase the electrical efficiency of conduction through an axon. As peripheral demyelination occurs, slowed conduction velocities are found on the EMG studies.

How does tetanus get to the central nervous system?

1. Travels by blood to the cerebrospinal fluid and then is absorbed to the spinal cord.
2. Travels retrograde from the peripheral nerve terminal to the cell body from which it passes transsynaptically to bind to cells in the spinal cord.
3. Travels with Schwann cells to the soma where protein synthesis is inhibited.
4. Tetanus toxin does not travel to the CNS.

Answer: 2

It was suggested in the early 1900s that the toxin ascended the axons to the spinal cord. Later, hematogenous spread was felt to be more likely. However, autoradiographic investigations have demonstrated retrograde transport as the major mean of spinal cord deposition of toxin. Once in the motor neuron soma, toxin must pass transsynaptically to nerve terminals having inputs on these cells. It has been suggested that these predominantly inhibitory terminals are then blocked, leading to the uncontrolled excitation of the alpha motor neuron. These inhibitory terminals may be glycinergic. As a result, unopposed excitation occurs and the result is clinical tetanus.

Which toxin(s) inhibits release of neurotransmitter presynaptically?

A. Tetanus
B. Botulism
C. Diphtheria

Answer: A and B

Both products of clostridial bacteria, these two toxins inhibit release of neurotransmitter; in the former, glycine or GABA appear to be inhibited from release, causing unopposed excitation of the alpha motor neuron. In the latter, the blocked release is acetylcholine from the alpha motor neuron.

■ REFERENCES

1. Adams RD: Disease of muscle. Harper & Row, Hagerstown, Md., 1975.
2. Allen N: Solvents and other industrial organic compounds. In PJ Vinken, GW Bruyn, eds., Handbook Clinical Neurology, Vol. 36, pp 361-390. North-Holland Publishing Co., Amsterdam, 1979.
3. Allen RW, Ecklund AW: Botulism in North Dakota. J. Am. Med. Assoc., 99:557-559, 1932.
4. Anden NR, Grabowska M, Strumbom U: Different alpha-adrenoreceptors in the central nervous system mediating biochemical and functional effects of clonidine and receptor blocking agents. Arch. Pharm. 295:43-52.
5. Arnon SS, Chin J: Clinical spectrum of infant botulism. Rev. Infect. Dis. 1: 614-621, 1982.
6. Arnon SS, Midura TF, Damus K, Thompson B: Honey and other environmental risk factors for infant botulism. J. Pediatr. 94:331-336, 1979.
7. Baker AB, Nolan HH: The central nervous system in diphtheria. J. Ner. Ment. Dis. 100:24-28, 1944.
8. Bennett JV: Tetanus. In PD Hoepich, ed., Infectious Diseases. Harper and Row, Hagerstown, 1972.
9. Bowman CG, Bonventue PF: Studies on the mode of action of diphtheria toxin. J. Exp. Med. 131:659-663, 1970.
10. Cherington M: Botulism—ten year experience. Arch. Neurol. 30:432-438, 1974.
11. Critchley M: Postdiphtheric chorea. Br. J. Child. Dis. 21:188-194, 1924.
12. Eyrich K, Agostini B, Schulz A, Muller E, Noetzel H, Reichenmiller NZ, Weimersk T: Clinical and morphological studies of skeletal muscle changes in tetanus. Ger. Med. Mth. 12:469-474, 1967.
13. Gargarosa EJ: Botulism. IN PD Hoeprich, ed., Infectious Diseases, Harper & Row, Hagerstown, Md., 1972.
14. Gupta OK, Saksena PN, Gupta NN: A clinical study of 856 patients with diphtheria. Ind. J. Ped. 40:93, 1975.
15. Haaland KY, Davis LE: Botulism and memory. Arch. Neurol. 37:657-658, 1980.
16. Habermaun E: Tetanus. In PJ Vinken, GW Bruyn, eds., Handbook of Clinical Neurology, Vol. 33, pp. 491-510. North-Holland Publishing Co., Amsterdam, 1978.
17. Hughes JM, Blumenthal JF, Merson MH: Clinical features of types A and B food borne botulism. Ann. Intern. Med. 95:442-445, 1981.
18. Jelsma F: Cervical intramedullary cyst due to corynebacterium diphtheria gravis. J. Neurosurg. 38:78-84, 1973.
19. Kaeser HE, Muller HR, Friedrich B: The nature of tetraplegia in infectious tetanus. Europ. Neurol. 1:17-21, 1968.
20. Lupton MD, Klawans HL: Neurologic complications of diphtheria. In PJ Vinken, GW Bruyn, eds., Handbook of Clinical Neurology, Vol. 33, pp. 479-488. North-Holland Publishing Co., Amsterdam, 1978.

21. Miyasaki K, Okada K, Muto S, Itokazu T, Matsui M, Ebisawa I, Kagabe K, Muro TK: On the mode of action of tetanus toxin in rabbits. Jap. J. Exp. Med. 37:217, 1967.
22. Risk WS, Bosch PE, Kimura J, Carrcilla PA, Fischbeck KH, Layzer RB: Chronic tetanus. Muscle Nerve 4:363-366, 1981.
23. Rolleston JD: Diphtheric paralysis. Arch. Pediatr. 30:335-337, 1913.
24. Simpson LL: Action of botulinal toxin. Rev. Infect. Dis. 1:656-659, 1979.
25. Takano K, Kano M: Gamma bias of muscle poisoned by tetanus toxin. Arch. Exp. Path. Pharmacol. 276:413-417, 1973.
26. Tsueda K, Oliver PB, Richter RW: Cardiovascular manifestations of tetanus. Anesthesiology 40:588-592, 1974.
27. Waksman BH: Experimental study of diphtheric polyneuritis. J. Neuropathol. Exp. Neurol. 20:35-45, 1961.
28. Weinstein L: Tetanus. N. Engl. J. Med. 289:1293, 1973.

CHAPTER 9

Animal Poisons and Venoms

MOST animal toxins of neurologic significance affect the cholinergic system, either through enhancement or blockade (Table 9.1). As a rule, injuries from bees, snakes, scorpions and ticks are more common during summer months when campers and vacationers may inadvertently encounter these animals. In the case of snakes, it is especially important to attempt to identify the snake species, since potent antivenene are now developed against specific poisons. The exotic marine toxins are not discussed in this section, but exhaustive reviews are available [23]. The only mammals with envenomating capacities are the Australian platypus (males only) and possibly two families of forest shrews, none applicable to this text.

BEES AND WASPS

Hymenoptera is the order of insects having four membranous wings, including bees, wasps, hornets and yellow jackets. Neurotoxic manifestations of such stings appear to be by and large immunologic in nature. The acute allergic reactions including bronchial spasm, laryngeal edema, tissue edema and circulatory collapse have neurologic complications only as secondary phenomena. Hypoxic brain damage leading to a depressed level of consciousness and occasional generalized seizures may occur [18].

Of more significant neurologic significance are the delayed immunologic reactions that may follow various insect stings. A progressive radiculomyelopathy has been reported after a hornet's sting and at autopsy the patient demonstrated demyelination of peripheral nerves as well as patchy demyelination in the spinal cord [13]. A similar case has been described where numbness and

Animal Poisons and Venoms

TABLE 9.1. Animal Toxins

Animal	Clinical features	Pathophysiology
Bees, wasps, hornets	Paresthesias, progressive weakness days after sting	Delayed hypersensitive immune reaction—often demyelination of nerve axons
Snakes	Progressive weakness and paralysis	Combined presynaptic block of acetylcholine release and postsynaptic neuromuscular block. Also myotoxicity leads to muscle necrosis and myoglobinuria (if notexin is present)
Scorpion	Muscle rigidity, over excitement, hypertension	Enhanced release of acetylcholine and catecholamine
Tick	Progressive weakness and paralysis	Decreased release of acetylcholine presynaptically

weakness developed one week after a yellow jacket sting. Progressive quadraparesis and dermatomal sensory loss with hyperreflexia in the arms and hyperreflexia in the legs followed. Cerebral spinal fluid examination demonstrated marked elevation of protein and at autopsy, multifocal demyelination was found in the spinal cord, dorsal lateral medulla and optic nerves. Demyelination was also seen in the peripheral nerves. A further intriguing case of a patient presenting with the typical signs of multiple sclerosis that began within one month of a bee sting incident demonstrated the presence of circulating antibodies to CNS tissue. Pure peripheral neuropathies have also been described, as well as brachial plexopathies, all occurring weeks after a significant sting. Although the mechanism of such neurologic disorders is not established, the clinical presentation and pathologic changes of demyelination suggest a delayed type of hypersensitivity. Hymenopteral venoms contain numerous proteins which could incite a cross reaction with CNS protein similar to that seen with experimental allergic encephalomyelitis and neuritis. Alternatively, such venoms also contain phospholipases which might liberate encephalitogenic proteins.

SNAKE VENOMS

The important venomous snakes of the world belong to three major groups. In the Viperidae group are the true vipers as well as the pit vipers, a subgroup that dominates the population of venomous snakes in the New World and includes various rattlesnakes. The Elapidae, found on every continent except

Europe, include cobras, kraits, mambas and American coral snakes. The Hydrophiidae or sea snakes are found chiefly in Asian and Australian waters. Snake venoms are potent toxins to cardiac muscle and the coagulant pathways as well as to the neurologic system. The specific neurotoxicity of these venoms depends primarily on their action on the peripheral neuromuscular junction. Snake neurotoxins may act either presynaptically or postsynaptically and most venoms are chemically composed of both types. Presynaptic toxins (notexin and taipoxin) act to inhibit the release of acetylcholine from the presynaptic cell of the neuromuscular junction (Table 9.2). Postsynaptic neurotoxins produce a non-depolarizing neuromuscular block, but vary in the degree to which the block is reversible in the laboratory. They also differ in their relative ability to combine with nicotinic acetylcholine receptors in other parts of the nervous system. The two types of toxins, often working simultaneously, lead to a depression of cholinergic function at the neuromuscular junction. This peripheral mechanism of action can explain the clinical presentation and natural history of snake bites and there is little evidence that snake venoms act directly on the central nervous system [5]. They may also be myotoxic, with local necrosic effects at the site of envenomation.

The clinical course can be considered under four categories: a) local evidence of envenomation; b) preparalytic signs and symptoms; c) paralysis; d) other systemic effects of envenomation.

The local pain and swelling are especially common with viper, rattlesnake and cobra bites. Swelling will increase over 24 hours, and may extend over the entire bitten limb or trunk. Sanguinous blistering and local gangrene are secondary local complications.

Preparalytic neurologic signs may include headache, vomiting, loss of consciousness, parethesias locally, ptosis and external ophthalmoplegia [3]. The latter two signs are more or less regularly encountered from bites with the South American rattlesnake and Berg adder. Loss of vision is a common complication of snake bite but relates primarily to coagulation disturbances and hemorrhage into the retina [7].

The latent period between snake bite and the development of the paralytic signs and symptoms may vary from one to ten hours. Following the extraocular muscle and eyelid levator weakness, facial and jaw paresis develops. Swallowing and mouth opening become progressively compromised over hours with gradual development of diaphragmatic, intercostal and limb weakness [24]. Secretions pool in the pharynx, the weakened respiratory muscles fail, consciousness is lost and convulsions may occur. If respiratory paresis is not relieved, circulatory arrest ensues.

No sensory disturbance other than around the bite itself occurs. Other systemic effects of neurologic importance relate to coagulation deficits, and cerebral

TABLE 9.2

Notexin: 119 amino acids, MW 13,574
1. Presynaptic blockade of release of acetylcholine
2. Myotoxic, causing massive myoglobinuria
3. Phospholipase activity

Taipoxin: Sialo-glycoprotein, MW 45,600
1. Presynaptic blockade of release of acetylcholine
2. Myotoxic, causing massive myoglobinuria

---

and subarachnoid hemorrhage have been reported after bites from many varieties of venomous snakes [24]. Pathologically, alterations appear confined to the muscles, except for the secondary bleeding effects already mentioned. Widespread hyaline necrosis in skeletal muscles is seen, and varies from focal to massive and diffuse [19].

The treatment involves the use of antivenenes, either a high titer monovalent type if the species of snake is known or a polyvalent antivenene if the responsible species is in question. The antivenene, a reconstituted antiserum, is titrated against the patient's signs, and several hundred milliliters may be needed. The response of established muscle paralysis to antivenene infusion can give additional information regarding the type of toxin and snake. Antivenenes are most effective against postsynaptic neurotoxins, and a rapid response to antivenenes, even when polyvalent, suggests that the snake is one with primarily postsynaptic toxins (cobra, mamba, death adder). Antivenenes do not alter established paralysis induced by presynaptic neurotoxins (South American rattlesnake, elapids, and kraits).

It is important that the antivenene be administered as early as possible. If it is injected intravenously before major weakness is apparent, both pre- and postsynaptic toxic effects can be aborted. Other respiratory support measures and blood transfusions may also be required. Specific dosages of antivenenes can be found in reference sources [4].

If possible, the snake should be killed without damaging identifying marks about its head. This will allow for rapid identification and the proper prescription of an antivenom. Importantly, the head of an apparently dead snake must be handled with extreme care because it can still deliver a venomous strike for as long as one hour after being severed from the body. Additional management of snake-bite victims remains controversial. Some clinicians advocate application of ice packs to the snake bite area, although others feel that excessive cooling increases tissue damage. High dose corticosteroids have also been advocated, although the benefits of such medications have not been demonstrated.

BIOLOGICAL TOXINS

SCORPION STING

The manifestations of scorpion sting depend on the responsible species and may include both local and systemic complications [10]. Early local changes include regional pain and swelling followed within hours by the systemic reactions of excessive salivation, sweating, and abdominal pain. Hypertension, peripheral circulatory collapse and cardiac failure are complications that may be fatal. Neurological involvement includes skeletal muscle rigidity, convulsions and alteration of mentation, the latter two probably as secondary complications of hypoxia. Cerebral infarction relative to coagulopathy or hypotension has been reported [12].

Scorpion venoms contain peptides that have a variety of neurochemical effects, the most pronounced of which is an enhanced presynaptic depolarization with resultant release of neurotransmitter from synaptic vesicles [26]. Increased excretion of catecholamines has been demonstrated after scorpion sting and may relate to the primary effect of the venom or to a secondary sympathetic adrenergic surge [9]. Treatment is non-specific and focuses on maintaining respiratory and cardiac as well as coagulation function. Anticonvulsants may be necessary for seizure control.

TICK PARALYSIS

Tick paralysis is a flaccid ascending paralysis caused by the bite of certain female ticks. This disease was first reported by Hovell [11] in 1824 and has now been reported from many parts of the world. In North America it is caused by the ticks Dermacentor andersoni, Dermacentor variabilis, Dermacentor occidentalis, Amblyomma americanum and Amblyomma maculatum. Tick paralysis has been seen in 15% of the 50 states but is common only in states west of the Rocky Mountains (Washington, Oregon, Idaho, Montana, Colorado and Wyoming) and in British Columbia and Alberta, Canada [26]. The toxin producing this disease is presumably excreted in the saliva of the mature female tick during engorgement. Although persons of any age may be affected, small children are particularly likely to become paralyzed. The head and neck are the most common site for tick attachment, although any part of the body may be involved. There is some indication of an association between the proximity of the site of attachment to the brain and the severity of the disease [15].

Despite intensive research, neither the nature of the neurotoxin nor the exact mechanism of its action is understood. Some believe that the toxin causes a failure in the liberation of acetylcholine at the neuromuscular junction while other investigators feel that the toxin causes a generalized depression of all excitable tissues including the neurons of the spinal cord and brainstem [22].

Within five to six days after the tick attaches to a person, the patient develops vague complaints such as restlessness, irritability, fatigue and muscular pain. Within the next 24 hours he develops an ascending flaccid paralysis which usually starts in the lower limbs, is symmetric and is associated with a loss of deep reflexes. He will, at this time, have difficulty in walking and may fall while attempting to stand. During the next few days the paralysis ascends to involve the trunk, arms, and neck [22]. If the tick is not found and removed, a number of patients will show continued progression with eventual involvement of the brainstem and cranial nerves. There may be paralysis of the sternocleidomastoid and lingual musculature, dysphagia, dysarthria, facial paralysis and ocular weakness. Eventually the patient dies of a respiratory paralysis. Convulsions may occur terminally and are believed to be due to hypoxia [26].

Sensory findings are usually absent and the sensorium is uninvolved. There are no signs of systemic involvement such as alterations in the temperature, blood, and sedimentation rate. The cerebrospinal fluid is also characteristically normal. In a patient described by Lagos and Thies, there was evidence of cerebellar involvement with ataxia of all limbs [15]. Occasionally purely local paralysis occurs.

The course of tick paralysis depends on how soon the tick is found and removed. If it is removed prior to the onset of bulbar symptoms, improvement occurs within hours and is complete by one week. If bulbar symptoms have begun, death often occurs despite intensive therapy.

SPIDERS, TARANTULAS AND GILA MONSTERS

Spiders that cause the most significant neurotoxic syndromes belong to the genus Lactrodectus, with the black widow spider the most prominent member. Black widow spiders build their webs in sheds and wood piles and slight provocation will cause the female to aggressively bite her victim. Initially there is sharp pain at the site of inoculation followed within 15 minutes by severe local cramps. The venom causes the forced release of acetylcholine with tetanic spasms initially, followed eventually by transmission blockade and paralysis after depletion of synaptic vesicles. During the acute excitatory phase, atropine can be used to control the cardiac muscle effect and gradual recovery will occur naturally over two days. The major toxic protein of black widow spider venom is latrotoxin. The venom includes other proteinaceous and nonproteinaceous products. The latrotoxin binds to the presynaptic membrane of the neuromuscular cholinergic neuron and causes a marked increase in the number of miniature end plate potentials. Ultrastructural studies during this early excitatory phase show synaptic vesicles fusing with the presynaptic plasma membrane. Later the nerve terminals swell and synaptic vesicles are only minimally detectable. Lethal doses of spider venom range from 0.5 to 10 mg/kg in mice. The female black widow spider's mark of red spot or hour glass is readily visible. Other neurotoxic signs include paresthesias, fasciculations, tremor and hyperreflexia during the excitatory phase. Antiserum 2.5 ml intramuscularly can be used, but often only hot baths and intravenous calcium and magnesium for cramping relief will be necessary. Fatalities do occur (2.5-6%). The venom related to tarantula bites probably is similar to that of black widow spider [14].

Gila monsters predominantly inhabit the southwest portions of the United States. The lizards are not aggressive and they bite only upon provocation or when they are in a confined setting. The pharmacology of the neurotoxin is not known, although it appears to stimulate smooth muscle. The clinical syndrome associated with gila monster bites include generalized weakness and diplopia. No antivenom is available.

FISH TOXINS

A distinction may be made between two classes of fish neurotoxins. In one group, the animals can deliver a toxin to an assailant or potential prey by means of a venom apparatus. Such animals include sting rays and stonefish. The second group is toxic to man only when he ingests the fish and examples of this type include puffer fish, sunfish, and morays. Sharks and certain rays overlap into both groups, possessing predatory venoms as well as endogenous poisons [20].

Fish venoms appear to be rather specialized in composition, differing in chemical structure from other animal venoms. They tend to deteriorate rapidly especially at warm temperatures, a fact that has therapeutic importance. The major venomous fish is the sting ray and its venom has been partially analyzed with ten amino acids identified so far. Crude venom extract includes, besides the toxic protein, serotonin, and phosphodiesterase. The venom appears to act primarily as a vasoactive agent and may have direct effects on skeletal and cardiac muscle. Low concentrations cause unpredictable vasodilatation or vasoconstriction. In experimental animals, bradycardia occurs with atrial-ventricular block of first, second, or third degree. Higher doses induce cardiac standstill which may relate to direct toxic effects on the pacemaker [21].

Clinical manifestations of sting ray bite include intense pain at the site of laceration and rapid swelling. Syncope, anxiety, and sweating may occur although the pharmacologic mechanism of muscle involvement is not known. Treatment involves placing the injured area, usually a limb, in hot water to enhance toxin degradation, maintenance of blood pressure and treatment of arrhythmias. If the bite is extensive, antibiotics and surgical debridement are helpful [21].

Stonefish are the second major group of venomous fish. These rather bizarre appearing animals are indigenous to the South Pacific but have been maintained in aquariums by fish enthusiasts as well. The principal action of stonefish venom is a direct toxic effect on muscle, resulting in paralysis of cardiac, involuntary and skeletal muscles. The venom is non-dialyzable and the lethal portion contains a high concentration of aromatic amino acids. The molecular weight approximates 150,000.

The precise pharmacologic mechanism of myotoxicity is not clear. Direct depolarization of skeletal muscle has been suggested based on work with experimental animals dying of respiratory arrests after envenomation. Action potentials from phrenic nerve recordings show that respiratory movement ceases before central respiratory activity is affected, and before nerve conduction velocities are changed. Further biochemical studies suggest that cholinergic release is not significantly altered so that direct muscle toxicity seems most probable [1].

Clinical features after stonefish envenomation include local pain so intense that the victim often writhes and thrashes about. Necrosis and sloughing at the wound site is much more common than with other fish envenomations and appears to relate to high concentrations of hyaluronidase in the venom. Respiratory depression is felt to be the usual cause of death, although direct cardiac muscle toxicity may also play a role [1].

A vivid description of the syndrome associated with probable tetrodotoxin exposure is found in Captain Cook's sea journal, where he describes the events related to dining at sea:

> Having no suspicion of its being of a poisonous nature, we ordered it to be dressed for supper; but very luckily, the operation of drawing and describing took up so much time that it was too late, so that only the liver and roe were dressed, of which the two Mr. Forsters and myself did but taste. About three o'clock in the morning, we found ourselves seized with an extraordinary weakness and numbness all over our limbs. I had almost lost the sense of feeling; nor could I distinguish between light and heavy bodies of such as I had strength to move, a quart pot, full of water and a feather being the same in my hand [6]

An antivenene has been developed against the deadly stonefish and antivenene administration accompanies the general therapeutic measures, warming the wound region to inactivate the toxin and providing respiration. Stonefish antivenene is the first to be developed against a fish venom and has reduced the morbidity related to stonefish poison. Laboratory evidence demonstrates that this antivenene can neutralize all observable toxic effects with laboratory animals. Because many victims cannot attest with certainty that the responsible fish was a stonefish, absolute statistics on the clinical benefits of antivenene have been difficult to obtain. The antivenene does not appear to be effective against other fish venoms and no cross protection is afforded against sting rays [17].

Fish that are poisonous when consumed have been recognized since the

Renaissance. The more important toxins identified in various species are tetrodotoxin and ciguatoxin. Tetrodotoxin is found in puffer and sunfish (Tetroodontiformes). These fish have a wide distribution including both the warm and temperate ocean waters. The toxin is the only fish toxin with a tentatively established structure. The empirical formula is felt to be $C_{11}H_{17}O_8N_3$. This simple dimer has a molecular weight of less than 1000. It is, however, one of the most potent known toxins exceeded only by botulinum toxin, palytoxin and ricin. Pharmacologically, it acts on the conduction of somatic motor and sensory nerves, on sympathetic nerves, on medullary centers and on muscle. Tetrodotoxin paralyzes the membrane sodium pump, preventing usual increases in permeability to sodium ions, but leaving potassium permeability unaltered [2]. It affects particularly preganglionic cholinergic and somatic motor nerves. There is apparently no specific effect on cholinesterase activity. In muscle, the toxin effects direct blockage of excitability. Respiratory compromise may be caused by combinations of the above deficits, as well as direct medullary center depression [2]. Clinical manifestations of such toxicity include rapid development of weakness over the first hour after ingestion of fish. Hypotension, pallor, and respiratory compromise follow. Treatment is symptomatic and there is no known antidote.

The other major fish toxin is ciguatoxin, widespread in the Pacific and West Indies. Unlike tetrodotoxin which is found almost exclusively in easily recognized fish species, ciguatoxic fish cannot be identified by their outward appearance; the poison is carried by hundreds of species and is unpredictable in its distribution, so that a species may be poisonous on one side of an island and perfectly harmless on the other. Furthermore, the areas of poisonous fish are constantly changing, making the risk of poisoning high even to endogenous people [16].

It appears that ciguatoxin must be an acquired substance harmful to man, but not harmful to the fish themselves. Both herbivorous and carnivorous fish may be ciguatoxic, so that a substance common to all fish diets has been implicated. Evidence suggest that the blue-green algae group and possibly filamentous algae are responsible.

Pharmacologic analysis of ciguatoxin demonstrates that the toxin acts in part by neuromuscular junction blockage, probably presynaptically since muscle contractions after direct stimulation remain unaffected. The toxin may have an effect on calcium activity and membrane function. Further details are not clear. Demyelination in peripheral nerve and central nervous system has also been reported.

Clinical morbidity usually relates to respiratory compromise, hypotension and generalized weakness. In animal studies, respiratory failure appears to relate to a central depression. The administration of calcium and magnesium along with aggressive forced respiratory support are advocated. Minimal and often

Animal Poisons and Venoms

unrecognized intoxication with perioral dyesthesias and a sense of vague weakness passing after an hour is probably common in the Virgin Islands and other sea areas [24]. Such "restaurant" syndromes occur with significant frequency in such vacation or resort areas, and are more likely recognized by the endogenous population than by visitors, including physicians.

■ STUDY QUESTIONS

The origin or neurologic dysfunction related to bee stings is primarily due to:
1. Toxin infiltration of subcutaneous sensory nerves
2. Immunologic reactions
3. Direct medullary depression
4. Cholinergic underactivity resembling botulism

Answer: 2

Hymenoptera induce immune allergic reactions, and the ones of most neurologic consequence are usually delayed hypersensitivity. Progressive demyelination of peripheral and/or central nervous system can resemble Guillain-Barré (if the peripheral system is involved) or remotely, multiple sclerosis (if the central nervous system is exclusively involved). The other answers have no relation to insect stings.

Naturally occurring venoms and poisons have served as superb tools for the study of the cholinergic system. Match the toxin with its effect on the cholinergic synapse.

1. Botulinum	A. Inhibits presynaptic release
2. Black widow spider venom	B. Enhances presynaptic release
3. Alpha bungaro toxin from the cobra	C. Blocks postsynaptic receptors
4. Beta bungaro toxin from the cobra	D. Stimulates postsynaptic receptors
5. Scorpion venom	E. None

Answer: 1-A; 2-B; 3-C; 4-B; 5-B

Agents that inhibit acetylcholine release include botulinum toxin (see bacterial toxin), and notexin and taipoxin, the latter two being frequent constituents of snake venoms. Agents that provoke tetanic-like activity with enhanced mild neurojunction function and severe contractions include black widow spider venom, beta bungaro toxin, and probably scorpion venom. These are associated with severe muscle rigidity and pain. Therapeutically, guanethidine also enhances release of acetylcholine and is used to counteract botulinin toxin. Alpha bungaro toxin blocks the acetylcholine receptor and has been used extensively to study the pathophysiology of myasthenia gravis, where a naturally occurring antibody similarly blocks the post-junctional cholinergic receptor, causing weakness and fatigability of muscle function.

Which general body systems other than neurologic are affected by venom?

1. Renal and hematopoetic
2. Cardiac and hepatic
3. Hepatic and renal
4. Cardiac and hematopoetic

Answer: 4

Cardiac toxicity includes destruction of cardiac muscle and the induction of lethal arrhythmias. Hematopoetic involvement focuses primarily on a severe coagulopathy.

Tic paralysis clinically resembles:

A. Tetanus
B. Ingestion of plants with centrally active anticholinergic property
C. Multiple sclerosis
D. None

Answer: D

Tick paralysis is a progressive, flaccid, often ascending paralysis occurring most commonly in children. The disease resembles Guillain-Barré syndrome and botulism in that such patients are weak, and often have cranial nerve involvement and absent tendon reflexes. Unlike these two disorders, however, tick paralysis is reversible with the removal of the causative female tick. Also, unlike Guillain-Barré, the CSF does not typically show a pronounced elevation of protein.

This clinical picture does not resemble the three choices given. Tetanus is associated with prominent stimulus sensitive contractions and muscle rigidity. Centrally active anticholinergic plants may demonstrate some weakness, mental agitation, delirium, and the systemic signs of antimuscurinic activity predominate. Multiple sclerosis associated with demyelination of the central nervous system is associated with prominent sensory abnormalities and spastic weakness.

■ REFERENCES

1. Austin L, Gillis RG, Youatt G: Stonefish venom: Some biochemical observations. Aust. J. Exp. Biol. Med. Sci. 43:79-90, 1965.
2. Banner AH, Helfrich P, Scheuer PJ, Yoshida T: Research on ciguatera in the tropical Pacific. Proc. Gulf Caribb. Fish Inst., 16th Ann. Session, 84-98, 1963.
3. Bouquier J-J, Guibert J, Dupont C, Umdenstock R: Les piqures de vipere chez l'enfant. Arch. franc. Pediatr. 31:285-295, 1974.
4. Buckley E, Porges N (eds.): Venoms. Am. Assoc. Adv. Sci. Pub. No 44, Washington, D.C., 1956.
5. Campbell CH: The effects of snake venoms and their neurotoxins on the nervous system of man and animals. In RW Hornabrook, ed.: Topics on Tropical Neurology. Philadelphia, FA Davis, 259-293, 1975.

6. Cook J. A voyage towards the South pole and round the world performed in his Majesty's ship, the Resolution. London, W. Strahan and T. Cadell, 1777.
7. Davenport RC, Budden RH: Loss of sight following snake bite. Br. J. Ophthalmol. 37:119-121, 1953.
8. Engleberg NC, Morris JG, Lewis J: Cinguatera fish poisoning: a major common source outbreak in the U.S. Virgin Islands. An. Inter. Med. 98:336-337, 1983.
9. Gueron M, Weizmann S: Catecholamine excretion in scorpion sting. Isr. J. Med. Sci. 5:855-857, 1969.
10. Horen WP: Insect and scorpion sting. JAMA 221:894-898, 1972.
11. Hovell WH, cited by Abbott KH: Tick paralysis: A review: I., Mayo Clin. Proc. 18:39-49, 1943.
12. Jammikal JH, Srinivas HV: Hemiplegia following scorpion sting. Ind. J. Pediatr. 10:337-338, 1973.
13. Jellinger K, Spunda C: Aufsteigende Neuritis nach Insektevstich. Wien. Klin. Wschr. 13:81-84, 1953.
14. Kaplin JG: Neurotoxicity of selected biological toxins. In PS Spencer and HH Schaumburg, eds., Experimental and Clinical Neurotoxicology. Williams and Wilkins, Baltimore, 1980.
15. Lagos JC, Thies RE: Tick paralysis without muscle weakness. Arch. Neurol. 21:471-474, 1969.
16. Li KM: On demyelination from the effect of ciguatoxin. Quoted by TI Kosaki and HH Anderson: Marine toxins from the Pacific—pharmacology of ciguatoxin. Toxicon. 6:57-67, 1968.
17. Narahashi T, Moore JW, Scott WR: Tetrodotoxin blockage of sodium conductance increase in lobster giant axon. J. Gen. Physiol. 47:965-974, 1964.
18. Rodichok LD, Barron KD: Neurologic complications of bee sting, tick bite, spider bite and scorpion sting. In PJ Vinken and GW Bruyn, eds., Handbook of Clinical Neurology, Vol. 37, pp. 107-114. North-Holland Publishing Co., Amsterdam, 1979.
19. Rowlands JB, Mastaglia FL, Kakulas BA, Hainsworth D: Clinical and pathological aspects of a fatal case of mulga (Pseudechis australis) snake bite. Med. J. Aust. 1:226-230, 1969.
20. Russell FE: Marine toxins and venomous and poisonous marine animals. Adv. Mar. Biol. 3:255-384, 1965.
21. Russell FE, Barritt WC, Fairchild MD: Electrocardiographic patterns evoked by the venom of the stingray. Proc. Soc. Exp. Biol. Med. 96:634-635, 1957.
22. Schmitt N, Bowmer EJ, Gregson JD: Tick paralysis in British Columbia. Can. Med. Assoc. J. 100:417, 1969.
23. Southcott RV: Marine toxins. In PJ Vinken and GW Bruyn, eds., Handbook of Clinical Neurology, Vol. 37. North Holland Publishing Co., Amsterdam, 1979.
24. Warrell DA, Barnes HJ, Piburn MF: Neurotoxic effects of bites by the Egyptian cobra (Naja haje) in Nigeria. Trans. Roy. Soc. Trop. Med. Hyg. 70:78-79, 1976.

25. Warwick JE, Albuquerque EX, Diniz CR: Electrophysiological observations on the action of the purified scorpion venom, Tityus-toxin on nerve and skeletal muscle of the rat. J. Pharmacol. Exp. Ther. 198: 155-157, 1976.
26. Weingart JL: Tick paralysis. Minn. Med. 50:383, 1967.

CHAPTER 10

Botanical Toxins

WIDE varieties of plants contain toxins of neurologic importance. The ingestion of colorful but dangerous berries and flowers is especially common in young children, although adults are not unusual victims of inadvertent mushroom toxicity. The growing enthusiasm for indoor gardening has brought new color and beauty into the home, but in a single six-month sampling, over 3,500 cases of plant toxin exposures were recorded in children five years old and younger. Almost half of these cases were infants under the age of one. The following section outlines the number of hazardous plants associated with specific neurologic complications.

MUSHROOMS

Poisoning by mushrooms dates far into history. The wife and children of Euripides (5th century B.C.), as well as the emperor Claudius (54 A.D.) were among probable victims of lethal intoxication. From a diagnostic viewpoint, mushroom toxicity may be divided into two plant groups, those with early toxic signs occurring within 6 hours after ingestion, and those with a delayed toxic onset (6–40 hours) (Table 10.1, Figure 10.1).

Mushrooms causing early signs of toxicity may induce a variety of clinical syndromes. Agitation, muscle spasms, ataxia, mydriasis, and convulsions are the severe neurologic complications. The mental changes usually predominate and begin within one hour after eating the mushroom. Patients appear intoxicated and are sometimes thought to be drunk or to have taken an anticholinergic overdose. Their agitation and confusion helps to distinguish this mushroom intoxication from ingestion of primary hallucinogenic mushrooms of the psilocybe genus (see below). Amanita (A. muscaria and A. pantherina), the prototype of

BIOLOGICAL TOXINS

TABLE 10.1. Poisonous Mushrooms [7]

Scientific name	Popular names	Area of distribution	Habitat	Occurrence	Toxin(s)
1. Amanita muscaria	Fly-agaric	Northern hemisphere, but locally (introduced?) in South Africa, South America, Australia, and New Zealand	In deciduous and coniferous woods; fairly common. Particularly under birch (Betula) and pine (Pinus), but occasionally under other trees.	Summer, autumn	cyclic polypeptides
2. Amanita pantherina	Panter cap	Temperate zone of northern hemisphere, but also (introduced?) in South Africa	Fairly common in woods, often near oak (Quercus)	Summer, autumn	Atropine-like toxins
3. Amanita phalloides	Death-cap	Temperate zone of northern hemisphere, also locally (probably introduced) in southern hemisphere	Particularly under oak (Quercus), but occasionally also under other trees. Common	Summer, autumn	Cyclic polypeptides
4. Amanita virosa	Destroying angel	Temperate zone of northern hemisphere	In coniferous and deciduous forest on acid soil, often with beech (Fagus) or spruce (Picea). Rather rare	Late summer, autumn	Cyclic polypeptides
5. Coprinus astramentarius	Inky cap	Temperate zone of northern and southern hemispheres	On wood, mostly on stumps or buried wood. Common	Summer, autumn	Coprine
6. Gyromitra esculenta	False morel	Temperate zone of northern and southern hemispheres	In coniferous forest, especially on sandy soil. Rather common	Spring, early summer	Gyromitrin

Botanical Toxins

mushrooms in fairy tales, with a scarlet red hood and white dots (see Figure 10.1), has strong neurotoxic effects based on its concentrations of ibotenic acid, muscazon, and muscimol. These agents are anticholinergic, and also may alter gabanergic and serotonergic function. Additional indol compounds not yet identified may account for hallucinations often encountered with intoxication with such mushrooms, although other investigators feel this effect is mediated through central anticholinergic mechanisms [8]. No specific antidote is available, and A. pantherine carries a mortality rate of 10-20 percent after ingestion.

The genera Inocybe and Clitocybe are usually small, brown and white mushrooms growing in the grasslands and open areas. They contain muscarine and cause cholinergic excitation at all parasympathetic nerve endings except those of neuromuscular junctions and nicotinic sites. Patients develop severe sweating, salivation, lacrimation with myosis, blurred vision, and hypertension. Gastric lavage often will allow recuperation of mushroom bits that facilitate diagnosis. Atropine treatment has decreased mortality.

Coprinus atramentarius, or Inky Cap, is a common mushroom generally considered edible, although its consumption in combination with alcohol results in a severe toxic reaction [24]. Even when alcohol is ingested days after the mushroom, the patient may become symptomatic, suggesting a delayed excretion of the neurotoxic chemical. Most cases occur after ingestion of cooked Inky Caps, so that the toxin may be activated or enhanced by temperature elevation. The intoxication syndrome closely resembles that seen with alcohol and disulfiram ingestion and involves facial flushing, paresthesias, and severe nausea and vomiting with hyperventilation. Fatalities have occurred and esophageal rupture and cerebral edema were found at autopsy. Since the reaction is dose related, gastric lavage can be life saving. In most cases, spontaneous recovery occurs. The toxin Coprine is a derivative of cyclopropanone and acts like disulfiram to increase acetaldehyde blood levels [5].

The specific mushrooms with hallucinogenic properties belong primarily to the genus psilocybe, and contain indole psilocybin and psilocicin. Psilocybe mushrooms are small slender-stalked mushrooms with a blue-green cap color occurring in most hallucinogen varieties. The ingestion of fresh or dried (uncooked) mushrooms equivalent to oral doses of 3-5 mg of psilocybin provokes altered mood and heightened activity within 30 minutes. With further ingestion, increased visual sensitivity, delusions, and hallucinations, usually on the background of a clear sensorium without confusion, will develop. Recovery is usually complete after twelve hours without significant "hang over". These hallucinogenic chemicals are further discussed in chapter 14. Four cases of accidental ingestion of psilocybin by children have been reported; in these patients high fever and seizures occurred and one child died. In adults, however, aside from the psychotomimetic properties, other acute or chronic neurotoxic signs have not been established.

BIOLOGICAL TOXINS

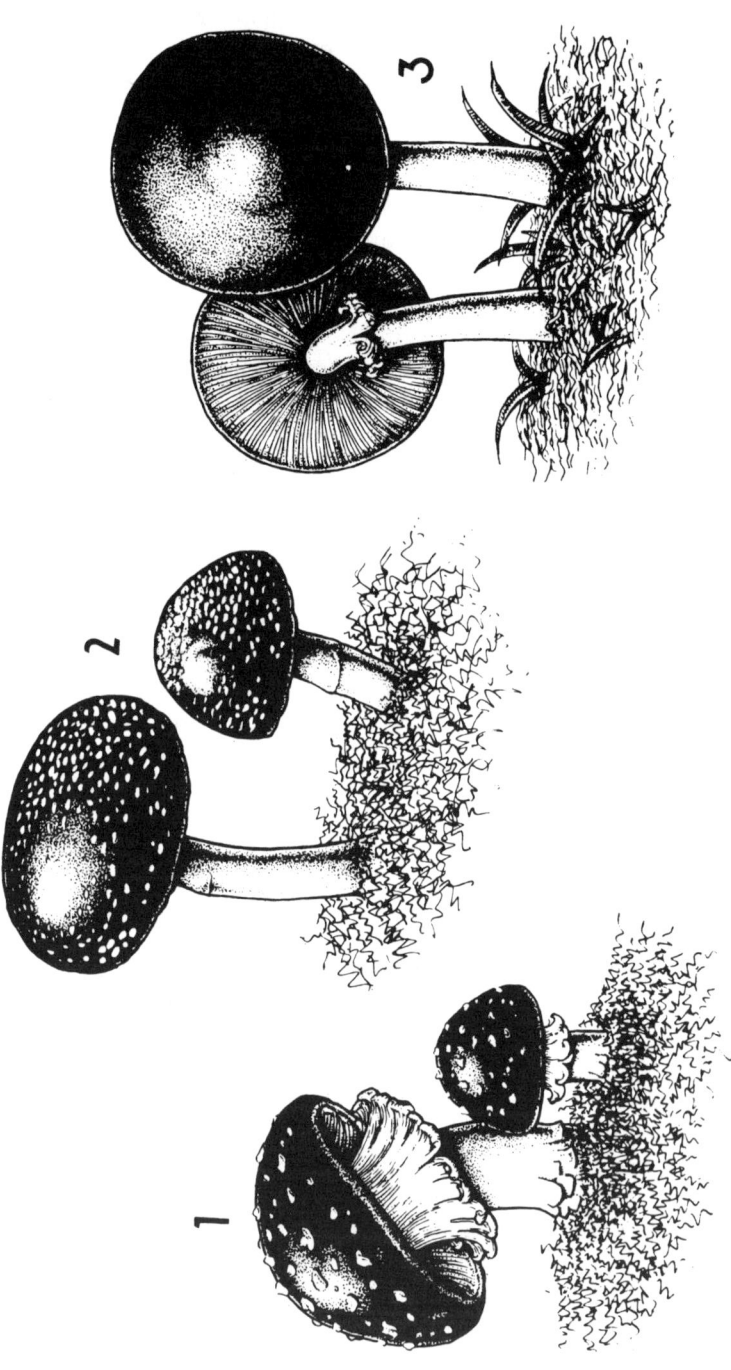

Botanical Toxins

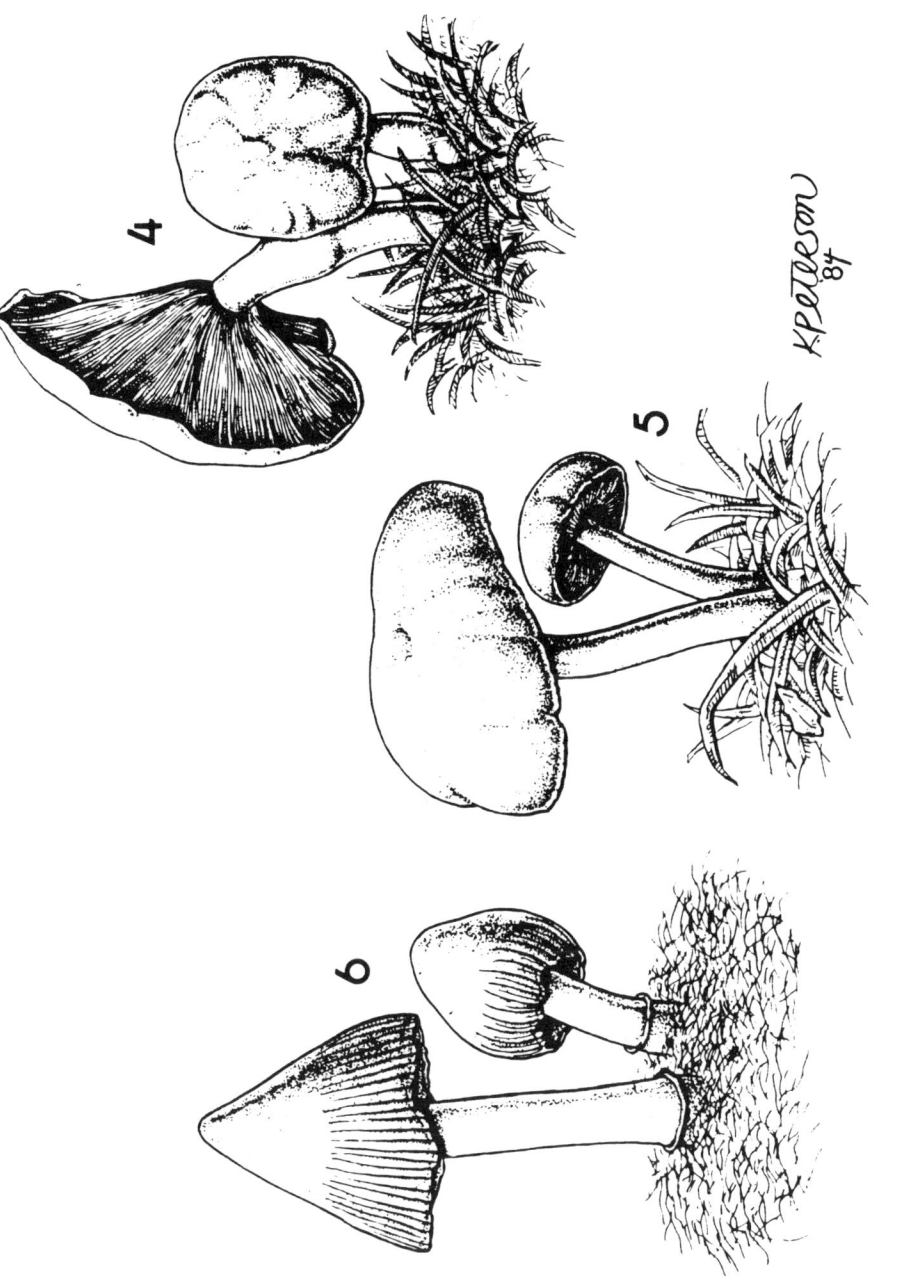

Figure 10.1. (1) Amanita muscaria, (2) Amanita pantherina, (3) Amanita phalloides, (4) Inocybe, (5) Clitocybe, (6) Coprinus.

BIOLOGICAL TOXINS

There are two major groups of mushrooms causing intoxication with delayed neurologic responses, Gyrimitra, which causes neurologic symptoms probably as a direct result of neurotoxic effects, and Amanita phalloides, which gives neurologic symptoms secondary to hepatic damage. Gyromitra esculenta or False Morel is a tempting early spring mushroom with fatality rates ranging from 15-35 percent. Within 8 hours after ingestion, headache and severe nausea occur, with progressive vomiting, watery diarrhea, and abdominal pain. Hepatosplenomegaly occur after 1-2 days, with increases in serum transaminases and icterus. Drowsiness, irritability, ataxia, and coma may follow with frequent, poorly controlled seizures. Although the mental changes may well relate to a hepatic encephalopathy, the presence of seizures suggests that the toxin may have direct neurologic effects. At autopsy, massive cerebral edema is the usual neurologic finding. The therapy has been non-specific with maintenance of fluid-electrolyte balance and hypertonic solutions in the presence of signs of cerebral edema. Since the toxin and its metabolites all appear to be water soluble small molecules, hemodialysis is a sensible therapy and has been used with significant success [22].

Amanita phalloides causes neurologic symptoms as a secondary effect of hepatic damage, with patients dying in hepatic coma. These Amanita mushrooms are responsible for about 95 percent of fatalities associated with mushroom ingestion, reaching globally several hundred per year [18]. The mushrooms have white gills and a cup at the base of the stem. Since these mushrooms so closely resemble non-toxic varieties, the risk of inadvertent poisoning is high. Two toxin groups, amatoxins and phallotoxins, both cyclopeptides, act to alter protein syntheses and disrupt cell membranes. There is no established specific effect on neuronal or glial tissue. The clinical course begins 6-8 hours after ingestion with massive emesis and bloody cholera-like diarrhea. While patients often die during this phase from electrolyte imbalance, the most dangerous phase of hepatorenal failure does not occur for three to five days. Secondary neurologic manifestations include a gradual decline of mental status with confusion, asterixis, and eventually hepatic coma and death [8]. Treatment involves hemodialysis, often with exchange transfusion, although mortality rates are 30-40 percent; when acute liver failure appears, 70 percent or more patients fail to survive [28]. Recently, thioctic acid, available from the National Institute of Health as an investigational product, has been used with success; the sulfhydryl group of the drug may combine with polypeptides of the mushroom, or the drug may act to protect the Krebs cycle function.

ANTICHOLINERGIC PLANTS

A large group of poisonous plants belong to the anticholinergic alkaloid group, and Table 10.2 includes some samples. After the ingestion of the plant, fever, visual disturbances, burning mouth, thirst, hot dry skin, headache, confusion, dilated pupils, severe hallucinations, and confusion result. The syndrome should be treated, once recognized, by the induction of vomiting with syrup of ipecac or gastric lavage. Physostigmine has been demonstrated in reversing the anticholinergic toxicity of tricyclic antidepressants and bella donna alkaloids so that in the appropriate cases, this agent should be considered for use. For adults and children with the above medication toxicity, 1-3 mg is usually administered slowly intravenously; an effect is usually seen within 20 minutes. The dose can be repeated. Duration of action is usually 15-30 minutes. An overdose of physostigmine can cause cholinergic crisis with increased salivation and respiratory distress. Atropine should always be on hand as a reversing antagonist. Physostigmine is not used in the presence of asthma, gangrene, diabetes, cardiovascular disease, or obstruction of the intestines or urogenital tract.

JAMAICAN VOMITING SICKNESS

This illness resembles Reye Syndrome clinically and is felt to relate to ingestion of unripe ackee, a fruit indigenous to West Africa and first brought to Jamaica in 1778. Until 1970, canned ackee was available in the United States. The responsible plant toxin is believed to be a hypoglycin A, which inhibits several short chain acetyl CoA dehydrogenases, thereby altering glycolysis and gluconeogenesis, amino acid metabolism, and fatty acid oxidation. Specific neurotoxicity appears to relate to hypoglycemia and the accumulation of short chain fatty acids centrally [31].

The clinical syndrome involves severe vomiting, followed by mild to moderate body twitching, progressing into generalized seizures, coma, and death [13]. The sequence may extend from hours to several days. The disease affects primarily children aged 2-10 years and is especially prevalent in those who are malnourished. It is unusual in adults, but when it does occur the clinical picture is different, with signs of agitation and delirium, ataxia, nystagmus, ptosis, and diffusely increased tendon reflexes. Neuropathologic changes include marked cerebral edema and hyperemia of the brain and meninges without specific microscopic changes [19]. Treatment involves electrolyte management and rapid administration of glucose to correct the severe hypoglycemia. Mortality before glucose administration was introduced in 1954 was 80 percent; no more recent statistics are available [31], although it is agreed that control of hypoglycemia has reduced mortality. Glycine administration has been suggested on the theoretical grounds that it will enhance conjugation of toxic metabolites. This treatment has been effective in reversing toxicity in hypoglycin A-treated rats but has not yet been tested extensively in humans.

BIOLOGICAL TOXINS

CHICKPEA (Lathyrism)

In certain areas in Europe and India, spastic paraplegia has been observed in man and animals following consumption of different varieties of the chickpea, Lathyrus. Two potent neurotoxins, alpha amino beta oxalyaminopropionic acid and alpha amino gamma oxalylaminobutyric acid, may be involved in the production of human lathyrism [34]. The ensuing condition is thought to result from toxic interference with oxidative de-amination of amino groups of peptide-bound lysine [6]. High manganese content in the chickpea also appears to play some role in the mechanism of the action of these toxins [23].

Chickpea ingestion is associated with toxic neurologic signs when it accounts for more than one-third of the caloric intake [30]. Men are more frequently affected than women, and the symptoms are fairly uniform. The onset is sudden, and the first ill effects are apparent on awakening in the morning. Initially, there is pain in the lumbar region, and the lower extremities feel stiff and weak. A slight fever may accompany these symptoms. During the next several days, marked diminution in strength develops, often accompanied by paresthesias. The legs become spastic and exhibit a clonic tremor. If the condition is severe, the upper extremities may also be involved. There may also be muscle atrophy and a marked sensory deficit with paresthesias, lightening pain, and decreased tactile, heat, and pain sensitivity. Ataxia with loss of tendon jerks is infrequent. Sphincter control is usually retained unless the involvement is extensive. Within one to two weeks, the pain and paresthesias usually disappear. There may be some recovery of muscle power following the initial attack, but spastic scissors-gait and pes cavus tend to persist. In some instances, relapses occur. Although spastic paraplegia is the most common neurotoxic effect, polyneuropathy may also be present. Peripheral mononeuropathy may also be present.

Neuropathologic findings involve primarily anterolateral sclerosis in the thoracolumbar cord with loss of axons and myelin [7]. Cortical lesions including senile plaques and neurofibrillary tangles in Ammon's horn may be found, although whether they are pathophysiologically related to the chickpea ingestion or incidental findings is not known. Experimentally, lesions of large blood vessels similar to those in copper deficiency have been produced, as well as peripheral neuropathic lesions [6,10].

KHAT

The bush-like plant *Cathaedulis*, also known as khat, grows naturally in Eastern Africa and Southern Arabia. Its fleshy leaves are chewed by millions of inhabitants who know the plant for its euphoric effects and its ability to reduce fatigue. Although not common in the United States, khat can easily be grown as

Botanical Toxins

a household plant, and this form of toxicity may increasingly be seen in immigrants, college students from north Africa and Arabia, and American visitors who have recently traveled in these regions. Khat induces amphetamine-like sympathomimetic and central stimulant effects, including elevated blood pressure, hyperthermia, insomnia, and a gregarious, often pressured speech [15]. Sociopsychiatric problems associated with Khat use include decreased economic productivity, depression, especially after cessation of use, and impotence. Of neuropsychiatric concern is a toxic manic-like psychosis that may occur and resembles the psychotic and overactive sympathetic state characteristic of amphetamine, cocaine, and other centrally active sympathomimetic agents. The leaves of the khat plant contain three major compounds; cathin, cathinome, and norephedrine. The former two substances closely resemble amphetamine in chemical structure [11].

BOTANICAL DEPRESSANTS AND CONVULSANTS

No plant in the United States is only a CNS depressant, but usually will also contain various resins causing cardiac and gastrointestinal irritation [17]. Andromedotoxin, veratrine, solanine, and taxins are the most important depressants, and are found in such plants as death camass, lambkill, sheep laurel, mountain laurel, and calico bush (Table 10.2). A peaceful progressive drowsiness and eventual coma without convulsion or mental irritability follows ingestion. No specific antidotes are known and the neuropharmacologic mechanisms of action of these agents are not well delineated. Respiratory and cardiac support during the intoxication phase will usually be followed by full recovery.

The convulsant plants vary in potency and may cause both acute and chronic toxic signs. The Cicuta species includes the extremely potent water hemlock, containing a human lethal dose within a single rhizome. The responsible cicutoxin is an unsaturated alipatic alcohol and induces, within one hour after ingestion, severe, usually generalized, seizures that may progress to status epilepticus. It has been suggested that cholinergic overstimulation is the pharmacologic basis of the convulsions [29]. Respiratory failure and anoxia are the usual cause of death. No specific antidote is available and supportive measures and oxygenation are the modes of therapy. The short acting barbiturate, thiopentane sodium, has been recommended because of its rapid actions and its possible anticholinergic effect [29]. In survivors, a peculiar retrograde amnesia that may include days prior to the toxic ingestion has been described [17].

Less common convulsants include various berry plants: Chinaberry, moonseed, pinkroot, and Carolina allspice. The latter contains calycanthine, which is similar to strychnine. Again, no specific antidotes are available and identification and respiratory support are the basic therapeutic aims. In the case of strychnine-like toxins, isolation of the patient from external stimuli is important.

TABLE 10.2. Poisonous Plants

Anticholinergic plants
Bittersweet
Black henbane
Black nightshade
Deadly nightshade
Jerusalem cherry
Jimson weed
Lantana, Red Sage, Wild Sage
Potato leaves, sprouts, tubers
Wild tomato

Depressant plants
Calico bush
Death camass
Lambkill
Mountain laurel
Sheep laurel

Convulsant plants
Carolina allspice
Chinaberry
Moonseed
Pinkroot
Water hemlock

Cyanogenic glycoside plants
Hydrangea macrophylla—Hydrangea
Pyrus sylvestris—Apple
Prunus americana—American plum
Prunus caroliniana—Cherry laurel
Prunus cerasus—Cultivated cherry
Prunus persica—Peach
Prunus serotina—Wild black cherry

A final group of patients exposed to convulsant plant toxins are those who consume plant extracts or various aqueous decoctions. Juniper, white cedar, and cypress contain volatile oils in which thujone or related substances constitute the primary toxic agent. Unlike the other two groups, acute ingestion of these decoctions even in a single large dose rarely causes neurologic signs; instead, chronic toxicity after daily ingestion of teas or brews is more clinically important. Personality changes and progressive seizure disorders have been described [3].

ERGOTS

The role of ergots in human history is at least as old as the cultivations of grain, particularly rye. The word "ergot," first used in France, is now generally used to describe the chemical compounds produced by the fungus Claviceps purpurea. This term means "spur", and is based on the resemblance between the curved dark purple sclerotium of the fungus and the spur of a cock. The fungus itself infects many grains, but has a predilection for rye, and is most plentiful during wet, rainy years or under boggy growing conditions [2].

As obstetrical agents, ergots may have been used as long as 3000 years ago by the ancient Chinese. Certainly the powers of these "sun baked rye kernels" were well-recognized by medieval midwives and physicians in Europe when rye cultivation became widespread after the advent of the Christian era. Other ergot properties, their ability to cause profound central nervous system alterations with dementia, psychosis and convulsions, sometimes accompanied by severe vascular disease with resultant gangrene and necrosis, were not attributed to the fungus for many centuries. Possibly the first record epidemic of ergot poisoning occurred in Athens in 4300 B.C.E., during the summer of the second year of the Peloponnesian War. The Athenians, but not the Spartans, were afflicted with a plague, the symptoms of which included lividness, severe internal heat, necrosis of toes and fingers, blindness, a severe dementia, and psychosis. An epidemic of gangrenous ergotism certainly occurred in Duisberg, Germany in 857, and following that, historians inform us that multiple episodes of "the fire plague", or "Ignus Sacer", afflicted the peasantry throughout the middle ages.

Perhaps the most vivid description of the medical changes associated with probable ergotism is that of St. Anthony of Egypt. As an early Christian hermit, he was afflicted by apparent ergotism but survived. Thus, he was believed to have had special power over the disease, which subsequently acquired the name St. Anthony's Fire. Prior to his affliction, St. Anthony is reported to have retired to meditate in solitude, subsisting only on bread. In the midst of his retreat, he was visited by devils and demons taking the form of lions, serpents, scorpions, and other frightening creatures which seemed to come through the walls of his hermitage to attack him. He is reported to have been of clear mind and to have survived the terrors of these hallucinations when he fled and changed his diet [16].

More recently, in 1961, the epidemic of Pont-Saint-Esprit in France reawakened the public and scientists to the curious and morbid consequences of possible ergot toxicity. Although never proven, the possibility or ergotism was suggested by the clinical presentation of the population and the definitive tracing of toxicity to the town bakers. Organic mercury poison also was considered.

The clinical features of ergotism are neuropsychiatric and vascular. From careful analysis of documents by doctors, artists, and historians, Girard has summarized the likely presentation of natural ergotism from plant contamination: burning dysesthesias, prominent hallucinations on an otherwise clear sensorium, insomnia, and gangrenous lesions of the distal extremities [12].

Far more common and well documented is medicinal ergot poisoning. Ergot drugs are prescribed for the management of migraine headaches, and new ergot preparations are currently used to treat Parkinson's disease. Acute poisoning is rare, but has occurred when large amounts of ergots were ingested in an attempt to provoke abortion. The symptoms consist of sudden vomiting, diarrhea, tingling dysesthesias over the skin, confused delirium, and unconsciousness. Migraneurs represent the largest group of patients exposed to ergot drugs. Importantly, while an antimigraine dose may be relatively standard for most sufferers of migraine, fever, hepatic disease, preexisting vascular disease, and septic states may all render a patient more sensitive to ergot preparations than he or she would ordinarily be. In fact, ordinarily, migraine patients appear relatively resistant to ergot toxicity. Friedman et al. (1980) reported a four year study of over 1,000 patients who were taking ergotamine, where side effects occurred in only ten percent and all were transitory, disappearing with reduction or cessation of the medication [9]. The syndrome of chronic ergot toxicity includes burning dysesthesias, hallucinations, gangrenous lesions, and often insomnia. The new antiparkinsonian ergot drugs (bromocriptine and pergolide) have dopaminergic properties and hence abate the Parkinson's disease, but are also associated with hallucinations and insomnia; in the case of bromocriptine, skin lesions in the distal extremities are also encountered, with erythema, edema, and tenderness. The problem simulates cellulitis or thrombophlebitis, but quickly responds to withdrawal of the bromocriptine. Chorea is also seen with these latter ergots.

The weekly dose of ergotamine tartrate is usually 8 milligrams total, and patients who ingest quantities in excess of this are likely to develop an additional neurologic syndrome—ergotamine rebound headache. In this case, the next headache is promoted by withdrawal from the last dose of ergotamine. This phenomenon can occur with great subtlety and can be misdiagnosed as recurrent migraine. For this reason, it is important that the frequency of ergotamine tartrate be determined in all patients experiencing chronic migraine-like headaches [27].

The treatment of ergotism involves the complete withdrawal of the ergot drug or source. In the case of impending gangrene or vascular constriction, pharmacologic agents that maintain adequate profusion to the affected parts are indicated; anticoagulants, low molecular weight dextran and potent vasodilatory drugs. Potent vasodilators such as ethyl alcohol, amyl nitride and sodium nicotinate have each been used in single case reports. Since ergots have both serotonergic and dopaminergic properties, agents blocking receptor sites (methysergide for the serotonergic system and neuroleptics like chlorpromazine or haloperidol for the dopaminergic system) might be specific antidotes. This, however, has not been demonstrated clinically.

CYANIDES

Hydrocyanic acid is one of the most rapidly acting poisons known. This feature has led to its frequent use as a suicidal or homocidal agent.

Free hydrocyanic acid or cyanogenetic glycosides are produced by chokecherry trees and other plants, and accidental poisoning has followed the ingestion and chewing of the toxic seeds. The cyanides are general protoplasmic poisons producing asphyxia by initial brief stimulation of the central nervous system that is rapidly replaced by paralyzing action. Cyanide intoxication also occurs accidentally during fumigation, electroplating, gold or silver ore extraction, and during other industrial procedures employing this poison.

Cyanide induced demyelinating lesions have been reported in experimental animals [14]. These do not appear to be due to the inhibition of the respiratory enzymes but rather the result of disturbance in the myelin metabolism.

Within 10 minutes after ingestion, some individuals will give a loud cry, lose consciousness, exhibit generalized convulsions and die within two to five minutes. Most often, the toxic effects appear more slowly, with some agitation, salivation, anxiety, confusion, and nausea, usually without vomiting. These symptoms are rapidly augmented by vertigo, headache, unsteady gait, and a feeling of stiffness in the lower extremities, followed by sudden unconsciousness, violent convulsions, and, at times, opisthotonos. The breathing is stertorous, the face is flushed, and then cyanotic; and the pupils are dilated. The respirations frequently cease before the heart stops and death usually ensues within 15 minutes to one hour. Recovery may occur when treatment is instituted rapidly [4]. If the patient survives the first hour, recovery is usual. Vomiting is then frequent, and for several days the patient may experience weakness, unsteady gait, headache, difficulty in speaking, and drowsiness. Patients have survived following ingestion of 6 mg of potassium cyanide, although as little as 0.13 mg has proved lethal.

After inhalation of toxic concentrations of gaseous hydrocyanic acid, nausea, vomiting, and difficulty in breathing lead to unconsciousness, and within 10 minutes there is respiratory failure and death. When smaller amounts of the gas are inhaled, the individual may lose consciousness.

A chronic form of cyanide intoxication has been suggested [26], manifested by a vague malaise and hemiparesis, visual disturbances, girdle pains, ataxia, and balancing dysfunction. Vertigo, speech difficulties, and periods of unconsciousness have also been observed.

Chronic cyanide intoxication has also been implicated in the etiology of "tropical amblyopia" and "tropical ataxic neuropathy". The source of the intoxication is believed to be cassava derivatives. Cassava is the tuberous root of a shrub-like plant, Manihot palmata, which contains a high concentration of glycoside. It yields cyanide by the action of hydrolase activated by handling, heating, or bruising the tubers. Farmers and housewives in closest contact with cassava are most frequently affected [21]. Lima beans also contain cyanogenic glycosides. Clinically this chronic intoxication is manifested by optic atrophy, bilateral nerve deafness, myelopathy with implications of posterior and lateral columns, either singly or together, and polyneuropathy [20]. The lower limbs are most frequently involved and show marked weakness and wasting. An occasional patient reveals mental changes and occasionally cerebellar findings. One third of the patients gave a history of recurrent mucocutaneous lesions such as angular stomatitis, painful glossitis, and scrotal dermatis (Table 10.2). The syndrome may well relate to general nutritional deficiency rather than to a specific effect of cyanide.

The patient will usually recover spontaneously from poisoning due to inhalation if he can be brought into the open air before respiration ceases. Artificial respiration is imperative if there is interruption of breathing. The spinal fluid is normal but plasma and urinary thiocyanide levels are high. Increasing use of nitroprusside as an agent to control hypertension has led to new iatrogenic cyanide toxicity. For this reason, nitroprusside maximal dosage has been suggested as 3.5 mg/kg or 10 micrograms/kg/minute.

Treatment of acute cyanide poisoning involves the induction of vomiting with syrup of ipecac or gastric lavage. For severe symptoms, a cyanide antidote package is available which includes amyl nitrite, sodium nitrite, and sodium thiosulfate. Sodium nitrite produces a high concentration of methemoglobin which competes with cytochrome oxidase for the cyanide ions. The actual detoxification is achieved by the infusion of thiosulfate which, under the catalysis of rhodanase, reacts with cyanide to form thiocynate. This latter product is excreted largely unchanged.

The recommendations made by the National Poison Center network are as follows: one ampule of sodium nitrite is administered every 15-30 seconds by inhalation until the amyl nitrite solution is ready. If systolic blood pressure drops below 80 mm/Hg, the amyl nitrite is stopped. Once the sodium nitrite is given the amyl nitrite can be stopped in all cases. When sodium nitrite is administered intravenously for adults, 10 ml of a three percent solution are administered over 2-5 minutes. Again, if blood pressure falls to below 80 mm/Hg, the nitrite solution must be stopped. In children weighing less than 25 kg, the dose must be recalculated based on the patient's hemoglobin and weight. Once the sodium nitrite is administered, the sodium thiosulfate in a 25 percent solution is administered intravenously with 50 ml given over 10-20 minutes. Clearly, since both sodium nitrite and amyl nitrite in excessive doses induce dangerous methemoglobinemia such substances are not without risk. The amounts found in a single cyanide antidote package, however, are not excessive for an adult. Again, calculations for children may be different. Excessive methemoglobinemia may be treated with methylene blue.

SPANISH RAPESEED OIL

A recent devastating epidemic in Spain was caused by the ingestion of denatured rapeseed oil. Eighty percent of the patients reported by the toxic epidemic syndrome study group had neurologic manifestations [33]. An oil not widely used in the United States, rapeseed oil comes primarily from India, Europe, Canada and Pakistan. In 1970, its estimated world production was 2,090 million short tons, less than cottonseed or peanut oil but more than olive or sesame seed. Along with soy bean and sunflower oil, rapeseed is largely responsible for the huge increase in edible vegetable oils over the past 30 years. Over 330 deaths were attributable to the toxic product in Spain and over 20,000 people were variably affected.

The clinical picture of intoxication was biphasic. Initially, patients suffered with nonspecific symptoms and signs including fever, headache, pruritis, and dyspnea with laboratory abnormalities including eosinophilia, altered liver enzymes and occasional thrombocytopenia. The second phase, about one month later, involved neuromuscular dysfunction with prominent dysesthesia and myalgias in the extremities. Weakness and muscle atrophy followed while the prominent respiratory symptoms apparent earlier tended to wane. Chronic problems other than the neuromuscular deficits included scleroderma-like lesions, Raynaud's syndrome and weight loss. Gradual improvement in muscle tenderness occurred after several months but in 65% of patients, significant chronic muscle atrophy was apparent. In 32%, the atrophy was severe and in 19% respiratory insufficiency was probably directed related to the weakness. Generalized areflexia was a further common residual. Nerve conduction velocities performed on patients with active disease were most compatible with an axonal problem [33].

Three percent of patients clinically showed evidence of central nervous system involvement. Encephalopathy with either global cerebral depression and somnolence or with focal hemispheric signs occurred in one half of these patients (1.5 percent). In such cases, the encephalopathy spontaneously resolved. In rare instances convulsions occurred and occasionally, fleeting focal abnormalities suggestive of thromboembolic transient ischemic attacks were seen. Increased intracranial pressure with bilateral papilledema and no focal signs was an additional presentation.

Detailed muscle and nerve biopsies have been analyzed in many afflicted patients, and the neurologic area most prominently involved is peripheral nerve. Perineuritis and later fibrosis of the perineurium were distinctive. Demyelination of axons occurred in late cases and distal nerves were more frequently affected than proximal although the same pathologic changes were qualitatively found diffusely. In those cases where the central nervous system was examined, anterior horn cells in the spinal cord as well as cranial nerve and pontine nuclei showed chromatolysis [23A].

Two distinct muscle abnormalities were reported as well. In the earlier phase where myalgia was the major clinical feature, inflammatory infiltrates of the muscle, muscle spindles, and intramuscular nerves were apparent. Later, after atrophy became the major abnormality, there was intense endomysial fibrosis without significant inflammation. This atrophy related most likely to the primary neuropathic alterations.

The lesions found in the nervous system were similar to those found in systemic organs. It has been suggested that the free radicals and precursors of arachidonic acid in the toxic oil may have precipitated the disease. Secondary involvement with prostaglandins and mast cell activation may have contributed to the inflammation and thrombotic alterations that followed. Even though high levels of IgE in the serum of patients experiencing the toxic syndrome have been documented, the clinical and pathologic findings did not easily resemble those seen with other allergic diseases. Since aniline was often used to denature the oil, an etiologic role of this compound has also been suggested [25].

CURARE

The arrow poisons used by the natives of certain river valleys in South America have long been known for their efficacy in paralyzing enemy victims. Extracted from a variety of bush ropes or vines growing in the dense jungles, curare can be combined with other plant juices and evaporated into a gummy substance with a consistency suitable to adhere to the arrow point. Bernard demonstrated the peripheral effect of the drug at the myoneural junction and early experiments using a tourniquet demonstrated that the victim can be saved by preventing the spread of the poison and by forcing respiration during the acute intoxication [1].

Curare alkaloids, in the form of tubocurarine, are now widely used in anesthesia to promote muscular relaxation. The drug blocks the postsynaptic receptor sites to acetylcholine at the myoneural nicotinic junction. Small rapidly moving muscles, such as those of the fingers, toes, jaw, eyes and ears are involved early followed by those of the trunk, neck and limbs. Ultimately, intercostal muscles and the diaphragm are paralyzed and respiration then stops. Hypoxia related to respiratory paralysis may cause terminal convulsions, although the observable manifestations may be minimal because of the paralysis. Since the duration of action of tubocurarine is transient, respiratory support is life saving.

D-tubocurarine and other quaternary neuromuscular blocking agents cannot effectively cross the blood-brain barrier, so that their toxic effects relate directly to peripheral neuromuscular blockade. Nicotinic receptors are also located on autonomic ganglion cells so that blood pressure decrease and tachycardia may occur [18].

These agents are rarely the cause of botanical poisoning, and are much more frequently used in anesthesia. Importantly, patients with myasthenia gravis or susceptible to malignant hyperthermia are especially susceptible to toxic reactions to curare prepared in doses that would cause only muscle relaxation in the rest of the population. In patients with myasthenia gravis, tiny doses of curare preparations can lead to life threatening muscular weakness. Patients with a familial tendency to malignant hyperthermia can develop life threatening hyperthermic crisis when exposed to halothane and curare drugs. Severely elevated body temperatures and rigidity follow and the patient must be treated in an emergency manner with rapid cooling and control of usually present acidosis. Procainamide which antagonizes the forced release of calcium into the muscle cells can be used to reverse the hyperthermic reaction. The patient with myasthenia gravis already has antibody active against postsynaptic cholinergic receptors, so even low doses of a blocking agent can cause precipitous weakness and even death.

D-tubocurarine is inactive after oral administration as evidenced by the impunity of flesh killed by curare poisoned arrows. When D-tubocurarine is injected intravenously, the action begins to wear off in about twenty minutes. Some residual effects are still discernable approximately three hours after the administration. In man, about one-third of the administered dose of D-tubocurarine in excreted in the urine over a period of several hours.

■ STUDY QUESTIONS

A 23-year-old college student comes to the emergency room with a three week history of clumsy legs, weakness, and dyesthesias of all distal extremities. He also has had cramping abdominal pains and diarrhea. The extremities are not painful, but feel heavy and tingling throughout the day and night. The history indicates that the patient recently worked on a farm over the summer harvesting and spraying fields. A vegetarian, his diet includes farm grown wheat germ, vegetables, and produce. The history is compatible with:

A. Ergot toxicity
B. Arsenic toxicity
C. Cyanide toxicity
D. Jimson weed toxicity

BIOLOGICAL TOXINS

Answer: B

The gastrointestinal symptoms and likely peripheral neuropathy in this patient along with the history of farm work should recall arsenic toxicity. Ergot toxicity would be expected to cause excruciatingly painful extremities and/or mental changes. Cyanide-containing plants can cause acute toxicity after ingestion or a chronic disorder characterized by visual disturbances, gait difficulty, and often myelopathic signs. Jimson weed provokes anticholinergic crises with significant abdominal distention and constipation gastrointestinally and delirious hallucinatory behavior.

A second vegetarian notices progressive visual and gait disorder over a six month period. He has been reading at the medical library and fears that he may have multiple sclerosis. His diet has been exclusively lima and kidney beans, occasional alfalfa sprouts, and carrot juice with goat's milk. Which of the following statements is true?

A. Lima beans have a high concentration of cyanogenetic glycosides.
B. Myelopathy and optic atrophy are not compatible with the diagnosis of multiple sclerosis.
C. Carrot juice and hypercarotenemia are likely causes of his disability.
D. Goat's milk has a protective effect against alfalfa sprout sulhydryl chelation.

Answer: A

Lima beans and cassava derivatives have been identified as a source of potential cyanide intoxication, where patients present with optic atrophy, a myelopathy and often polyneuropathy. The patient's clinical presentation is completely compatible with a diagnosis of multiple sclerosis, and, in animals, demyelinating lesions have been identified after cyanide exposure. Peripheral neuropathy is not typical of multiple sclerosis and the patient's history would suggest that a dietary cause could explain the patient's problems. Carrot juice contains a high concentration of vitamin A, and over-ingestion of vitamin A has been associated with the distinct neurologic syndrome of pseudotumor cerebri where headaches and increased intracranial pressure occur. This is not the presentation in the above case. The last response is nonsensical and has no scientific basis.

Match the mushroom with the correct response:

1. Amanita muscaria
2. Clitocybe group
3. Coprinius Atramentarius (inky cap)

A. Toxicity seen only with alcohol ingestion
B. Toxicity related to cholinergic overactivity
C. Toxicity related to cholinergic underactivity

Answers: 1-C; 2-B; 3-A

In spite of its name, muscaria, there is only a small and clinically insignificant concentration of muscarine in this mushroom and most toxicity involves anticholinergic effects both systemically and centrally. Hallucinations and delirium are the typical neurologic problems of these ibotenic mushrooms. In contrast, the clitocybe group causes cholinergic excitation peripherally, although the muscarine toxin does not act centrally. Inky cap is a safe and edible mushroom, and becomes toxic only when consumed along with alcohol. The alcohol provokes a cataclysmic disulfiram-like reaction. The toxic compound inhibits the conversion of acetaldehyde to acetate. The high levels of acetaldehyde provoke the symptoms of severe headache and abdominal pain. The alcohol does not have to coincide with the mushroom ingestion, and alcohol can precipitate toxicity hours or even days after the mushroom has been eaten.

The following is/are true regarding mushroom ingestion:

A. Non-poisonous mushrooms have a thin filmy skin that identifies them as non-toxic.
B. Most poisonous mushrooms can be detoxified by simmering ten minutes and draining well.
C. Toxic and non-toxic species may exist in the same genus.
D. A given genus may be more or less toxic depending on the environmental conditions in which it grows.

Answers: C & D

There is no easy distinguishing feature of non-toxic versus toxic mushrooms. Cooking and draining in no way assure safety, and there is no truth to the common adage that the mushroom is safe if the silver utensil cooked with the mushroom does not tarnish. The toxicity of various mushrooms will change depending on the individual who ingests them and the area of the world where they are found.

■ REFERENCES

1. Bernard C: Lecons sur les effets des substances toxiques. Paris, Balliere, 1857.
2. Bove FJ: The Story of Ergot. S. Karger, New York, 1970.
3. Brauch F: Das klinische bild der Thujaven giftung. Zeit. Klin. Med. 19:86-92, 1932.
4. Chen KK, Rose CL: Nitrite and thiosulfate therapy in poisoning. JAMA 149: 113-122, 1952.
5. Coldwell BB, Genest K, Hughes DW: Effect of C. atramentarius on the metabolism of ethanol in mice. J. Pharm. Pharmacol. 21:176-182, 1969.
6. Coulson WF, Lenker A, Bottcher E: Lathyrism in swine. Arch. Path. 87: 411-413, 1969.
7. Denny-Brown D: Neurological conditions resulting from prolonged and severe dietary restrictions. Medicine 26:41-48, 1947.
8. de Wolff FA: Neurologic aspects of mushroom intoxication. In PJ Vinken and GW Bruyn, eds., Handbook of Clinical Neurology, Vol. 37, pp. 529-536. Amsterdam, North-Holland Publishing Co., 1979.

9. Friedman AP: Migraine: Pathophysiology and pathogenesis. In, PJ Vinken and GW Bruyn, eds., Handbook of Clinical Neurology, Vol. 5, pp. 37-95, Amsterdam, North-Holland Publishing Co., 1980.
10. Ganapathy KT, Dwivedi MP, Nagrajan V, Dikshitulu VN: Experiments on chicks feed on lathyrus sativus. Indian J. Med. Res. 51:865-867, 1963.
11. Giannini AJ, Castellini S: Manic like psychosis due to khat. J. Toxicol. 19: 455-459, 1982.
12. Girard PF: Le mal des ardents ou le feu Saint-Antoine. In M. Baucher, ed., Conférences lyonnaises d'Histoire de la neurologie et de la psychiatrie, pp. 47-88. Oberval, Lyon, 1982.
13. Hill KR: Vomiting sickness of Jamaica: A review. West Indian Med. J. 1: 243-246, 1952.
14. Hurst EW: Experimental demyelination of the central nervous system. Aust. J. Exp. Biol. Med. Sci. 18:201-204, 1940.
15. Kennedy JG, Teague J, Fairbanks L: Khat use in North Yemen and the problem of addiction. Cult. Med. Psychiatry 4:311-317, 1980.
16. Klawans HL, Tanner CM, Goetz CG: Psychiatric reactions to ergot derivatives. In K. Fuxe and D. B. Calne, eds., Dopaminergic Ergot Derivatives and Motor Function, pp. 405-414. Pergamon Press, New York, 1979.
17. Lanye KF, Fagerstrom R: Plant Toxicity and Dermatitis. Williams and Wilkins, Baltimore, 1968.
18. Litten W: The most poisonous mushrooms. Sci. Am. 232:91-102, 1975.
19. Moran NC, Dresel PE, Perkins ME, Richardson AP: Pharmacological actions in andromedo toxin. J. Pharmacol. Exp. Ther. 110:415-416, 1954.
20. Osuntokum BO: An ataxic neuropathy in Nigeria. Brain 91:215-224, 1968.
21. Osuntokum BO, Monekasso GL, Wisson J: Cassava diet and a chronic degenerative neuropathy: An epidemiological study. Nigerian J. Sci. 3:3-15, 1969.
22. Poplawski A, Bulhak W, Juchnicka Z: Hemodializa w leczenu zatruc muchomorem sromotnikowym i fie strzenica kasztanowata. Pol. Tyg. lek 29:583-586, 1974.
23. Prasad LS, Sharon RK: Latharism. In PJ Vinken and GW Bruyn, eds., Handbook of Clinical Neurology, Vol. 36, 505-514. North-Holland Publishing Co., Amsterdam, 1979.
24. Ramsbottom J: Mushrooms and Toadstools. London, Collins, 1972.
25. Ricoy JR, Cabello A, Rodriguez J, Tellex I: Neuropathological studies of the toxic syndrome related to adulterated rapeseed oil in Spain. Brain 106: 817-835, 1983.
26. Sandberg CG: A case of chronic poisoning with potassium cyanide. Acta Med. Scand. 181:233-238, 1967.
27. Saper JR: Chronic headaches. In WJ Weiner and CG Goetz, eds., Neurology for the Non-Neurologist, pp. 58-73. Harper and Row, Philadelphia, 1982.
28. Scheminzky C, Kircher W: Zur therapie der knollenblatterpilzvergiftung beim kinde. Paed. Paedol. 91:14-23, 1973.
29. Starreveld E, Hope CE: Ciguatoxin poisoning. Neurology 25:730-734, 1975.

30. Strong FM: Lathyrism and oratism. Nutr. Rev. 14:65, 1956.
31. Tenaka K: Jamaican vomiting sickness. In PJ Vinken and GW Bruyn, eds., Handbook of Clinical Neurology, Vol. 37, pp. 511-540. North-Holland Publishing Co., Amsterdam, 1979.
32. Thompson TM: Accidental cyanide poisoning. Occup. Med. 4:419-424, 1947.
33. Toxic Epidemic Syndrome Study Group: Toxic epidemic syndrome. Spain 1981: Lancet 2:697-702, 1982.
34. Weaver AL: Lathyrism: A review. Arthritis Rheum. 10:470-474, 1967.

IV.
Iatrogenic and Medicinal Toxins

CHAPTER 11

Neurological Drugs

THE drugs prescribed to treat nervous system dysfunction are associated with neurotoxic problems which can often obscure diagnosis, complicate patient management, and limit or alter prognosis. Because most neurologic diseases are chronic, drugs are used over long periods of time, provoking acute, subacute, and chronic toxic syndromes. Drugs used in four major areas of neurology are discussed below: epilepsy, Parkinson's disease, myasthenia gravis, and spasticity. Drugs used in other conditions are discussed in other chapters: neuroleptics (Chapter 12), Ergots (Chapter 10), pain medications (Chapter 13), amphetamines and analeptics (Chapter 14).

■ ANTICONVULSANTS

Anticonvulsant medications are used primarily for epilepsy control, but neuropathies, other painful syndromes, dystonias and dyskinesias are also treated with these drugs. The toxic syndromes associated with their use may be acute, subacute or chronic, appearing only after months or years of exposure. For more extensive details or discussions of less frequently used drugs in this class, the reader is referred to more comprehensive texts dealing exclusively with these agents [33,40].

PHENYTOIN

Phenytoin, one of the most effective anticonvulsants, can induce significant nervous system toxicity. The incidence of side effects estimated from 12-38% of patients increases if blood levels extend far beyond the therapeutic range. When the drug is first introduced, even low doses can be associated with some complaints of neurologic dysfunction. Since there is poor correlation between the dose of PHT (mg/kg) and the presence of side effects, blood levels have been used to establish therapeutic and toxic "windows." Even these ranges are not absolute and moderate reversible toxicity may appear even when blood levels remain in the therapeutic range of 10-20 µg/cc. Guidelines suggesting that nystagmus appears at 20 µg/cc, ataxia and slurred speech at 30 µg/cc, and mental changes at 40 µg/cc are approximate. Since blood determination of PHT calculate total drug and not the active non-protein bound fraction, variation may largely be due to this transport factor. The effects of drug/drug interactions are also discussed below. Most side effects are related to the blood level of phenytoin and hence may be acute, subacute or chronic depending on how the patient has taken the medication to attain the toxic blood levels.

Clinical Features

Nystagmus may be seen even when the blood phenytoin level is in the normal range. As levels pass beyond 20 µg/cc, nystagmus becomes prominent, especially with lateral gaze accompanied by a fine postural tremor, often with a resting component. When ataxia appears, the patient may stagger as he walks because of trunkal imbalance; the extremities are less involved. The mental changes vary widely from impaired memory and somnolence, which is usual, to a wild toxic delirium with exhilaration and euphoria.

Once the drug levels pass 40 µg/cc, more severe vestibulocerebellar and mental changes usually occur. Vertigo and vomiting disable the patient and progressive lethargy prevails. In retarded patients, the decline in function may initially suggest a progression of their underlying neurologic disease.

Glaser described another form of encephalopathy associated with PHT therapy which was selective to higher cortical activity without preliminary involvement of the vestibulocerebellar systems. Increased seizure activity, mental changes often with focal abnormalities, hemianopsias and unilateral weakness of sensory deficits occurred [40]. This rare syndrome, seen primarily with drug levels outside the therapeutic antiepileptic range, resolved with discontinuation of the drug.

A further rare but prominent phenytoin toxic syndrome includes a variety of involuntary movement disorders. Facial grimacing and lingual-buccal choreic dyskinesias may occur as well as wild and flailing ballistic movements, dystonias and myoclonic asterixic movements. Blood levels may range from 30-90 µg/cc. The pharmacologic bases of these various movements may not all be the same. Chorea is felt to relate to increased activity of striatal dopaminergic systems although phenytoin's effect on these neurons and receptors is unclear. Unlike another drug induced form of chorea, neuroleptic-induced tardive dyskinesia, phenytoin chorea is regularly reversible after drug cessation. These dyskinesias may be more frequent in patients with prior early life anoxic encephalopathy with extrapyramidal signs [23].

Although the prominent neuropathy associated with PHT is unrelated to blood levels, a reversible neuropathy that promptly clears with drug withdrawal can occur [10]. This neuropathy is associated with slowed conduction velocities that revert to normal as the blood level returns toward 20 μg/cc. Other signs of toxicity need not be present [33]. Even in the therapeutic range, clinical neuropathic changes can occur rarely.

These PHT intoxication syndromes are caused by a dose increment that changes the pharmacokinetics of phenytoin to a non-linear curve. In this way, even a seemingly small increase (100 mg tablet daily) can suddenly precipitate clinical intoxication and elevated blood levels. In protein deficiency states, a "normal" blood level may in fact become toxic since more free PHT circulates; serum albumin levels below 3 gr/dl are associated with adverse reaction three times more frequently than when the albumin levels are higher [4]. The subcellular target of PHT toxicity is unknown.

The above syndromes fit the model of traditional toxic complications, whereby PHT levels outside the therapeutic range precipitate dose dependent signs. There are some data, however, from patients maintained within the 10-20 μg/cc ideal blood levels, suggesting possible cognitive alteration related to the drug at therapeutic level. Significant methodological problems exist in these studies where seizures are obvious complicating factors and the frequency of blood levels not always consistent. To date, it is not established whether exposure to PHT per se is dangerous to cognitive functioning. Folate levels are often decreased in patients on PHT (and other anticonvulsants) and folate deficiency has been implicated in the pathogenesis of some forms of dementia [31]. The direct role of folate deficiency, seizure control and behavioral alterations is unsettled.

A number of syndromes have been described that occur in association with PHT use, but do not correlate with the blood level of the drug. After long term exposure to phenytoin, a patient may develop a mild neuropathy unrelated to blood drug level but instead correlated with age and duration of PHT exposure. The incidence of such neuropathy varies (8-50%) depending on whether EMG or clinical techniques are used in diagnosis. The neuropathy, when clinically detectable, is bilateral, primarily sensory and associated with loss of the deep tendon reflexes in the lower extremities. The pathogenesis is unknown and vitamin B-12 and folate serum levels can be normal in these subjects. Swift et al. have suggested that the neuropathy is not a direct effect on phenytoin, having found the prevalence of neuropathy in epileptic patients on phenytoin no greater than those not receiving the drug [36].

Two other irreversible changes occur in seizure patients exposed to chronic phenytoin, cerebellar degeneration and mental deterioration. Unlike neuropathy which does not occur as an accompanying feature of epilepsy and therefore may well relate to its treatment, these two alterations in fact can occur with chronic and poorly controlled seizures and anoxia. Establishing a drug-effect relationship for these two syndromes has therefore been difficult.

Animal studies performed by Dam failed to demonstrate direct phenytoin-induced cerebellar changes. However, human cases of controlled epilepsy or epileptics on chronic phenytoin who do not have major convulsions and resultant gross anoxia have demonstrated marked Purkinje cell loss [9,14,32]. In Ghatak's patient, the blood phenytoin levels whenever examined were in the therapeutic range. Furthermore, cerebellar pathology occurred in the absence of hippocampal involvement, suggesting that hypoxia could not be the primary factor. Whether the cerebellar alterations related to seizure activity itself without hypoxia has not been settled.

Multiple factors have been proposed to explain the chronic mental alterations with which many epileptics suffer: the underlying neurologic lesion responsible for the seizures; the frequent seizures; hypoxia related to the seizures (and sometimes their management); social ostracism; and drugs. Vallarta reported irreversible mental dysfunction in 9 patients on phenytoin and one on mephenytoin [38]. The changes were varied and included stubborn and destructive behaviors, confusion, withdrawal, antisocial changes and psychosis. After cessation of the anti-epileptic agents, the patients did not all revert to their pre-medication personalities, but showed new mental deficits. None had further progression after drug cessation. Other reports have not established a clear relationship between drugs and long term mental changes.

Practical Management

Drug absorption by the oral routes is slow (6-12 hr) due to limited solubility of phenytoin in the gastrointestinal tract. In low doses, elimination is linear but at higher doses zero-order kinetics predominate so that high plasma concentrations and symptoms will last longer than the expected adult half-life of 24 hours. Children and black males seem to metabolize phenytoin more rapidly than white males.

To decrease absorption in the acutely intoxicated subject, emesis or lavage and activated charcoal (30-50 gr for a child, 50-100 gr for an adult) and a saline cathartic can be used. Efforts to improve renal clearance by diuresis or changed pH have not been successful. Dialysis has been reported to lower the plasma levels although the high protein binding suggests that it should not be highly effective. Fluid and electrolyte balance, as well as cardiac arrhythmias must also be controlled. Phenytoin withdrawal seizures also may occur, so that in ambulatory patients with side effects, the drug should be tapered and stopped over a few weeks.

Neurological Drugs

PHENOBARBITAL (See Hypnosedatives (Chapter 13))

PRIMIDONE

Primidone is a drug with primary anticonvulsant properties which is metabolized to two additional anticonvulsants, phenobarbital and phenylethyl malanic acid (PEMA). Sedative effects and mild ataxia occur in approximately 20% of patients and may be disconcerting enough to the patient and the physician to necessitate switch over to another drug. Most of the unpleasant neurological effects, however, are seen soon after initiation of treatment and gradually self-resolve. As with phenobarbital, these problems include sedation, nystagmus, nausea and trunkal ataxia. If the patient has already received phenobarbital or phenytoin, the sedative effects of primidone are less, suggesting cross tolerance that may be related to pharmacokinetic changes as well as cortical adaptation. The relative amounts of primidone and its metabolites can be changed by phenytoin or carbamazepine, so that these latter drugs can precipitate toxic phenobarbital effects by shifting the metabolism and decreasing the primidone:phenobarbital ratio. With renal insufficiency, primidone and PEMA levels are high with low phenobarbital levels; with hepatic disease, primidone levels rise, since the drug is not effectively converted to its metabolites.

Abrupt cessation of primidone leads to no immediate consequences, but like phenobarbitol, tremor, irritability and withdrawal seizures occur 5-9 days later. Since the parent drug is rapidly cleared, these effects do not appear to relate to primidone itself [33,3].

Treatment focuses on the same principles as described for phenobarbital. Dialysis can be useful here in eliminating the short-acting primidone before its biotransformation to long-acting phenobarbital and PEMA.

CARBAMAZEPINE

Carbamazepine has numerous side effects associated with its use, some of them similar to those associated with phenytoin and phenobarbital, some particular to carbamazepine. Reported to occur in one-third of exposed patients, these effects are usually mild and in only 5% is drug cessation required. The potential prominent bone marrow suppression has no direct neurotoxic syndrome associated with it.

Mild neurologic side effects, like those seen with other anticonvulsants, include sedation, nystagmus and ataxia. Since this drug is so often used as adjunctive therapy to phenytoin, phenobarbital or primidone, establishing carbamazepine as the causative agent of these signs is not straightforward. Carbamazepine has been advocated to have less depressant effects than other anticonvulsants and is, therefore especially useful in patients with altered mood and behavioral changes related to other drugs. However, carbamazepine can itself be depressing or alternatively be associated with intense irritability [25]. Its effects on sodium and fluid balance can induce secondary headache and mental confusion.

Carbamazepine induces diplopia, which can be a highly useful clinical sign of early toxicity. Distinct from nystagmus, this diplopia generally develops as the blood level moves slightly out of the therapeutic range of 5-9 $\mu g/cc$. When blood levels are not readily or frequently available, the clinician and patient can use this monitor with relative reliability.

Carbamazepine has been associated with involuntary movement disorders of several varieties. Joyce and Gunderson reported oral facial dyskinesias with nystagmus and ataxia after massive overdose of carbamazepine and Crosley and Swender reported transient reversible dystonia [22,8]. These latter investigators suggested an interaction between carbamazepine and the central dopaminergic system. Since carbamazepine does not change dopamine or homovanillic acid levels in rat striatum, Jacome has suggested that the drug may alter cholinergic/dopaminergic balance by affecting primarily the cholinergic system [19]. Clearly these reactions appear more frequently in patients with preexisting brain damage and may occur with carbamazepine levels within the therapeutic range [24]. Curiously, carbamazepine is effective in the management of some forms of childhood dystonia and kinesiogenic choreoathetosis, a seizure disorder with involuntary extrapyramidal movements.

Other signs seen with acute overdose of carbamazepine include respiratory depression, increased seizure activity, myoclonus with asterixis, and hyper or hyporeflexia. Because of its similar structure to tricyclic antidepressants, some of these effects may be anticholinergic in origin. In two cases of acute carbamazepine intoxication, however, physostigmine did not reverse the neurotoxic signs [35]. The half-life of carbamazepine initially is 18-54 hours, but decreases after chronic use to 16-26 hours, perhaps because of enzyme induction. Total external ophthalmoplegia has also been reported.

Treatment of neurotoxic effects involves cessation of the drug and careful supportive care and observation in the acutely intoxicated subject. Because of cardiac arrhythmias, critical care monitoring is often needed for 24-48 hours. Since there is a relatively high amount of circulating free drug (25%), hemoperfusion has been successful in the management of acute severe intoxication [13]. Delayed gastric emptying that is typical for carbamazepine can probably help to prevent more frequent intoxication. Forced emesis, lavage and activated charcoal are additional adjuncts to therapy.

VALPROIC ACID

A relatively new anticonvulsant, valproic acid has gained wide acceptance in the management of absence seizures and other forms of epilepsy. It is often used in association with other anticonvulsants, especially phenobarbital, making conclusions regarding its pure toxicity more difficult. Sedation can be prominent when used with phenobarbital, since phenobarbital plasma levels rise when valproate is added [5]. Clinicians must use caution when adding valproate in a patient on barbiturates. A decrease in the phenobarbital dose and frequent drug level checks will assist in the transition period. When used alone, there may be mild sedation, ataxia, slurred speech and nightmares. In an acutely intoxicated infant where sedation was extreme with unconsciousness and pinpoint pupils, naloxone (0.01 mg/kg) intravenously reversed the neurotoxic signs within 3 minutes. Steiman suggested that naloxone reversed the acute encephalopathy by acting as a gabaminergic antagonist [6].

The most lethal effect of valproate is the hepatotoxic reaction that can occur after chronic use. Elevation in SGOT, SGPT, and alkaline phosphatase may be transient and inconsequential, but may also be the first signs of fulminant liver failure. When present, tremor and asterixis, increased seizures and hyperammonemic encephalopathy may occur [1]. Although most cases of tremor and asterixis have associated liver failure, well documented instances without hepatic disease are described, suggesting that the effects can be seen as part of a primary neurotoxic syndrome related directly to valproate. These signs may occur when the plasma levels are in the therapeutic range, and the postural tremor, although it resembles essential or familial tremor, does not universally respond to propranolol therapy [25].

Recent additional concern has developed over whether valproate induces neural tube defects and spina bifida in infants. Because only abnormal births are usually reported, it has been difficult to estimate the precise incidence of this defect in the valproate exposed fetus relative to the general population.

DRUG-DRUG INTERACTIONS

Although anticonvulsants are not unique or particular in their drug-drug interactions, they are better studied than many other drug classes. Usually, such interactions involve either an altered availability of drug due to absorption, distribution, metabolic or excretory changes, or to direct synergism or antagonism of two drugs on nervous tissue or other body systems. In the former instance, changes in clinical response are associated with change in plasma drug levels, while in the latter, clinical response may vary with stable plasma drug concentrations. In Table 11.1, several of the former interactions are listed. The changes are related primarily to enzyme induction, and competition for transport mechanisms. Phenobarbital is especially associated with hepatic enzyme induction and changes in many nonneurologic drug concentrations. In Table 11.2, some of these drugs are listed along with the net behavioral effect of the added phenobarbital.

TABLE 11.1 Drug–Drug Interactions [30]

Drug A	Interacting drug B	Resultant plasma concentrations of drug A
Carbamazepine	Phenobarbital	Decreased
	Phenytoin	Decreased
	Propoxyphene	Increased
Clonazepam	Primidone	Increased
Phenytoin	Ethanol	Decreased
	Phenobarbital	Decreased
	Chloramphenicol	Increased
	Benzodiazepines	Increased
	Disulfiram	Increased
	Isoniazid	Increased
	Methylphenidate	Increased
	Naproxen	Increased
	Phenothiazines	Increased
	Phenylbutazone	Increased
	Salicylate	Decreased
	Sulfonamides	Increased
	Valproate	Decreased
	Tolbutamide	Decreased
Primidone	Phenytoin	Decreased
	Isoniazid	Increased
	Carbamazepine	Decreased
Phenobarbital	Phenytoin	Increased
	Valproate	Increased
Valproate	Phenytoin	Decreased
	Salicylate	Increased
	Primidone	Decreased
	Carbamazepine	Decreased

■ ANTIPARKINSON DRUGS

Parkinson's disease patients ingest two classes of drugs, those that augment striatal dopaminergic function and those that antagonize central muscarinic cholinergic activity. The two classes cause different profiles of neurotoxicity. Dopaminergic drugs cause chorea, nausea, vomiting, and dystonia. Anticholinergic drugs cause prominent blurred vision, bladder dysfunction and constipation. Both classes, however, can provoke significant mental changes in parkinsonian

TABLE 11.2. Effect of Phenobarbitol on Other Drugs [33]

Drug	Induced biochemical change	Probable net result
Chloramphenicol	Stimulates metabolism	Decreased antibiotic effect
Chlorpromazine	Stimulates metabolism	Decreased antipsychotic effect
Furosemide	Impairs absorption reduces renal sensitivity	Decreased diuretic effect
Griseofulvin	Stimulates metabolism Impairs absorption	Decreased antifungal effect
Coumadin/Warfarin	Stimulates metabolism	Increased coaguability enhances bleeding if phenobarbital withdrawn

patients. Although the classic behavioral alterations induced by dopaminergic drugs are different from anticholinergic induced defects, there is overlap, making the detection of the provoking agent and subsequent patient management significantly challenging. Also, as indicated in Table 11.3, some symptoms of drug toxicity including falling, sleep abnormalities, and cramps, can be seen in the untreated parkinsonian patient as a manifestation of the disease itself.

ANTICHOLINERGIC DRUGS

Anticholinergic drugs are used predominantly in the control of tremor in Parkinson's disease. The most common side effects of anticholinergic drugs are dryness of the mouth, blurred vision, constipation and bladder dysfunction. The dry mouth is due to a reduced flow of saliva. Blurred vision is predominantly due to poor convergence and patients complain predominantly that they can not see well as they read. Distant vision is much less affected because of the cycloplegic actions of anticholinergics. They may precipitate glaucoma, although if the glaucoma is already under treatment anticholinergics can usually be used. The constipation that plagues Parkinson's disease patients is aggravated by anticholinergic drugs since peristalsis is inhibited. Similarly, the anticholinergic effects of these drugs on bladder contractility can cause patients to have trouble initiating voluntary urination. Acute urinary retention can occur in men with prostate hypertrophy.

Anticholinergic drugs can induce cognitive changes. Amnesia is dose-related and any drug which acutely blocks central muscarinic cholinergic receptors

TABLE 11.3.

Problem	Disease	Medications
Stiffness	X	
Shaking (tremor)	X	
Falling	X	X
Reversed sleep pattern	X	X
Cramps	X	X
Nightmares		X
Twitching or jerking movements		X

causes a defect of short term memory, believed to result from blockade or hippocampal cholinergic neurons. The acute effects of these agents on cognition may be different from their chronic effects. In an ongoing study of patients with dystonic disorders who received many times the daily anticholinergic dose of the typical Parkinson's disease patient, the author and his colleagues have found that chronic treatment with gradually increasing doses of the drug has not caused a statistically significant decrease in memory function as compared to baseline (unpublished). If this observation is also true for Parkinson's disease patients, the relative paucity of serious memory loss in these patients can be explained.

Many clinicians feel that significant drug induced disorders of memory and dementia-like syndromes occur primarily in those patients with an associated underlying cognitive disability. For this reason, anticholinergic treatment should not be initiated if signs or symptoms of memory loss are present. Patients with memory deficits should be given no anticholinergic agent, or only very small doses of these drugs. Family members should be cautioned that changes in memory may occur after treatment is initiated. If a patient who is taking anticholinergic drugs develops memory deficits, removal of the drugs may provide complete relief of this problem. When withdrawing an anticholinergic drug for any reason, however, it is best to taper dosage over several days, since abrupt withdrawal causes a rebound worsening of parkinsonian symptoms.

In high doses, anticholinergic drugs also can induce a toxic delirium with agitation, fearful hallucinations and confusion. Hallucinations are further discussed later in the chapter.

In addition to these mental changes, ataxia, dysarthria, nausea, and drowsiness occur with anticholinergic drugs and relate to central nervous system toxicity. In severe overdose, stupors, delirium and coma occur. Although anticholinergic drugs act to help abate the resting tremor of Parkinson's disease, they may in fact induce a tremor when intoxication occurs. This latter movement disorder is most marked when the patient holds his hands out in front of him or performs an action, and therefore contrasts with the resting tremor of parkinsonism. Asterixis and fasciculation of muscles may also occur [2].

DOPAMINERGIC DRUGS

Since the primary neurochemical alteration in Parkinson's disease is decreased presynaptic synthesis of dopamine in the nigro-striatal pathway, dopaminergic drugs are the mainstay of therapy. Three classes of agents are available, amino acid precursor therapy (levodopa or carbidopa/levodopa combination), indirect agonists like amantadine and possibly bupropion and direct acting agonists, including bromocriptine and experimental drugs like pergolide. The neurotoxic side effects of these drugs are probably quite similar and can be discussed as a group. Because the treatment may differ with each side effect, practical management recommendations are included individually, and discussion of drug holidays follows at the end of the section.

Clinical Features and Practical Management

Dyskinesias

Dyskinesias induced by dopaminergic drugs are commonly associated features of antiparkinsonian therapy. These dyskinesias are usually choreiform movements of the limbs, hands, trunk, and lingual-facial-buccal musculature. Irregular muscle contractions of the abdominal and thoracic regions may occur, causing gasping and interrupted speech. These movements contrast with drug induced dystonias, discussed separately. The incidence of levodopa-induced dyskinesias relates most prominently to the duration of high dose levodopa therapy. Dyskinesia occurs in 40 to 80% of patients being treated chronically with levodopa. Direct acting agonists are also associated with the induction of and the exacerbation of dyskinesias. Anticholinergic drugs may exacerbate ambient chorea, but do not appear to cause chorea by themselves [17].

The mechanism underlying dopaminergic drug induced dyskinesia is unknown. Some investigators have suggested that the nigral striatal denervation, the anatomic substrate of Parkinson's disease, may be likely to contribute to the sensitivity of the brain to dopaminergic drugs and the later induction of dyskinesia. This denervation hypersensitivity theory would imply that parkinsonian patients are at a higher risk for dyskinesias than a nonparkinsonian population treated with the same drugs. Since levodopa and direct acting agonists in high doses are only used in Parkinson's disease, this theory is difficult to test in humans. In animal experiments, however, normal animals given chronic levodopa do in fact develop hypersensitivity to the drug with lower thresholds for stereotypic behavior. If the denervation were the primary pathophysiologic factor, one would expect prominent dyskinesias shortly after a patient with severe parkinsonism was treated with levodopa and fewer dyskinesias in a patient with only mild parkinsonism treated for the same duration of time. In fact, the duration of levodopa therapy seems to be the most prominent risk factor for the development of dyskinesia.

In many cases of chorea, the movements are of cosmetic importance without a significant medical morbidity. In this case, patients and the families prefer the enhanced drug effect to control their parkinsonism and are not concerned significantly about the often unsightly involuntary movements. However, when the movements interrupt normal breathing and speaking patterns or when the jerking movements are severe enough to interfere with balance and proper ambulation, these movements become medically significant. The respiratory dyskinesias can be so severe as to cause persistent respiratory alkalosis that is poorly compensated metabolically. In such cases, therapy must be directed towards the correction of this side effect of dopaminergic therapy [39].

To control dyskinesias is to reduce the drugs. All dopaminergic drugs are associated with dyskinesias although most data have been accumulated for levodopa. The daily dose of levodopa or direct or indirect acting agonists can be reduced by 10 to 25% over a 24 hour period to see if involuntary movements cease without a significant exacerbation of the parkinsonism. More substantial drug reductions will usually cause the patient to become too parkinsonian to function. These mild reductions in one or more drug can often given the patient relief from chorea and not compromise functional independence. When small reductions of dopaminergic drugs do not bring about a significant abatement of the chorea, more substantial reductions are necessary, in the form of a drug holiday. Guidelines are outlined at the end of this section.

Another potential therapy for the control of drug-induced dyskinesias would be to alter the cholinergic balance in the striatum. If chorea relates pathophysiologically to enhanced dopaminergic activity of striatal cells, it is reasonable to suggest that augmentation of cholinergic activity would functionally antagonize this dopaminergic supersensitivity. Centrally active cholinergic drugs like physostigmine when given parenterally do in fact abate levodopa-induced dyskinesias transiently. However, the parenteral use of this drug is not practical for chronic control of dyskinesias and hence other oral agents like phosphatidyl choline (Lecithin) and choline chloride have been tested. These agents have not universally helped the control of dopaminergic drug-induced dyskinesias [21]. A final therapeutic approach would be to treat these patients with a dopaminergic blocking agent. However, patients with dopaminergic blockade will likely become more parkinsonian so that this is of no practical use. Patients with significant dyskinesias should not in general be treated with neuroleptic agents. The development of more selective dopaminergic receptor site blocking agents may offer future benefits to chorea patients.

On/Off Phenomenon

The on/off phenomenon is a term used by clinicians to describe the irregular motoric fluctuation of patients with Parkinson's disease who are treated with dopaminergic drugs. Although some degree of fluctuation in motor performance in parkinsonian patients was described even prior to levodopa, including "kinesia paradoxica," wild and irregular motor fluctuations have become much more frequent since levodopa has been in common use. Different clinicians define on/off differently; some restrict it to wild motor fluctuations that occur unpredictably and others include end of dose waning of effect that progressively plagues almost all parkinsonian patients receiving levodopa for more than 5 years. It is the author's belief that true on/off is much more a clinical feature in patients who have been treated for 3-5 years and that this wild fluctuation gradually abates, and that the patient is left with "wearing off" episodes that occur at end of dose as his disease progresses and treatment is more prolonged.

Numerous hypotheses have been advanced to explain the on/off phenomenon. Duvoisin suggested that on/off is related to progressive loss of nigral neurons with secondary axonal collateral sprouting. More recently, Nutt et al. have demonstrated that irregular fluctuations in motor function can be reduced by bypassing absorption mechanisms in the intestinal tract with constant intravenous infusion of levodopa [29]. This procedure produced a stable clinical state lasting for 12 hours in all 6 patients studied. They found that high protein meals reversed the therapeutic effect of infused levodopa and suggested that dietary factors and absorption competition between large neutral amino acids and levodopa at the blood-brain barrier may play significant roles in explaining the fluctuating clinical response of patients with Parkinson's disease.

The practical management of the patient with significant on/off, currently focuses on an attempt to decrease the "pulses" of drug administration. Frequent small doses of medication that have short half-lives, like levodopa, and the introduction of long-acting direct agonists (bromocriptine and pergolide) have been associated with modest improvements in on/off. Patients may report a smoother drug effect if they ingest their levodopa 30 minutes before eating and avoid heavy or large meals.

Other Drug-Induced Movement Disorders: Dystonia and Myoclonus

Early morning dystonia, seen when levodopa levels are very low in the blood stream, can be significantly painful and disabling to patients with Parkinson's disease on chronic levodopa therapy. In fact, patients with this problem complain more of the dystonia usually than their parkinsonism. In most instances, the abnormal contorted foot spasm is first detected 2-6 years after starting on levodopa therapy and abates if the patient receives a drug holiday and receives no levodopa over several days. The dystonia usually develops when the patient first gets out of bed and starts to walk. It does not relate directly to the first dose of levodopa, or other dopaminergic drugs since it usually develops in the patient on chronic therapy whether he takes his levodopa or not. It slowly subsides over 1-2 hours whether or not the patient ingests dopaminergic drug. The dystonic foot posture is unilateral and develops more frequently on the side of the major parkinsonian signs.

In some instances, baclofen has been used (5-40 mg/daily) with some success in the abatement of the dystonic foot postures, although patients may complain that baclofen exacerbates their parkinsonism. Other forms of dystonia that do not occur early in the morning may also plague patients with Parkinson's disease. These may take the form of a torticollic posture, trunkal dystonia or oral facial dystonic disorders. When these postures occur, anticholinergic drugs often will abate them and at the same time help in the control of the parkinsonian tremor. Levodopa-induced myoclonus has also been described. These patients suffer from involuntary lightninglike jerks usually when resting at night prior to sleep. These movements can be disturbing both to the patient and to his spouse who may be precipitously awakened. Methysergide (2 mg at bedtime), a serotonergic antagonist, can reduce or stop the myoclonic jerking and a reduction in levodopa also abates the problem [23].

Nausea and Vomiting

One of the most frequent problems with chronic dopaminergic therapy is nausea and vomiting. This side effect is not solely gastrointestinal but relates also to stimulation by dopaminergic drugs at dopaminergic receptor sites in the area postrema. This region of the medulla is not protected by the blood-brain barrier so that systemic dopamine or peripherally active dopaminergic drugs will cause nausea and vomiting. Prior to the addition of carbidopa to levodopa (Sinemet®), significant nausea was reported in up to 80% of patients on levodopa. Since carbidopa (peripheral dopa-decarboxylase inhibitor) has been added to levodopa, peripheral levodopa is not transferred into dopamine and medullary stimulation and resultant nausea can now be avoided. Levodopa itself does not have an effect on the vomiting center of the medulla. It has been estimated that 100 mg daily of carbidopa inactivates all peripheral dopa-decarboxylase although some patients may remain highly susceptible to dopamine and require more carbidopa. In the event that a patient on carbidopa/levodopa combination does not receive enough carbidopa to control nausea, carbidopa may be obtained from the manufacturer (Merck, Sharp and Dohme) to be given separately along with Sinemet®. Also, domperidone has recently been studied for the control of continued nausea and vomiting in patients on Sinemet®. This drug acts to block dopamine receptor sites but cannot cross the blood-brain barrier.

Cognitive and Sleep Changes

Parkinson's disease patients often suffer with significant mental alterations that may relate directly to the Parkinson's disease (especially dementia and depression), or to their medications. In Table 11.4, mental changes associated with antiparkinsonian drugs are listed. Since dementia can be seen as part of the underlying disease as well as a sign of intoxication, the management of patients with this mental change can be especially complicated.

Chronic treatment with levodopa has been postulated to cause dementia, but this is probably not accurate. Early assessments of the effects of levodopa on cognitive function in Parkinson's disease reported enhanced cognitive function as well as improved motor function in treated patients. Cognitive improvement has been described to include improvement in tests of immediate memory, IQ, and verbal learning.

Six sleep abnormalities in Parkinson's disease patients receiving chronic medication have been studied by Nausieda and his colleagues: difficulty maintaining sleep, excessive daytime sleepiness, vivid dreams or nightmares, nocturnal vocalizations, nocturnal myoclonus and somnambulism [28]. Of these, the most prominent complaint is that of disrupted sleep. In these patients, falling asleep is not difficult, but the patient awakens frequently and is unable to fall back to sleep. Total sleep time in 24 hours is usually adequate, since there is also daytime hypersomnia. These symptoms generally precede other sleep abnormalities. Of 100 patients studied, 74 complained of sleep disruption, alone or associated with other sleep abnormalities.

Subsequently, vivid dreams, nightmares, and nocturnal vocalizations tend to occur together. Patients report dreams that are especially vivid. They often have a prominently frightening component, or they may be perceived as ridiculously funny. Somnambulism is very rare.

Although these all appear to relate to chronic treatment with levodopa, or possibly other dopaminergic drugs, the actual pharmacologic abnormality is not certain. In many patients, reduction of daily levodopa dosage or avoidance of levodopa after 8 or 9 p.m. until morning may cause symptom resolution. In other patients, treatment with amitriptylene, a tricyclic antidepressant with prominent serotonergic properties in a single bedtime dose of 25 to 100 mg, will increase nocturnal sleep, decrease dreams, and decrease daytime sleepiness. Rarely, patients will be helped by hypnosedatives, but often these drugs cause a paradoxical agitated confusion, so that they should be used cautiously in this

TABLE 11.4. Mental Alterations Possibly Related to Antiparkinson Drug Therapy

1. Cognitive deterioration
   a. Dementia
   b. Inattention
   c. Confusion and Agitation

2. Sleep disruption
   a. Insomnia
   b. Excessive Daytime Napping
   c. Vivid Dreams/Nightmares
   d. Nocturnal Vocalizations
   e. Myoclonus
   f. Somnambulism

3. Hallucinations
   a. Toxic Delirium
   b. Hallucinations with Clear Sensorium
   c. Psychosis

population. A final approach to therapy for severe sleep disorder is temporary withdrawal of levodopa or "drug holiday" (see below).

Hallucinatory Syndromes

It is well known that both aminergic and anticholinergic drugs can induce hallucinations in nonparkinsonian patients. Since Parkinson's disease patients are exposed chronically to both classes of drug as part of their therapy, hallucinations are a frequent and often disabling therapeutic complication. Hallucinations usually require decreases in medicine doses and consequently suboptimal control of Parkinson's disease. Three separate types of hallucinatory syndromes occur: the toxic delirium of anticholinergic overdosage, hallucinations occurring in the presence of a clear sensorium, and psychosis.

The toxic delirium produced by anticholinergic drugs is a symptom of overdosage, and does not necessarily relate to duration of therapy. In general, elderly persons and persons with preexisting cognitive deficits are more likely to suffer symptoms of anticholinergic toxicity at "therapeutic" doses. The hallucinations accompanying this syndrome are typically vague and disturbing. Visual hallucinations predominate, and these are often poorly formed, described as dark spots or crawling insects. Patients also show prominent memory loss, with confusion and characteristic autonomic signs of anticholinergic toxicity (tachycardia, intestinal ileus, urinary retention, mydriasis and anhidrosis with fever and flushed, dry skin).

In most cases, however, slow withdrawal and discontinuation of anticholinergics and supportive care will restore the patient. Some investigators have reported good responses to the cautious administration of intravenous physostigmine, a centrally active cholinesterase inhibitor, in anticholinergic overdosage. This therapy should be reserved for only the most severely affected patients, since it has its own potential morbidity, and should be given only in an intensive care unit.

A specific hallucinatory syndrome occurring in the presence of a clear sensorium has been recognized in parkinsonian patients receiving chronic dopaminergic therapy. These hallucinations occur after months of therapy and, if they occur acutely the patient usually has an antecedent history of psychosis. The majority of patients with hallucinations also suffer from sleep disorder (90% in Nausieda's study above). Tanner and her colleagues found hallucinations in 33% of 775 patients with idiopathic Parkinson's disease [37]. In this and previous studies, hallucinations were most commonly purely visual (86%), less commonly visual and auditory (7%) or visual and olfactory (4%), and least commonly purely auditory (3%). Typically, the content of the hallucination is familiar to the patient, such as a relative or close friend who is no longer living, or a former pet. Once patients are aware of the possibility of drug-induced hallucinations, they are able to easily identify their visions as unreal phenomena. For this reason, all patients receiving chronic therapy with dopaminergic agents should be aware of the possibliity of developing hallucinations [15].

If the patient is receiving amantadine, the onset of a hallucinatory syndrome should prompt a check of renal function. Amantadine is not metabolized, and its clearance is purely renal, so that patients with even mild degrees of renal impairment may develop high blood levels of amantadine and subsequent hallucinations. If the hallucinating patient is receiving an anticholinergic agent, tapering this drug over a period of several days may allow resolution of symptoms. Similarly, modest reduction in the total daily dose of levodopa or a direct acting dopamine agonist will control hallucinations in many patients. Bromocriptine is a dopamine receptor agonist which also stimulates serotonin receptors. Bromocriptine is associated with an increased incidence of hallucinations, possibly as the result of its serotonergic activity, and this drug should be reduced if patients taking it develop hallucinations.

If hallucinations do not resolve with modest dosage reduction, or if parkinsonian disability cannot be tolerated on daily doses which are not associated with hallucinations, a drug holiday should be considered.

In a few patients, hallucinations are accompanied by paranoia or by a confusional state. Early studies by Moskovitz and her colleagues demonstrated an orderly progression from vivid dreams to benign hallucinations to psychosis in some parkinsonian patients receiving chronic therapy [27]. Psychosis is not, however, an inevitable sequela of drug-induced hallucinations, and other patients suffer from paranoia or confusion at the onset of their hallucinations, without apparent progression. Treatment of these drug-induced symptoms is mandatory, usually with appropriate drug holiday. If symptoms are severe and unremitting, a neuroleptic agent may be needed. Such a drug, however, may produce parkinsonism in normal patients and is likely to exacerbate Parkinson disease. For this reason, phenothiazine compounds (including prochlorperazine, chlorpromazine, and fluphenazine) and butyrophenones such as haloperidol should be avoided when possible in psychotic parkinsonian patients, in order to avoid aggravation of Parkinson's disease. A highly anticholinergic neuroleptic, thioridazine, may be useful in these extreme cases where a neuroleptic is needed.

Drug Holidays [16]

In patients receiving chronic antiparkinson drugs who develop side effects, the logical management is a reduction in drug dose. Anticholinergics cannot be stopped precipitously. Levodopa is usually reduced by 1/2 or 1 tablet of Sinemet® to control the side effects. Unfortunately, this reduction may be associated with increased motoric disability, forcing the patient and doctor to choose between compromised motor control without side effects or motoric independence with toxicity. In this situation, where neither choice is acceptable, a drug holiday is recommended. This drug free period is emotionally and physically trying for the patient and his family, but after 5 drug free days, a slow reintroduction of medication often allows the patient to gain more drug efficacy on less drug and be free from side effects for several months. A drug holiday is outlined below:

1. Hospitalization required.
2. Patients and families must be emotionally prepared to find the patient significantly parkinsonian during the holiday.
3. Dopaminergic drugs are stopped without tapering. For chorea and cognitive changes, anticholinergic drugs are tapered and stopped. For other chronic side effects, anticholinergic drugs are maintained at about 50% the preholiday dose.
4. Active physical and respiratory therapy must be maintained with emphasis on the prevention of aspiration pneumonia, pressure neuropathies, and thrombophlebitis. Low dose heparin may also be administered.
5. Patients remain off drugs for 4-7 days. Medicine is then started at a low dose and increased each 2-4 days, aiming to discharge the patient at about half the preholiday dose. The entire drug holiday requires 2-3 weeks.
6. In patients with mild side effects, a weekend outpatient holiday can be useful where patients stop dopaminergic drugs 2 consecutive days each

week. Anticholinergic drugs are maintained. This chronic outpatient management does not require hospitalization.

DRUGS FOR MYASTHENIA GRAVIS

Two drug classes have been used in the management of patients with myasthenia gravis, peripherally acting cholinesterase inhibitors and steroids. The former drugs act to increase the activity of acetylcholine at the neuromuscular junction receptor site. The latter compounds have antiinflammatory properties and may alter the synthesis of the abnormal antibodies that are intimately related to the pathogenesis of the disorder. Both classes of drugs are associated with significant neurotoxicity.

CHOLINESTERASE INHIBITORS

The hallmark of cholinergic overactivity, like underactivity, is progressive weakness, so that the complaint of weakness does not help in the differentiation between over or under medication with cholinesterase inhibitors. In the case of the elderly myasthenic who usually suffers predominantly with bulbar weakness (difficulty speaking and swallowing), drug excess will resemble myasthenia through several mechanisms: excess activity of acetylcholine at the neuromuscular junction leads to depolarization blockade; excess drug also increases salivation; and bronchial constriction provokes the symptoms of shortness of breath and difficulty swallowing. Features that do help differentiate over- from undermedication include autonomic changes like nausea, vomiting, colicy abdominal cramps and diarrhea, seen with drug intoxication. Muscular twitching over the entire body also is an additional characteristic feature of cholinergic excess. Agents that act only at the periphery do not cause central nervous system toxicity although occasionally physostigmine is used in the management of myasthenics. If over-medicated with physostigmine, the patient will have, in addition to the above symptoms, confusion, ataxia, respiratory depression and possibly seizures. The vasomotor and cardiovascular effects of physostigmine are more than those seen with peripherally acting agents suggesting that these signs are related to combined central and peripheral toxicity [18].

Whenever a patient with myasthenia gravis who is receiving cholinesterase inhibitors comes to the emergency room short of breath, the physician must decide whether he is over or under medicated. A therapeutic edrophonium (Tensilon®) test may be helpful but the medication must be given in tiny (1 mg) increments in order to avoid a precipitation of cholinergic crisis. Vital capacity taken after each increment may demonstrate progressive improvement when the patient is undermedicated or progressive respiratory decline if overmedicated.

Practically, however, the therapeutic Tensilon test is often inconclusive and the patient must be hospitalized and cholinesterase inhibitors stopped for a drug free observation period of 12-48 hours. If it is clear that the patient is overmedicated, cessation of cholinesterase inhibitors should be continued and atropine (1-2 mg) may be given to hasten the patient's recovery. In most instances, however, cessation of cholinesterase inhibition and observation with respiratory support is sufficient.

STEROIDS

Steroids are potent antiinflammatory agents used in the treatment of myasthenia gravis and multiple sclerosis as well as temporal and cranial arteritis. Three neurotoxic syndromes are associated with steroid compounds: increased intracranial pressure (pseudomotor cerebri), toxic encephalopathy and myopathy.

Infants are more likely than adults to develop steroid related, increased intracranial pressure, hydrocephalus and papilledema. This syndrome may occur while patients are receiving steroids, or after withdrawal. The pathophysiology of this syndrome is unknown although it has been suggested that it relates to water intoxication [33]. When it occurs, patients have been treated for weeks or months with steroid compounds.

In contrast, steroid-induced toxic encephalopathy may occur within days of steroid introduction. The behavior is varied and markedly fluctuant, ranging over 24 hours from momentary euphoria to depression to fully developed psychosis. Depersonalization and motoric retardation may make these patients difficult to manage during the intoxicated phase. Paranoia with visual and auditory hallucination and markedly delusional thinking may predominate [14].

Although this syndrome typically occurs early in the course of steroid therapy, cases exist where mental decline developed after more than 3 months of treatment. Doses of medication do not clearly correlate with symptoms although as a general rule the encephalopathy is more frequent in high dose treatment groups. Patients with a prior history of psychiatric care or depression may be at higher risk for encephalopathy than other patients. Suicides have occurred, making this encephalopathy a significant source of potential morbidity. Treatment focuses on withdrawal of the steroid and supportive medical and psychiatric support. Sometimes steroids can be reintroduced later without reappearance of the problem.

When medications are needed neuroleptics will control psychosis and tricyclic antidepressants can abate the depression. Lithium has also been effective and has been used prophylactically prior to reintroduction of steroids in patients who previously became encephalopathic on steroid drugs.

A therapeutic dilemma develops when a patient with systemic lupus erythematosis or other vasculitis becomes psychotic while receiving steroids. Is the psychosis part of the vasculopathy or a toxic effect of the drug? If the steroids have only recently been started, the effect may likely be drug-induced. When associated focal neurologic abnormalities are present (hemiparesis, hemianopia), however, the psychosis probably relates to the primary disease or to other metabolic or infectious causes. If significant doubt exists, stopping the drug is probably more hazardous than treating the psychosis empirically with neuroleptics.

Steroid myopathy, characterized by proximal weakness and atrophy, appears unrelated to the actual duration of drug treatment [7]. In experimental animals, fluorinated steroids cause the most profound lesions. Biopsies from humans show mild fiber atrophy with dark sarcolemmal nuclei but significantly little inflammation or frank necrosis. This finding helps in differentiating steroid myopathy from the intensely inflammatory necrotic lesions seen in various collagen vascular disorders for which the drug is often prescribed. Type II fibers appear to be selectively affected with steroid myopathy.

Because the steroid compounds alter coagulation factors, secondary hypercoaguable states can occur, resulting in embolic disease. Rapid withdrawal of steroids induces the behavioral manifestations clinically seen in Addison's disease. These are secondary phenomena and are not directly related to drug neurotoxicity.

■ ANTISPASTICITY AGENTS

Besides the benzodiazepine drugs discussed in Chapter 12, two other major muscle relaxants are currently used. Balcofen is an analogue of the putative neurotransmitter GABA, although unlike GABA, it easily crosses the blood-brain barrier. It is used effectively to control dystonic cramps and spasticity, especially in multiple sclerosis, the condition for which it is specifically approved. It is unlikely that the clinical effect is due directly to GABA agonism or antagonism; glutamate or substance P may be the more likely transmitter systems altered by baclofen at the spinal cord level. Three types of neurotoxic syndromes are seen with baclofen: a global encephalopathy, a withdrawal encephalopathy, and weakness, as an accentuation of the normal drug therapeutic effect on muscle tone.

The toxic encephalopathy usually begins with increased somnolence and confusion, and can progress to coma. This may occur acutely after a high overdose or as a subacute problem after many weeks of medication. Pupillary changes are inconsistent and both myosis and mydriasis have been reported. Seizure activity and myoclonus as well as combative hallucinatory agitation can also occur visually during the late stages of unconsciousness [19].

Hypoventilation can be life threatening and may relate to baclofen-induced muscle relaxation or to effects on central ventilatory drive. In the acutely intoxicated patient, bradycardia and hypothermia complicate the neurologic picture. Gastric lavage and diuresis will promote the excretion of the active drug. Atropine (600 µg i.v.) has reversed bradycardia, hypotension and hypothermia in one report [12]. Multiple seizures can be treated with traditional anticonvulsants. Single, short seizures do not require specific medication, but may be managed by careful attention to airway and vital function maintenance. Baclofen should not be stopped precipitously, but tapered over several days or a few weeks [19].

Withdrawal hallucinations, manic behavior and seizures can also occur when baclofen is precipitously stopped. For this reason, slow tapering of the drug over a few weeks is recommended. The pharmacologic basis for the two encephalopathic syndromes are unclear and may not be directly related to one another.

The toxic effects of baclofen on muscle tone include hypotonia and weakness. These may occur as overdose phenomena, but increased weakness is a frequent complaint of patients on baclofen at therapeutic doses. Many spastic patients require their increased tone to maintain their ambulatory function, since the spasticity supports their weight. In such cases, a decrease in tone is associated with poorer function. On the other hand, spastic patients with excrutiatingly painful flexor spasms will often find the increased weakness an acceptable side effect. Along with hypotonia, decreased reflexes often occur. In patients with spasticity who receive baclofen and complain of increasing weakness, the baclofen dose should be tapered by 25-50%. They may be able to tolerate this lower dose with more comfort and less hypotonic disability.

Dantrolene is a unique muscle relaxant, different from baclofen and the benzodiazepines. It affects skeletal muscle directly by decreasing the amount of calcium release from sarcoplasmic reticulum. It is used to treat muscle spasms, spasticity, and the muscle rigidity of malignant hyperthermia, and neuroleptic malignant syndrome. Its major systemic toxicity is hepatic. Of neurologic significance, weakness is a prominent complaint in patients receiving dantrolene, probably related to the same direct muscle activity that abates the painful spasms and hypertonicity. If weakness occurs in patients receiving dantrolene, the drug should be decreased in dose to approximately 50%. Often the complaint will resolve and the patient will maintain the original beneficial effects. Mental alterations may include euphoria, lightheadedness, dizziness and fatigue. These are usually seen early when the drug therapy is initiated and often will self-resolve even on maintained doses.

Neurological Drugs

▪ STUDY QUESTIONS

Which of the following Parkinson disease patients will likely benefit from a drug holiday?

A. A patient with chorea and nausea 2 hours after each levodopa dose.
B. A patient with resting tremor and bradykinesia prior to his afternoon levodopa.
C. A patient with hallucinations and increasing bradykinesia.
D. A patient with resting and intention-postural tremors.

Answer: C

Discussion: The indication for a drug holiday in Parkinson's disease is the simultaneous presence of signs indicating over and under medication. In this case, temporary cessation of drug and later reinstitution of low dose therapy often will enhance the antiparkinsonian effects without precipitating hyperdopaminergic side effects. Hence, the patient with increasing bradykinesia, indicative of under medication, and hallucinations, indicative of over medication, is a reasonable candidate for drug holiday. Patient A has only signs of over medication and could be managed with a lower dose of drug; patient B has only signs of under medication and can be treated with more drug. Patient D has multiple tremors and may be helped by treating the resting tremor with anticholinergic drug and the postural-intention tremor with a beta-noradrenergic blocking agent.

A patient with myasthenia gravis who is over medicated with cholinesterase inhibitors can be short of breath and thereby resemble myasthenia gravis itself. Why?

A. Cholinesterase inhibitors induce medullary stimulation and hyperventilation.
B. Cholinesterase inhibitors cause bronchoconstriction.
C. Cholinesterase inhibitors act like botulinum toxin.
D. Cholinesterase inhibitors cause increased salivation.

Answers: B and D

Discussion: Shortness of breath is a common complaint of the over medicated elderly myasthenic. Anticholinesterase agents provoke bronchoconstriction, increased flow of oral secretions, and also provoke direct depolarization blockade of respiratory muscles. The agents used to treat myasthenia gravis do not cross the blood–brain barrier and hence, would not induce medullary alterations. These agents increase cholinergic function in direct contrast to botulinum toxin that inhibits the release of acetylcholine.

A patient with a known right occipital lobe focal seizure disorder has been treated with an unknown antiepileptic agent. Which of the following clinical signs suggest acute overmedication.

A. Nystagmus

B. Ataxia
C. Parkinsonism
D. Extreme Sedation
E. Increased seizures
F. Aphasia

Answers: B, D and E

Discussion: Nystagmus is seen even when patients are in the therapeutic range of their anticonvulsants and is not necessarily indicative of toxicity. Parkinsonism is not a side effect of anticonvulsants, although another extrapyramidal sign, chorea, is associated with phenytoin or carbamazepine ingestion. Aphasia, indicative of focal left frontal or temporal-parietal is not directly related to anticonvulsant use. On the other hand, ataxia with falling, extreme sedation, and an increase in seizure activity can all indicate over medication. The increase frequency of seizures with high doses of anticonvulsants can be particularly confusing since they are in fact prescribed specifically to abate seizures.

Match the anticonvulsant with the prominent side effect.

A. Chorea
B. Sedation
C. Hyperactivity
D. Tic douloureux

1. Carbamazepine
2. Phenytoin
3. Phenobarbital
4. Valproic Acid

Answers: A-1 and 2; B-all; C-3; D-None

Discussion: Chorea is a curious movement disorder associated with carbamazepine and phenytoin use and usually seen in patients who have a prior history of chorea (Sydenham's chorea or lupus chorea). Sedation is a complicating side effect of all anticonvulsants and no medication is totally free of this problem. Hyperactivity is seen with barbiturate drugs, especially in children. The exact mechanism whereby a sedating drug can cause paroxysmal hyperactivity is not known but many pediatric neurologists will prescribe mebarol rather than phenobarbital for seizure control in a child who can not tolerate the phenobarbital and yet requires barbiturate anticonvulsant therapy. Tic douloureux is a form of intense facial pain of sudden and lancinating character that is often treated with carbamazepine but is not associated as a side effect with any of the anticonvulsants.

■ REFERENCES

1. Batshaw ML, Brusilow SW: Valproate-induced hyperammonemia. Ann. Neurol. 11:319–321, 1982.
2. Bianchine JR: Drugs for Parkinson's disease. In: AG Gilman, LS Goodman, and A Gilman, eds., Pharmacological Basis of Therapeutics, pp. 475–494. Macmillan, New York, 1980.
3. Bleyer WA, Marshall RE: Barbiturate withdrawal syndrome in a passively addicted infant. J.A.M.A. 221:185–186, 1972.
4. Boston Collaborative Drug Surveillance Program: Diphenylhydantoin side effects and serum albumin levels. Clin. Pharmacol. Ther. 14:529–532, 1973.

5. Bruni J, Wilder B, Perchalski RJ, Hammond EJ, and Villarreal HJ: Valproic acid and plasma levels of phenobarbital. Neurology 30:94–97, 1980.
6. Burckart CJ, Ternullo SR: Anticonvulsants. In: VA Skoutakis, ed., Clinical Toxicology of Drugs. Lea & Febiger, Philadelphia, 1982.
7. Coomes EN: Corticosteroid myopathy. Ann. Rheum. Dis. 24:465–467, 1965.
8. Crosley CJ, Swender PT: Dystonia associated with carbamazepine administration: experience in brain-damaged children. Pediatrics 63:612–615, 1979.
9. Dam M: The density and ultrastructure of Purkinje cells following diphenylhydantoin treatment in animals and man. Acta Neurol. Scand. (Suppl) 49: 3–65, 1972.
10. Dobkin B: Reversible subacute neuropathy induced by phenytoin. Arch. Neurol. 34:189–190, 1977.
11. Duvoisin RC: Variations in the "on-off" phenomenon. In: F McDowell and A Barbeau, Advances in Neurology, Vol. 5, Second Canadian-American Conference on Parkinson's Disease, pp. 337–340. Raven Press, New York, 1974.
12. Ferner RE: Atropine treatment of baclofen overdose. Postgrad. Med. J. 56: 865–866, 1980.
13. Gary NE, et al: Carbamazepine overdose: treatment with hemoperfusion. Nephron 27:202–203, 1981.
14. Ghatak NR, Santoso RA, McKinney WM: Cerebellar degeneration following long-term phenytoin therapy. Neurology 26:818–820, 1976.
14. Glatzel J, Penin H: Klinisch-elektroencephalographische verlaufsuntersuchung einer. Psychose narch hoch dosierter ACTH. Arch. Psy. Nerven 209: 365, 1967.
15. Goetz CG, Tanner CM, Klawans HL: Pharmacology of hallucinations induced by long-term drug therapy. Am. J. Psychiatry 139:494–498, 1982.
16. Goetz CG, Tanner CM, Klawans HL: Drug holiday in management of Parkinson's disease. Clin. Neuropharmacol. 5:351–364, 1982.
17. Goetz CG, Weiner WJ, Klawans HL: Treatment of the choreas. In: A Barbeau, ed., Disorders of Movement, pp. 29–42. Lippincott, Philadelphia, 1981.
18. Grob D, Johns RJ: Treatment of anticholinesterase intoxication with oximes. Neurology 8:897–899, 1958.
19. Haubenstock A, Hruby K, Jager V, Lenz K: Baclofen intoxication: report of four cases and review of the literature. Clin. Toxicol. 20:59–58, 1983.
20. Jacome D: Movement disorder induced by carbamazepine. Neurology 31: 1959–1060, 1981.
21. Jankovic J: Management of motor side effects of chronic levodopa therapy. Clin. Neuropharmacol. (Suppl. 1) 5:19–28, 1982.
22. Joyce RP, Gunderson CH: Carbamazepine-induced orofacial dyskinesia. Neurology 30:1333–1334, 1980.
23. Klawans HL, Goetz CG, Bergen D: Levodopa-induced myoclonus. Arch. Neur. 32:331–334, 1975.

24. Logan WJ, Freeman JM: Pseudo-degenerative disease due to diphenylhydantoin intoxication. Arch. Neurol. 21:631-637, 1969.
25. Masland RL: Carbamazepine neurotoxicity. In: DM Woodbury, JK Penry, and CE Pippenger, eds., Antiepileptic Drugs, pp. 521-531. Raven Press, New York, 1982.
26. Mattson RH, Cramer JA: Tremor due to sodium valproate. Neurology 31:114-115, 1981.
27. Moskovitz C, Moses H, Klawans HL: Levodopa-induced psychosis. Am. J. Psychiatry 135:668-676, 1978.
28. Nausieda PA, Weiner WJ, Kaplan LR, Weber S, Klawans HL: Sleep disruption in the course of chronic levodopa therapy: early features of levodopa psychosis. Clin. Neuropharmacol. 5:183-194, 1982.
29. Nutt NG, Woodward WR, Hammerstad JP, Carter JH, Anderson JL: The "on-off" phenomenon in Parkinson's disease: relation to levodopa absorption and transport. N. Engl. J. Med. 310:483-487, 1984.
30. Pippenger CE: An overview of antiepileptic drug interactions. Epilepsia (Suppl. 1) 23:S81-S86, 1982.
31. Reynolds EH, Chanarin I, Matthews DM: Neuropsychiatric aspects of anticonvulsant megaloblastic anemia. Lancet 1:394-397, 1968.
32. Salcman M, Defendini R, Correll J, Gilman S: Neuropathological changes in cerebellar biopsies of epileptic patients. Ann. Neurol. 3:10-19, 1978.
33. Schmidt D, Seldon L: Adverse Effects of Antiepileptic Drugs. Raven Press, New York, 1982.
34. Sternberg A, Bierman T: Corticosteroids, pseudomotor cerebri. Arch. Derm. 92:746-747, 1965.
35. Sullivan JB, Rumack BH, and Peterson RG: Acute carbamazepine toxicity resulting from overdose. Neurology 31:621-624, 1981.
36. Swift TR, Gross JA, Ward C, Crout BO: Peripheral neuropathy in epileptic patients. Neurology 31:826-831, 1981.
37. Tanner CM, Vogel C, Goetz CG, Klawans HL: Hallucinations in Parkinson's disease: a population study. Ann. Neurol. 14:136, 1984.
38. Vallarta JM, Bell DB, Reichert A: Progressive encephalopathy due to chronic hydantoin intoxication. Am. J. Dis. Child 128:27-34, 1974.
39. Weiner WJ, Goetz CG, Nausieda PA, Klawans HL: Respiratory dyskinesias: extrapyramidal dysfunction presenting as shortness of breath. Ann. Intern. Med. 88:327-331, 1978.
40. Woodbury DM, Penry JK, Pippenger CE: Epileptic Drugs. Raven Press, New York, pp. 329-340, 1982.

CHAPTER 12

Psychiatric Drugs

THE symptoms of mental agitation, anxiety, and depression haunt industrial societies, and the medications used to treat them have become ubiquitous. The major tranquilizers, or neuroleptic agents, are usually prescribed for psychotic behavior where tranquilization and antipsychotic activity are needed simultaneously. Minor tranquilizers are used to treat the more common and widespread symptoms of anxiety. Hypnosedative agents technically should be prescribed for insomnia, although they are widely used as antianxiety agents as well. They are discussed in another chapter. Antidepressant medications fall into three major categories: tricyclic and newer generation antidepressant drugs, MAO inhibitors, and lithium carbonate. Modern society has been characterized as overmedicated, overtranquilized, and hence escapist because of these drugs. Others maintain that such agents are relatively inexpensive and effective means of contending with inevitable and normal stress with its accompanying discomfort and misery. The toxicity of these psychoactive drugs is important to discuss because of the frequency with which these agents are ingested and the variety and severity of drug effects and drug-drug interactions.

- **NEUROLEPTIC AGENTS**

    PHENOTHIAZINES AND HALOPERIDOL

    The neuroleptic agents or major tranquilizers include the phenothiazine drugs and the butyrophenone, haloperidol. Their antipsychotic activity probably relates to blockade of dopaminergic receptors, possibly at the level of the limbic system [34]. As a class, they are associated with a variety of important neurologic complications. These include sedative and autonomic ef-

IATROGENIC AND MEDICINAL TOXINS

TABLE 12.1 Neuroleptic Drugs

Phenothiazine Group	Daily Dosage Range (mg)	Dosage Equivalent to 300 mg Chlorpromazine
Aminoalkyl		
Chlorpromazine	100-1,000	300
Triflupromazine	20-150	100
Piperidyl		
Thioridazine	30-800	300
Mesoridazine	50-400	150
Piperazinyl		
Trifluoperazine	2-30	25
Perphenazine	2-64	28
Butaperazine	30-50	30
Prochlorperazine	15-125	60
Thiopropazate	6-30	30
Fluphenazine	0.5-20	6
Thioxanthenes		
Chlorprothixene	50-1,000	300
Thiothixene	10-60	30
Haloperidol	2-40	15
Clozapine	100-1,000	300

fects, acute dystonic reactions, akathesia, parkinsonism, and the late complication of tardive dyskinesia. The different classes of neuroleptics are listed in Table 12.1. Although the side effects discussed below occur with all drugs in the phenothiazine class, the incidence of certain ones is not equivalent in all chemical subclasses; Table 12.2 illustrates such differences in relative prevalence for autonomic dysfunction and acute and subacute extrapyramidal side effects.

TABLE 12.2 Side Effects with Different Phenothiazine Subclasses

Subclass	Hypotension	Acute and Subacute Extrapyramidal Complications (Dystonia and Parkinsonism)
Aminoalkyl	+++	++
Piperidyl	++	+
Piperazinyl	+	+++

Psychiatric Drugs

Clinical Features and Practical Management

Encephalopathy

Although sedation can be profound with initiation of therapy, there is only minimal respiratory depression in adults, and these drugs are relatively safe. Toxic confusional states may occur, especially in the elderly, an effect probably related to the anticholinergic effects of these drugs [31]. Autonomic changes include alterations in body temperature and mild anticholinergic signs. These drugs are felt to lower the seizure threshold and have been associated with exacerbation of preexisting epilepsy as well as the appearance of seizures de novo. The less potent, more sedative agents (i.e. the aminoalkyl group, chlorpromazine) are more likely to be associated with this phenomenon than the piperazine drugs or haloperidol [14].

Neuroleptics affect the central nervous system at multiple levels, although the effect on the reticular activating system is probably primary to their depressive neurotoxin activity in young children. Numerous cases of unexplained sudden death in infants have been attributed (without careful documentation) to the ingestion of neuroleptic drugs [34]. Since neuroleptics cross the blood-brain barrier, depressive activity and apneic spells may occur after birth in infants born to mothers regularly receiving neuroleptic medications.

The management of an acute encephalopathy caused by neuroleptics involves the general maintenance of life systems. If cardiac arrhythmias are present, phenytoin will reverse the quinidinelike A.V. conduction depression typical of neuroleptic drugs. The adult dose is 10 mg/kg intravenous over three minutes repeated every five minutes until arrhythmias cease or until a total dose of 1 gram is administered. Physostigmine may reverse anticholinergic toxicity.

Neuroleptic Malignant Syndrome

The neuroleptic malignant syndrome includes extrapyramidal signs and subsequent severe hyperthermia. Additional neurologic signs may include dysarthria and dysphagia, oculogyric crisis, opisthotonus and seizures. Autonomic dysfunction, in addition to the hyperthermia often includes pallor, diaphoresis, blood pressure instability, tachycardia, and tachypnea. Laboratory findings are usually normal, although there may be a transient elevation of serum aldolase or creatine kinase.

The neuroleptic malignant syndrome is attributed to neuroleptic agents, particularly long-acting preparations, and the symptoms usually begin soon after starting therapy, or after a recent increase in dosage. The syndrome differs from the well-known malignant hyperthermia, where the crisis is always precipitated by general anesthesia and changes in myoplasmic calcium. With malignant hyperthermia, often there is a family history of an autosomal dominant transmission. Neuroleptic malignant syndrome must also be differentiated from heat stroke, which can occur in patients on antipsychotic medications. Because of the prominent anticholinergic effects of many neuroleptic drugs, the normal sweating response to heat is diminished. Hence, if psychotic patients dress in excessively warm clothing, severe hyperpyrexia, stupor, and coma may occur. With heat stroke, however, the extrapyramidal signs so typical of neuroleptic malignant syndrome do not occur.

The pathophysiology of neuroleptic malignant syndrome is not clear. The rigidity and tremor in neuroleptic malignant syndrome can be profound and may well generate excessive heat. The patient's pallor suggests that peripheral vasoconstriction is occurring, so that a central defect in the control of heat loss may be active. It has been suggested that the neuroleptics alter hypothalamic dopamine receptors to precipitate the syndrome [18]. A similar syndrome has been reported in a patient with Parkinson's disease and a chronic psychiatric disorder treated with haloperidol for a chronic period of time. The syndrome developed when the patient's antiparkinsonian drugs were suddenly discontinued. In this case, however, it is possible that the sudden appearance of extrapyramidal signs and fever related to the sudden withdrawal from anticholinergic drugs.

As with other causes of hyperthermia, the treatment of neuroleptic malignant syndrome involves first, the patient's removal from the heat source. The neuroleptic should be stopped and the patient should be placed in a cooled environment. Ice packs about the body and ice water stomach lavage may be instituted. When the rectal temperature drops to 38 degrees centigrade, these dramatic efforts at cooling can be stopped, since patients have been reported to experience seizures when temperatures drop too rapidly. If the temperature rises, the measures are reinstated. Antipyretic agents are not recommended, since they usually are not active at the high temperatures seen in the hyperthermic patient. Aspirin should be withheld because of its effects on the coagulation system. When a patient recovers and is again severely psychotic, the question is whether to give another neuroleptic drug or switch over to a different class of psychoactive medication. Information is not available on cross-reactivity for patients with neuroleptic-induced malignant syndrome, but if a patient requires antipsychotic medication and has a history of such a reaction, hospitalization is recommended for the induction of the new drug.

Although the psychophysiology of neuroleptic malignant syndrome is felt to relate to central nervous system alterations, probably hypothalamic, dantrolene, an agent that acts at the muscle, will also decrease rigidity and lower body temperature. Doses range from one to ten mg/kg intravenous in four divided doses; the acid medium requires that the fluid volume of drug be large.

Levodopa, usually given in the form of carbidopa/levodopa combination and bromocriptine (usually 1.25 mg qid) can also be successful in rapidly returning excessive temperatures to the normal range and reducing the patient's prominent rigidity.

Dystonias

Acute neuroleptic-induced dystonias are seen early in the course of neuroleptic therapy and are often seen following a single parenteral dose of phenothiazine or haloperidol. The manifestations can be quite diverse, although the most common clinical signs involve the eyes and neck. Patients with oculogyric crises often complain of inability to move their eyes in the vertical plane as well as double vision, blurred vision, and, rarely, pain on attempted gaze. Most often, the eyes maintain a sustained upward gaze. The severe dystonic displacement of the eyes may itself be painful, as may other severe, acute contorting dystonias. The abnormal postures of the head and neck, including opisthotonos, in which the head and neck are in retrocollic position, give the patient a bizarre appearance. Other muscles may be involved in the acute drug-induced dystonias, but these are much less common [25].

The incidence of dystonia with different neuroleptics seems to parallel the differential incidence of drug-induced parkinsonism, the piperazine agents being the most hazardous [2]. Agents causing a high incidence of parkinsonism have a high incidence of drug-induced dystonia, while those associated with a low incidence of parkinsonism have a low incidence of dystonia. The simultaneous administration of anticholinergic agents is felt to decrease the incidence of neuroleptic-induced dystonia, and the acute administration of anticholinergic agents almost invariably reverses these dystonias. Physiologically, acute neuroleptic-induced dystonia is felt to represent a sudden disruption of basal ganglia function in some way related to dopamine. This alteration is most probably acute dopaminergic receptor blockade, since all offending agents are capable of blocking striatal dopamine receptors. The ability of anticholinergic agents to prevent and ameliorate these dystonias suggests that dopamine-acetylcholine balance is involved in these events. Acute therapy involves intravenous or intramuscular injection of an anticholinergic agent. This treatment will ameliorate the dystonia within minutes, but since the anticholinergic effect is short-lived, oral anticholinergic agents should be prescribed for the next 24-48 hours. If the patient's psychosis requires continued neuroleptic therapy, he should be placed on maintenance anticholinergic treatment for several weeks or switched to another neuroleptic (e.g. thioridazine) with a lower propensity to cause acute dystonia.

The ability of neuroleptics to elicit dystonia disappears to a great extent as the duration of therapy is extended. New dystonias are rare after the first few weeks, and dystonias that occur in the acute phase are usually no longer present after months of therapy. As a result, the anticholinergic agents used to treat and/or prevent dystonia can be decreased and withdrawn in most patients after 1-2 months of use. Drug-induced dystonias are most common in younger patients given prochlorperazine for vomiting and in young adults (especially between the ages of 20 and 40) being started on chronic neuroleptic therapy.

Although dystonias are generally considered an early side effect of neurologic therapy, tardive or late dystonia can occur as well. These movements occur after months or years of chronic neuroleptics and, although predominantly dystonic, usually also have fine choreic features intermixed.

The immediate treatment of drug-induced dystonia is the administration of an anticholinergic drug like trihexyphenidyl given intramuscularly or intravenously, 1-2 mg. Importantly, a long-acting oral dose must also be administered or the patient may return to the emergency room within a matter of hours with a return of his dystonia. Oral anticholinergics may be administered for 48 hours after the acute treatment (trihexyphenidyl 2 mg, 2-4 times daily). During the dystonic episode, reassurance and supportive comfort should be maintained. Respiratory function must be observed, although the episode is more frightening to observe and experience than it is medically dangerous. For tardive dystonia, withdrawal of neuroleptics is usually effective, although chronic treatment with anticholinergic drugs and sometimes reserpine (see section on tardive dyskinesia, below) may be needed.

Akathisia

Akathisia is a severe restlessness, subjectively associated with the feeling of intense anxiety. This neuroleptic side effect usually occurs within the first days of therapy, and, similarly to the dystonias, anticholinergic treatment rapidly reverses the syndrome. The pathophysiology of the syndrome is not understood, but may relate to acute imbalances between dopaminergic and cholinergic systems [30]. Akathisia resolves with withdrawal of the neuroleptic agent. If an anticholinergic drug is used to treat the akathisia, (trihexyphenidyl, 2-4 mg/day), it must be administered for several weeks with gradual withdrawal. Since akathisia is usually self-limited, lasting only weeks to a few months, these intermittent attempts to wean the patient from the anticholinergic drug will allow the patient to eventually discontinue anticholinergic therapy. Although akathisia is usually seen when the neuroleptic is first introduced, it may also occur whenever the dose of the drug is increased suddenly. A less common, late-onset akathisia has been described and is not responsive to conventional anticholinergic treatment. The pathophysiology of this latter condition has been suggested to be related to tardive dyskinesia.

Because akathisia is so discomforting to the patient, it is a frequent cause of noncompliance. The clinician must be careful to properly diagnose akathisia, since its motor manifestations can resemble those seen with psychotic agitation. In the latter condition, the physician would increase the antipsychotic drug, whereas akathisia would be only exacerbated by such therapy. If in doubt, the clinician may treat with a single dose of injectable anticholinergic drug (trihexiphenidyl, 1 mg intramuscular). This treatment should transiently reduce akathisia but would have no effect on agitation due to underlying psychosis.

Parkinsonism

Parkinsonism is a frequent side effect of neuroleptic agents. These agents block striatal dopamine receptors and thus that drug-induced parkinsonism is descriptively indistinguishable from Parkinson's disease. Usually this effect begins within the second to fourth week of neuroleptic therapy; rididity, resting tremor, bradykinesia, and postural reflex abnormalities may all be seen. Because of the slow clearance of phenothiazines, the syndrome may persist for up to months after discontinuation of therapy [30]. Generally older patients are more susceptible to the parkinsonian effect of neuroleptics than younger ones are.

The patient's early complaints in drug-induced parkinsonism relate usually to bradykinesia and tremor. The patient has difficulty rising from a chair or turning over in bed. His movements are slow, with particular difficulty walking through narrow doorways or pivoting to turn. Speech may become slow and hesitant. The tremor is seen when the patient is at rest and diminishes when he writes or eats. Occasionally a patient will complain of shaking inside his body even when the observer cannot see resting tremor externally. Because of postural reflex abnormalities, patients have poor balance and will fall either moving propulsively or retropulsively.

An anticholinergic drug (trihexyphenidyl, 2-8 mg/day) administered to control drug-induced parkinsonism is usually associated with a good effect. Some physicians administer amantadine, which has both anticholinergic and dopaminergic properties, although there is concern that amantadine could exacerbate the psychotic condition for which the neuroleptics are originally prescribed. Since drug-induced parkinsonism is self-limited to weeks or months, if an anticholinergic drug is used, it should be tapered every two months to reevaluate the patient's need for it. Anticholinergic drugs are associated with visual, bladder, and psychiatric side effects, and therefore such agents should only be used as long as they are needed.

Although drug-induced parkinsonism is indistinguishable from idiopathic Parkinson's disease, the former is reversible if the neuroleptic medication is stopped. It has been suggested that patients with subclinical idiopathic Parkinson's disease may be more likely to become clinically parkinsonian at low doses of neuroleptic medication than other patients, but there is no evidence that the neuroleptics actually cause or hasten the onset of idiopathic Parkinson's disease.

IATROGENIC AND MEDICINAL TOXINS

Tardive Dyskinesia

Tardive dyskinesias are abnormal, involuntary, usually choreic movements associated with chronic neuroleptic therapy. The movements often begin in the face and tongue (lingual-facial-buccal masticatory syndrome) and progress to involve the trunk and extremities. In some cases the diaphragm may be involved, and breathing and speech become irregular with grunting, gasping sounds [10,36]. The pathophysiology of tardive dyskinesia is suspected to relate to chronic dopamine receptor site blockade by the neuroleptics, with resultant striatal denervation hypersensitivity. The abnormal movements are often first noticed when the neuroleptic dose is decreased, presumably because the hypersensitive receptors are now no longer blocked, and therefore exposed to new concentrations of dopamine [25].

No consistent neuropathologic changes are seen in these patients, although the possibility remains that ultrastructural receptor site alterations occur [22]. Initially, following neuroleptic withdrawal, tardive dyskinesias may worsen because of better access of dopamine to striatal receptors. This exacerbation, however, is usually only a short-term effect. Tardive dyskinesias, in fact, are often reversible and may spontaneously remit following neuroleptic withdrawal. Large studies with long-term follow-up after the withdrawal of antipsychotic drugs have shown that patients can improve for up to two years after drug cessation, and that mildly affected patients are more likely to remit completely. While the syndrome may be reversible in some patients, residual or even progressive chorea can be seen in over half the patients with tardive dyskinesias [19].

First, the neuroleptic should be stopped if the psychiatric condition for which the drug was originally prescribed will permit. Patients who are receiving neuroleptic drugs for the treatment of depression or anxiety without a psychotic disorder should be switched to other medicines. In general, only those patients who are psychotic require these potent medications. If after a drug-free period of three months, the movements persist, medication treatment may be necessary. Reserpine, which depletes stored presynaptic dopamine, norepinephrine, and serotonin, has been moderately successful in doses of 1-5 mg/day. Side effects of reserpine include hypotension and a drug-induced depression. The hypotensive effects are seen early in the treatment, but the drug-induced depression must be monitored throughout the treatment. Both side effects are reversed by cessation of the reserpine therapy [25]. The use of cholinergic agonists, choline chloride, and lecithin remains experimental. Judicious use of neuroleptic agents in the lowest possible doses, with frequent "drug holidays" where patients receive no medication, may help to decrease the incidence of this drug-induced condition [24]. Treatment of tardive dyskinesia with neuroleptics themselves is clearly treatment with the presumed offending agent, and should be avoided. This short-sighted therapy may temporarily abate the pathophysiology of the condition, but serves to aggravate its pathogenesis.

Psychiatric Drugs

RESERPINE

Reserpine was the original neuroleptic drug, although it is not currently used to treat psychiatric illness to a significant degree. It is mostly used as an antihypertensive agent and it does induce a number of neurologic complications. With chronic use, reserpine can induce a parkinsonian syndrome that is indistinguishable from Parkinson's disease. Whether all patients are equally susceptible to the drug-induced parkinsonian syndrome of reserpine or whether reserpine is more likely to induce this syndrome in patients who will eventually develop Parkinson's disease is not known. Part of an adequate history on a patient with probable Parkinson's disease is to establish that he is in fact not receiving reserpine. The treatment of reserpine-induced parkinsonism is withdrawal of the causative agent, and within weeks the patient's clinical status should return to normal.

Depression is a significant and more frequent side effect of chronic reserpine therapy. It usually occurs weeks or months after the onset of treatment and can be so severe as to lead to death by suicide. Since reserpine depletes the brain of dopamine, norepinephrine, and serotonin, the precise neurotransmitter related to the depression is not known. In patients with hypertension, another drug can usually be found if the patient has a history of depression. In depressed patients with tardive dyskinesia, reserpine must be administered with great caution.

Hypotension is an additional secondary neurologic side effect. Also, the drug may worsen the vasospastic portion of migraine attacks (principally associated with the aura) although it tends to reduce the incidence of chronic migraine attacks [11]. Epileptic attacks have also occurred while patients were receiving reserpine, although these cases are anecdotal.

■ ANXIOLYTICS OR ANTIANXIETY AGENTS

BENZODIAZEPINES

Benzodiazepines are currently popular anxiolytic agents, and include diazepam (Valium), chlordiazepoxide (Librium), and Oxazepam (Serax). Flurazepam (Dalmane) belongs to this class of agents as well, but is used primarily as a hypnosedative. Diazepam is additionally used in conjunction with phenytoin to treat status epilepticus. The general mechanism of action of benzodiazepines appears to relate to depression of multisynaptic reflexes throughout the central nervous system [3]. They act as muscle relaxants on the basis of central mechanisms [7]. These drugs are known to effect neurochemical alterations as well, increasing brain GABA levels and decreasing norepinephrine and serotonin [8].

Although the therapeutic index of benzodiazepines is 10 to 30 times that of the barbiturates and hence their absolute toxicity is less, adverse reactions are seven times more frequent with benzodiazepines. This statistic apparently relates to the vast number of patients consuming these anxiolytic agents [15]. In almost all cases, patients have ingested more than one agent, so that the precise responsibility of the benzodiazepine drug is rarely established. When used intravenously, however, these agents have been associated with documented respiratory depression and death.

The most frequent toxic symptoms are increased drowsiness or paradoxical excitation. After large doses, exacerbation of neurotic depression has been reported and antisocial behavior, outbursts of temper, and hypnogogic hallucinations may occur [16]. Withdrawal seizures have been reported as well [20]. A peculiar appetite stimulation has been observed at therapeutic and toxic levels of these agents and may relate to hypothalamic alterations [21].

Dry mouth, tachycardia, dilated pupils, and depressed bowel sounds often occur early all due to anticholinergic effects of these drugs. Patients may then lapse into somnolence and later into coma. Addiction after chronic use of benzodiazepines has been reported [29], and a patient may be effectively treated for acute intoxication only to fall into a withdrawal syndrome. If diazepam is stopped after chronic ingestion of 100 mg over 40 days, withdrawal syndrome usually occurs. With chlordiazepoxide, withdrawal occurs if a patient stops the drug after chronic ingestion for 2-6 months at a dose of 300 to 600 mg/day. Withdrawal symptoms in both cases include excessive apprehension, anorexia, nausea, postural tremulousness, insomnia, confusion, and often hallucinations. In those cases, withdrawal syndromes must be handled in the hospital and barbiturates are usually substituted (see below).

Presently there is no specific therapy regarding the management of patients acutely intoxicated with benzodiazepine agents. Successful treatment includes emergency supportive measures and symptomatic therapy. Respiratory insufficiency is treated with assisted ventilation, and attention to fluid and electrolyte balance is of utmost importance. Hemodialysis and forced diuresis have not been proved effective. Since these drugs are often ingested simultaneously with other agents, the treating physician should obtain a blood drug screen and suspect that the patient has ingested other sedative hypnotic agents or tranquilizers. A patient may undergo withdrawal from the benzodiazepine and/or the additional agent. Usually, this may be managed using only a barbiturate substitution to cover all agents simultaneously. The calculation of the dose is usually based on 30 mg phenobarbital equivalent to diazepam 5 mg or chlordiazepoxide 25 mg. One-quarter of the benzodiazepine dose in the form of phenobarbital may be administered and increased if abstinence symptoms develop. A slow withdrawal over several days can then be effected from this dose [32].

MEPROBAMATE

Meprobamate was introduced as an antianxiety agent in 1955, and, although its specific antianxiety effects are equivocal, it is still a widely prescribed compound. It depresses polysynaptic reflexes in the spinal cord, an effect thought to contribute to its muscle relaxant properties. Additionally, it is a mild analgesic and enhances the analgesia effected by other drugs [12].

The major toxicity of meprobamate relates to sedation and ataxia. Doses of 1600 mg are associated with considerable learning impairment and slowed reaction time. Sedation is enhanced when meprobamate is consumed along with other drugs, including tricyclic antidepressants, monoamine oxidase inhibitors, and possibly ethanol. In these instances, or when mild overdosage occurs (blood concentrations 30-100 μg/cc, toxic signs include broad-based stumbling gait, slurred speech, vertigo, and drowsiness, which may progress to prolonged sleep. Blood levels of 100-200 μg/cc are associated with hypotension, respiratory depression, and coma. The lethal dose of meprobamate is generally in excess of 40 grams, although an anecdote of death after 12 grams has been reported. Hemodialysis has been advocated for rapid detoxification, and elimination can be enhanced with saline-furosemide therapy. In man, meprobamate ingestion has been associated with exacerbation of grand mal and myoclonic epilepsies.

Systemic side effects include hypotension, urticaria, and exacerbation of acute intermittent porphyria (AIP) [17].

■ ANTIDEPRESSANT AGENTS

TRICYCLIC ANTIDEPRESSANTS

Tricyclic antidepressants, prescribed specifically for the treatment of depression, have a relatively narrow therapeutic index and can be associated with acute and chronic toxicity of significant morbidity. The acute encephalopathy that is life-threatening can follow suicidal ingestion of high doses of medication or seemingly therapeutic doses of the tricyclic drug when it is consumed with additional drugs or with alcohol.

Clinical Feature and Practical Management

Acute Encephalopathy

The early clinical picture of acute encephalopathy includes agitation, confusion, mydriasis, and sometimes convulsions. Somnolence follows, often with hypoventilation; tremor and myoclonus may also occur. Most feared are the complex cardiac irregularities, tachycardia, atrial fibrillation, venticular flutter, and conduction blocks, all of which may fluctuate unpredictably and require frequent changes in medication therapy [6].

Pharmacologically, many of the acute toxic signs can be divided into anticholinergic and aminergic. The dry mouth, palpitations, tachycardia, loss of accommodation, and postural hypotension are typical antimuscarinic effects. Postural tremor and increased agitation may relate to noradrenergic overactivity. This latter activation appears to relate directly to the tricyclic antidepressant's inhibition of norepinephrine reuptake from the synaptic cleft. This blockade mechanism is also important in explaining the drug-drug interaction between guanethidine-type drugs and tricyclic antidepressants. Guanethidine antihypertensive medications are concentrated in the noradrenergic nerve; when the pump is blocked by the antidepressants, the uptake for the antihypertensive agent guanethidine is also blocked. Hence, treatment with a tricyclic antidepressant interferes with the therapeutic effects of guanethidine-type antihypertensive agents [33].

Myoclonus, suggested to relate often to alterations in serotonergic systems, is an additional acute neurotoxic syndrome associated with tricyclic antidepressants. Myoclonus is self-limited when the tricyclic antidepressant is stopped. In animal studies using myoclonus induced by 5-hydroxytryptophan, tricyclic drugs with major serotonergic activity (such as imipramine) potentiate the behavior, whereas amitriptyline does not. Data regarding the relative frequency of myoclonus with different tricyclic agents in man are not available.

When acute encephalopathy due to tricyclic antidepressants is encountered, general life-support measures must be maintained for the overdose patient. Continuous gastric lavage has been suggested, since these agents are secreted back into the stomach. Hemodialysis and peritoneal dialysis are not significantly effective because of four properties of these drugs: their rapid and firm protein binding, their rapid entry into the circulation, their stable fixation to tissues, and their poor water solubility. In two lethal cases, less than one percent of the drug could be recovered through dialysis.

Physostigmine, a centrally active cholinesterase inhibitor given 1 to 2 mg intravenously, often awakened the patient from coma. This finding suggests that much of the toxic mental alteration relates directly to central anticholinergic toxicity. Importantly, physostigmine may have to be given multiple times as the anticholinergic effect of the antidepressants may be too long-lasting to be overcome with a single dose. Physostigmine may be effective additionally in controlling cardiac atropine toxicity. However, the cardiac effects of acute intoxication are multidimensional; other drugs, including propranolol, may also be required. Curiously, the cardiac toxicity may be delayed and even 100 hours after hospital admission, sudden cardiac decompensation may occur in a patient seemingly in the process of recovery.

Tremor

Tricyclic antidepressants may also precipitate a more chronic neurotoxic syndrome, with tremor and sedation or insomnia. The tremor is usually postural or intentional and resembles that seen with amphetamine intoxication, hyperthyroidism, or lithium intoxication. The tremor may interrupt the patient's ability to hold his hands quietly outstretched and interfere with handwriting and other fine-motor tasks like eating. Drowsiness is a common symptom, particularly in the early stages of therapy. Amitriptyline is reported to be more sedating than imipramine. Such sedation may be desired in the agitated, depressed patient with insomnia, but can also be quite disabling to a younger, active patient [6]. These effects are similar but less traumatic than the life-threatening encephalopathy discussed above.

Excitation may also occur with antidepressant agents. Sometimes, this syndrome blends into a toxic confusional state, which probably relates to central anticholinergic toxicity. In these patients, there is additional confusion, difficulty concentrating, and irritability. Physostigmine can reverse the syndrome, often within minutes after an intravenous injection of 1 mg. Tricyclic drugs have also been associated with the exacerbation of schizophrenic symptoms in previously psychotic patients. Similar to the precipitation of mania in a patient with bipolar disease, this reactivation of psychosis may relate to the blockade of norepinephrine or serotonin reuptake typical of these drugs.

NEWER GENERATION ANTIDEPRESSANTS

The frequent side effects and slow onset of action seen with the traditional tricyclic antidepressants has led to a search for newer medications. New tricyclic drugs, as well as tetracyclic compounds and other agents, have been recently introduced (see Table 12.3).

Among the newer tricyclic drugs are trimipramine and amoxapine. The former drug has a similar side effect profile to imipramine and amytriptyline, although the frequency of toxicity may be lower [4]. Amoxapine (Ascendin®) has strong noradrenergic activity, as well as dopaminergic antagonist effects. The latter property suggests that drug-induced parkinsonism, dystonias, and akathisia could be significant side effects of this agent. Tardive dyskinesia, a long-term effect of dopaminergic blocking agents, could also become a potential toxic effect of this drug. At present, these extrapyramidal effects are of theoretic importance.

Tetracyclic compounds include maprotiline (Ludiomil®) and other agents currently used in Europe. Maprotiline has potent noradrenergic activity, moderate antihistaminic anticholinergic effects, and little if any serotonergic activ-

TABLE 12.3 Effects of Various Antidepressants on Neurotransmitter Systems

Drug	Serotonin	Norepinephrine	Dopamine
Traditional Tricyclic Agents			
Clomipramine	4+	0	0
Amitriptyline	4+	1+	0
Nortriptyline	2+	2+	0
Imipramine	3+	2+	0
Desipramine	0	4+	0
Newer Tricyclic Agents			
Trimipramine	4+	1+	0
Amoxapine	1+	3+	2−
Tetracyclic Agents			
Maprotiline	0	4+	0
Oxaprotiline	0	4+	0
Mianserin	0	2+	0
Serotonergic Reuptake Blockers			
Trazodone	3+	0	0
Zimelidine	4+	0	0
Fluoxetine	4+	0	0
Fluvoxamine	4+	0	0
Miscellaneous			
Nomifensine	0	3+	2+
Bupropion	0	0	1+
Alprozalam	0	0	0

0 = no significant effect; 4+ = marked increased effect; 4− = marked antagonistic effect

ity. These drugs have very few other anticholinergic properties, and hence are associated with a low incidence of blurred vision, urinary retention, and confusion [9].

Triazolopyridine derivatives, specifically trazodone, are unusual in that they are strongly serotonergic without prominent effects on the dopaminergic, noradrenergic, or cholinergic system. The major side effect associated with trazodone is sedation, which can be used therapeutically in agitated, depressed patients, but could conceivably become a major toxic effect in another situation. Headaches also have been reported. Recent reports of priapism threaten the wide use of this drug in males. The neurovascular origin of this effect is not clear. Zimelidine is a bicyclic compound that also acts as a serotonergic agent by blocking reuptake. Common side effects of this drug include hyperactivity, restlessness, tremor, and occasionally severe unremitting headaches [5].

Nomifensine inhibits both norepinephrine and dopamine reuptake, and may additionally be an anticonvulsant. Pharmacologically, it appears to have no anticholinergic effects, although dry mouth, tremulousness, and restlessness are significant side effects of this drug. The underlying biochemistry of such side effects is not known. Also, both manic episodes and psychotic symptoms have been exacerbated with this drug [23]. Bupropion, with dopaminergic properties, induces tremulousness, nervous excitement, and sometimes nausea and vomiting. It has been used successfully to treat parkinsonism and may be used in the future to treat depressed patients with Parkinson's disease [13].

MONOAMINE OXIDASE INHIBITORS (MAOI)

Monoamine oxidase is an intramitrochondrial enzyme responsible for the breakdown of intracellular dopamine, norepinephrine, and serotonin. The administration of an inhibitor of this enzyme leads to the potentiation of catecholaminergic and indolaminergic activity. Selective MAO inhibitors have been effective antidepressants, although significant toxicity is associated with their use. In most instances, MAO inhibitors have been replaced by newer antidepressant agents.

Acute poisoning with MAO inhibitors can lead to coma, high fever, and sometimes death. This syndrome can be seen with high doses of MAO inhibitor alone, and can also be induced by MAO inhibitors with tricyclic antidepressant drugs or with MAO inhibitors and tyramine products. Less common are interactions between MAO inhibitors and amphetamine or meperidine [4].

The hallmark of acute MAOI intoxication is hyperpyrexia, with fevers as high as 108°F. Coma, tachypnea, tachycardia, dilated pupils, and profuse sweating accompany. The syndrome usually occurs several hours after the ingestion of the drug. A patient who ingests large amounts of MAO inhibitors and appears clinically stable should not be discharged or viewed nonchalantly, since the clinical effects may not begin for several hours. A 24-hour observation period after potential toxic ingestion, therefore, is required [23].

Rapid recovery after hemodialysis has suggested that this is an effective means of therapy. Acidification of the urine will enhance the excretion of such drugs as phenelzine. Drugs like neuroleptic-blocking agents (haloperidol or chlorpromazine) may be useful since they block catecholaminergic receptor sites.

A second cataclysmic syndrome is the hypertensive crisis associated with the combined use of MAO inhibitors with tyramine products or other centrally active agents. Classically, the syndrome develops when a patient ingesting MAO inhibitors also eats well-ripened cheese, such as Camembert, cheddar, or liederkranz. Sudden severe headache, stiff neck, profuse sweating, and hypertension develop within minutes. Rarely, intracranial bleeding may follow. While cheese is the most typical precipitant, other foods such as chicken livers, chocolate, wine, and some forms of herring also can invoke this syndrome. Additionally, drugs like amphetamine, methylphenidate (Ritalin) and ephedrin, available in over-the-counter cold medicines, can participate in such a reaction. The treatment is usually alpha blocker, such as phentolamine, or chlorpromazine, a dopaminergic blocking agent. Finally, MAO inhibitors can react with tricyclic antidepressants and induce hyperpyrexia, sweating, convulsions, and occasionally death. The same encephalopathy can be seen with patients given intravenous or intramuscular doses of meperidine along with MAO inhibitors [25].

Much less cataclysmic, but also more common, are milder side effects related to MAO inhibitor ingestion. Mild dizziness, generalized weakness, dysarthria, and confusion may occur when patients receive therapeutic doses of MAO inhibitors. Occasionally, a patient ingesting these drugs will convert from a retarded hypoactive, depressed patient into an agitated or even hypomanic subject. Severe insomnia may also complicate MAO treatment.

LITHIUM CARBONATE

Lithium is well established as an efficacious agent in the treatment of manic depressive illness and some types of monopolar depression. Neurotoxic side effects are not rare and the most common and annoying effect is a fine postural or intention tremor. This tremor occurs in the vast majority of patients and at times can be quite disabling. In such individuals, the tremor appears to be either an exacerbation of preexisting benign essential tumor or precipitation of tremor de novo. Usually, reduction of the dosage will either eliminate the tremor, or significantly reduce its intensity. The beta-adrenergic blocker, propranolol, has proved beneficial in some cases [26].

EEG changes are also seen in lithium-treated patients, often when the serum level is in the normal range. Asymmetric slow activity and sharp waves have been described as well as a more diffuse bilateral slowing of background rhythms [27].

A toxic confusional state may occur in the absence of signs of toxicity and at relatively low serum lithium levels. This reaction is characterized by disorientation, confusion, lack of continuity of thought, memory loss, lability of mood, and reduced comprehension. The symptoms are usually preceded by a steady or precipitous rise in oral lithium dosage, often within the first few weeks of treatment, but may occur at serum lithium levels as low as 1.0 mEq/liter. The condition usually remits within a few days following reduction or withdrawal of the dosage. It has been suggested that patients with schizophrenia or pre-existing organic brain disorders are particularly susceptible to this complication [28].

Once the therapeutic or maintenance level of lithium has been established, it is necessary that the kidneys be able to excrete as much lithium as is administered. If the kidneys cannot handle lithium intake owing to excessive dosage or undetected renal insufficiency, accumulation and intoxication may result.

Psychiatric Drugs

Prodromal symptoms include nausea, vomiting, diarrhea, coarse tremor, drowsiness, ataxia, muscle twitching, and slurred speech. These symptoms may be present for four or more days before more severe problems occur, and are easily reversed by reduction of dosage or discontinuation of medication. As intoxication advances, there are increased neurological complications leading to impaired consciousness, ataxia, and, eventually, seizures and coma. Although most cases of lithium intoxication occur at serum levels exceeding 2.0 mEq/liter, some patients may become toxic at serum levels considered within safe limits. Neuropathy and alterations of auditory evoked potential responses have also been reported [26].

There is no specific antidote for severe lithium intoxication; effective treatment involves enhanced lithium excretion. Excretion is complicated by the fact that lithium passes relatively slowly through neural cell membranes. Administration of aminophylline and osmotic diuresis using mannitol or urea have been reported to increase lithium excretion, although results have been inconsistent. Hemodialysis has been employed successfully in a few cases. If treatment is inadequate or tardy, death may result, usually from pulmonary complications.

Until recently, it was thought that patients who survived severe lithium intoxication suffered no permanent neurological damage. However, reports during the past few years indicate that patients may suffer irreversible brain damage following acute intoxication. The basal ganglia and cerebellum are affected, and symptoms include ataxia, nystagmus, choreoathetoid movements, and hyperactive deep tendon reflexes [27]. Ultrastructural neuropathologic changes in monkeys with lithium toxicity included changes in the endoplasmic reticulum—both smooth and rough—that were believed to relate to accumulated lithium ion at the sodium pump sites along membranes. Marked changes were seen in the temporal lobes, basal ganglia, and hypothalamus [1].

■ STUDY QUESTIONS

An elderly lady is found in a dilapidated apartment and is rushed to the emergency room where the diagnosis of heat stroke is made. The history reveals that she is a chronic undifferentiated schizophrenic receiving depot fluphenazine each month. Which factors are important to the hyperthermic response?

1. The neuroleptic
2. The psychotic behavior and life-style
3. Both
4. Neither

Answer: 3

IATROGENIC AND MEDICINAL TOXINS

In most cases, both the neuroleptic and the patient's psychotic behavior precipitate the hyperthermia. Psychotic patients may overdress, even in warm weather. Furthermore, their poor adaptation to the society often results in their living in impoverished, unventilated surroundings, putting them at additional risk for heat exposure in the summer. If their psychosis provokes agitation, this may further elevate the basal temperature. The neuroleptics act to increase the body temperature during the summer by two mechanisms: first, they have anticholinergic activity and thus normal sweating responses may be blocked; furthermore, these drugs act at the hypothalamic level to render a patient "cold-blooded," i.e. the patient's body temperature will increase or decrease depending on the ambient environmental temperature. These combined features of environment and drug lead to the remarkable morbidity in the treated psychotic population during the heat of the summer.

Match the drug with the anticipated side effects:

1. Tricyclic antidepressant
2. Reserpine
3. Lithium

A. Myoclonus and agitation
B. Depression
C. Postural tremor
D. Parkinsonism

Answers: 1-A and C; 2-B and D; 3-C

Tricyclics often increase serotonergic activity by blocking reuptake. The serotonergic system is believed to be related to the pathophysiology of several forms of myoclonus, including postanoxic myoclonus and possibly infantile spasm, among others. Severe myoclonus, agitation, and delirium can be dangerous side effects of overdosage of antidepressants. Postural tremor may be seen. Reserpine is associated with drug-induced parkinsonism and depression; both may be dose-limiting. Lithium is associated with a fine postural tremor often when the drug is in the therapeutic range and becomes coarse and irregular as the drug accumulates.

Below are listed five neurologic complications of neuroleptic therapy. Indicate whether they are usually:

A. Acute, occurring minutes or hours or, at most, days after starting the drug.
B. Subacute, occurring days, weeks, or a few months after starting the drug.
C. Chronic, occurring after several months or years of drug treatment.

1. Dystonia
2. Parkinsonism
3. Chorea
4. Tremor
5. Oculogyric crises

Answers: 1-A; 2-B; 3-C; 4-B; 5-A

The acute neurologic side effects related to neuroleptic drugs are dystonia and akathisia. The contorted posture of dystonia is frightening to see or experience. An oculogyric crisis, with the eyes thrown back and the neck usually hyperextended, is only one example of a dystonic complication of neuroleptics. Recently, a late onset dystonia has been described as within the realm of tardive dyskinesia, but this is probably not common. Tardive dys-

Psychiatric Drugs

kinesia should be, by and large, considered a choreic or stereotypic disorder and is the major chronic side effect of neuroleptic drugs. The subacute problem associated with neuroleptic medications is parkinsonism, which may include any of the following: tremor, bradykinesia, rigidity, or postural reflex compromise.

MAO inhibitors are associated with:

1. Hyperthermia
2. Hypertensive crisis after eating strawberries
3. Depression
4. Tremor and agitation with small doses of amphetamine

Answers: 1 and 4

Hyperthermic responses, hypertension, especially in association with tyramine products (well-ripened cheese, pizza, chicken livers—but not strawberries) and a heightened sensitivity to all sympathomimetic products (amphetamine, Ritalin, or ephedrine) are among the neurotoxic signs associated with MAO inhibitors. Depression is treated, not provoked, except in rare instances, by this drug.

■ REFERENCES

1. Akai K, Roizon L, Liu JC: Ultrastructural findings of the CNS in lithium neurotoxicology. In I Roizin, H Shiraki, N Grcevic, eds., Neurotoxicology. Raven Press, New York, 1977.
2. Ayd FJ: Neuroleptics and extrapyramidal reactions in psychiatric patients. Rev. Can. Bio. 20:451, 1961.
3. Ban TA, Amin M: Hypnotics, minor tranquilizers and sedatives. In PJ Vinken and GW Bruyn, eds., Handbook of Clinical Neurology, Vol. 37, pp. 347-364. North-Holland Publishing Co., Amsterdam, 1979.
4. Brogden R, Heel RC, Speight TM, et al: Nomifensine: A review of its pharmacologic properties and therapeutic efficacy in depressive illness. Drugs 18:1-24, 1979.
5. Burgess CD, Montgomery S, Wadsworth J, et al: Cardiovascular effects of amitriptyline, mianserin, zimelidine, and nomifensine in depressed patients. Postgrad. Med. J. 55:704-708, 1979.
6. Chang SS, Davis JM: Toxicity of psychotherapeutic agents. In PJ Vinken and GW Bruyn, eds., Handbook of Clinical Neurology, Vol. 37, pp. 229-328. North-Holland Publishing Co., Amsterdam, 1979.
7. Cohen IM: Benzodiazepines. In FJ Ayd and B Blackwekk, eds., Discoveries in Biological Psychiatry, pp. 130-139. Lippincott, Philadelphia, 1970.
8. Cook L, Seginwald J: Behavioral analysis of effect and mechanism of action of benzodiazepines. In E Costa and P Greengard, eds., Mechanism of Action of Benzodiazepines, pp. 125-137. Raven Press, New York, 1975.
9. Feighner JP: New generation of antidepressants. J. Clin. Psychiatry 44:49-55, 1983.

10. Gerratt BR, Goetz CG, Fisher HR: Speech abnormalities in tardive dyskinesia. Arch. Neurol. 41:273-276, 1974.
11. Gilbert CJ: Reserpine for migraine. Headache 16:125-126, 1976.
12. Gilbert MM, Koepke HH: Relief of musculoskeletal and psychopathological symptoms with meprobamate. Curr. Ther. Res. 15:820-832, 1973.
13. Goetz CG, Tanner CM, Klawans HL: Bupropion-HCl in idiopathic Parkinson's Disease. Neurology 33:123-125, 1983.
14. Goodman LS, Gilman A: Pharmacologic Basis of Therapeutics, Macmillan New York, 1980.
15. Goth A: Medicinal Pharmacology. C.V. Mosby, St. Louis, 1972.
16. Greenblatt DJ, Shrader RI: Benzodiazepines. N. Engl. J. Med: 291, 1011-1013, 1974.
17. Harvey SC: Hypnotics and sedatives. In AG Gilman, LS Goodman, A Gilman, eds. Pharmacologic Basis of Therapeutics, pp. 339-375. Macmillan, New York, 1980.
18. Henderson VW, Wooten GF: Neuroleptic malignant syndrome. Neurology 31:132-137, 1981.
19. Hersohn HL, Kennedy PF, McGuire RJ: Persistence of extrapyramidal disorders and psychiatric relapse after long term phenothiazine therapy. B. J. Psychiatry 120:41-50, 1972.
20. Hollister LE, Motzenbecker FP, Degan RO: Withdrawal reactions from chloridazepoxide. Psychopharmacology 2:63-68, 1961.
21. Jarvik ME: Benzodiazepines. In LS Goodman and A Gilman, eds., Pharmacologic Basis of Therapeutics, pp. 151-203. Macmillan, London, 1970.
22. Jellinger K: Neuropathologic findings after neuroleptic long term therapy. IN L. Roisin, H Shiraki, N Grcevic, eds., Neurotoxicology, pp. 18-22. Raven Press, New York, 1977.
23. Kelwala S, Stanley M, Gershon S: History of antidepressants: Successes and failures. J. Clin. Psychiatry 44:40-48, 1983.
24. Klawans HL, Goetz CG, Perlik S: Tardive dyskinesia: Review and reupdate. Am. J. Psychiatry 137:900-908, 1980.
25. Klawans HL, Weiner WJ, Nausieda PA, Goetz CG: A Textbook of Clinical Neuropharmacology. Raven Press, New York, 1982.
26. Manocha M, Chokrovserty S, Nora R: Neurotoxicity of lithium therapy. Neurology 34:162, 1984.
27. Prien RF: Lithium in the treatment of affective disorders. IN HL Klawans, ed., Clinical Neuropharmacology, Vol. 3, pp. 113-130. Raven Press, New York, 1978.
28. Reilly E, Halmi KA, Noyes R: EEG responses to lithium. Int. Pharmacopsychiatry 8:208-213, 1973.
29. Rumack BH: Anticholinergic poisoning: Treatment with physostigmine. Pediatrics 52:449-451, 1973.
30. Simpson GM: Neurotoxicity of major tranquilizers. In L Roisin, H Shiraki, and N Grcevic, eds., Neurotoxicology, pp. 1-7. Raven Press, New York, 1977.

31. Simpson GM, Amuso D, Blair JH, Farkas T: Phenothiazine-produced extrapyramidal system disturbance. Arch. Gen. Psychiatry 10:199-208, 1964.
32. Skoutakis VA: Tricyclic antidepressants. IN VA Skoutakis, ed., Clinical Toxicology of Drugs, pp. 127-136. Lea Febiger, Philadelphia, 1982.
33. Sulser F: Mode of action of antidepressant drugs. J. Clin. Psychiatry 44: 14-20, 1982.
34. Thompson EA: Amitriptyline overdose. Drug Intell. Clin. Pharm. 7:451-458, 1973.
35. Van Rossum JM: Significance of dopamine receptor blockade for mechanism of action of neuroleptic drugs. Arch. Int. Pharmacodyn. Ther. 160: 492-494, 1966.
36. Weiner WJ, Goetz CG, Nausieda PA, Klawans HL: Respiratory dyskinesia, extrapyramidal dysfunction and dyspnea. Anat. Intern. Med. 88:327-331, 1978.

CHAPTER 13

Narcotics and Hypnosedatives

A widespread increase in the illicit use of hypnosedatives and narcotic drugs began in the 1960s. Public concern over the spread of such drugs beyond the college campus into high schools, grammar schools, and the working world resulted in the establishment of presidential committees, new legislation, and growing research support for the understanding of the biochemistry and physiology of drug addiction. An estimated 9 million Americans have used sedative drugs without medical supervision, and approximately 5½ million of them are aged 18-25. A variety of neurologic syndromes have been described in these victims of illicit drug exposure, as well as in patients given these drugs for medical or psychiatric purposes.

■ NARCOTICS

The strict structural requirements of opiates, their high potency, and their stereospecificity suggest that narcotics may in fact act at specific opiate receptor sites. Such opiate binding sites have been demonstrated in the central nervous system, specifically in those regions felt to be associated with pain transmission and with brain stem visceral reflexes including respiration [12]. Opiates additionally alter the activity of known neurotransmitter systems centrally, although consistent changes and a unifying concept of interaction have not been established [18]. Hypotheses linking together opiates and neurotransmitters have been suggested to explain narcotic tolerance on the basis of denervation hypersensitivity.

Narcotics and Hypnosedatives

HEROIN AND TRADITIONAL MORPHINE DERIVATIVES

Narcotic agents, whether naturally occurring or synthetically prepared, are associated with a variety of neurologic complications. Morphine is the most widely used medical opiate, and heroin, its diacetyl derivative, has become the major opiate of illicit drug abuse. Other opiate derivatives, pantopan, dihydromorphine (Dilaudid), levorphanol (Dromoran), meperidine (Demerol), and methadone share the general toxic properties of the opiate group, but vary in their onset and duration of toxic signs. It must be emphasized that opiate drug abusers may often be exposed to multiple other toxic agents, including septic conditions and drug adulterants as well as alcohol or hallucinogens. For this reason, some neurotoxic syndromes, especially in the case of heroin abuse, should be viewed more as potential hazards of drug abuse and its life-style than hazards of the pharmacologic agent itself. These secondary abuse syndromes include subacute bacterial endocarditis with multiple emboli and abscess formation, osteomyelitis and various infections. Additionally, a transverse myelitis and various forms of neuropathies and myopathies may occur. Although all these complications are most likely not related to direct opiate neurotoxic effects, they occur in the addicted population and are clinically important.

Clinical Features and Practical Management

Morphine overdose is especially common in circulatory collapse after the drug is administered more than once; while the patient is in shock, the drug remains at the site of the injection, but, once the blood pressure is reestablished, large amounts of morphine are suddenly absorbed and toxic signs may develop. Initially, there is a sensation of warmth and comfort progression to a dreamy confusion. The face flushes, but within approximately one hour, it pales as the pulse begins to slow. Lethargy progresses, reflexes are lost, the muscles relax and become flaccid. The pupils constrict to pinpoint size and fail to react to light although they dilate terminally. As the pulse slows, skin temperature declines, cyanosis becomes evident, and secondary anoxic seizures may develop, especially in children [10].

Neurorespiratory Depression

Respiratory complications of morphine relate primarily to its direct suppressive effect on brain stem respiratory centers [19]. The respiratory depression is evident even when the doses are too small to alter the level of consciousness, and abnormal respiratory patterns have been reported after therapeutic doses of the drug. These therapeutic doses actively suppress multiple respiratory functions including rate, minute volume, and tidal volume. The patterns of abnormal breathing range from slow but regular to periodic and eventually irregular breathing after the dose becomes higher. In man, death from morphine intoxication is almost invariably due to respiratory arrest.

Maximal respiratory depression occurs within seven minutes after intravenous morphine administration, but peaks at approximately thirty minutes after intramuscular and ninety minutes after subcutaneous administrations. The sensitivity of the respiratory center returns towards normal after two to three hours, although even after therapeutic doses, respiratory minute volume remains considerably below normal for four to five hours. The mechanism of respiratory depression relates to two major factors. First, narcotics cause a direct depression of both pontine and medullary respiratory centers, and rhythmicity and automaticity are disturbed. This effect appears to be primary to the brain stem and not related to depressed afferent input since even electrical stimulation of the brain stem centers fails to elicit normal responses. Second, the brain stem chemoreceptivity declines so that increases in pCO_2 fail to induce reflex hyperventilation. This loss of chemosensitivity is selective and hypoxia remains at least a partly effective respiratory stimulant. This fact has therapeutic significance in that the hypoxic drive may be the only factor maintaining automatic respiration in a patient; inadvertent overoxygenation will remove this drive and may cause total apnea. The combined effects of these two depressant factors, direct brain stem depression and loss of chemosensitivity, are life-threatening. An additional, less understood, factor that aggravates respiratory compromise in morphine-intoxicated patients is an alteration of voluntary control of breathing. After large doses of morphine, patients breathe if instructed to do so, but if left unstimulated, they become relatively apneic. The pathophysiology of this effect relates presumably to the drug's preferential activity on brain stem centers with descending cortical influences left predominantly intact. Natural sleep also produces a decrease in medullary center pCO_2 sensitivity, so that the effects of morphine and sleep are addictive. These pharmacologic findings help to explain the historical treatment of morphine intoxication which included forced arousal, constant and deliberate reminding of the patient to breathe, and above all, prevention of sleep.

Not all narcotic agents are equivalent to morphine in their effects on respiratory depression. Death from respiratory depression is exceedingly rare after codeine administration, while heroin is felt to be even more potent in its depressive effects on respiration than morphine.

No natural or synthetic narcotic is free of respiratory depressive effects and all are dangerous to varying degrees. Other morphine effects that are not directly respiratory, but that may secondarily compromise ventilation include the induction of central vomiting and suppression of the cough reflex. Both increase the risk of aspiration and subsequent inadequate ventilation. Opiates as a class have an additional bronchoconstrictive effect.

During recovery from morphine overdose, there is gradual improvement in respiration and in the depression of consciousness. Coma will lighten into a prolonged sleep lasting hours, interrupted by waking periods where the patient is lucid but often complains of headaches. Relapses may occur and are felt to be due to reabsorption of morphine previously excreted into the intestinal tract. The ordinary fatal dose of morphine is generally considered to be 120-240 mg, although individual responses vary: death from therapeutic doses has occurred, although some addicts tolerate up to one gram of morphine daily.

Present treatment of morphine overdose centers on the use of the narcotic antagonist (naloxone) 1 cc (0.4 mg) given intravenously at 5-minute intervals until the patient awakens. Failure to obtain significant improvement after three doses suggests that other nonopiate drugs have also been administered or that other concomitant disease processes may be active [8].

Heroin is synthetically prepared by acetylation of both hydroxyl groups of morphine, resulting in diacetyl morphine. It is utilized in large amounts principally for its euphoric effects and is often the drug most sought by addicts. The analgesic and euphoric properties of heroin are greater than those of morphine; excitement often accompanies the euphoric state. Respiratory depression, however, is also greater with heroin and is a continual and predictable hazard of heroin abuse. The drug is rapidly absorbed from the mucous membranes, hydrolyzed completely in the body, and excreted as morphine. Heroin crosses the blood-brain barrier more rapidly than morphine, with brain levels peaking 15 minutes after intravenous administration. Once within the brain, heroin is metabolized to morphine.

The most serious neurologic-respiratory complication of heroin abuse is the acute toxic narcotic syndrome, which accounted for more than one-half the deaths in narcotic users reported for New York City in 1974. Clinically, the syndrome is characterized by severe hypoventilation with increasing lethargy, coma, constricted pupils, and massive pulmonary edema [18].

The pathophysiology of this catastrophic syndrome remains obscure. Formerly considered to relate exclusively to overdosage, it appears that multiple factors are probably important. Overdosage in the strict sense does occur, especially with long-acting methadone where the user readministers the heroin because there are no acute effects. When the heroin finally does peak, the patient is exposed to a double dose, with the dangerous hazards of respiratory toxicity. However, not all respiratory complications can be explained by high central nervous system narcotic levels. Addicts are sometimes found with injection needles still in place and witnesses have described very rapid, fatal responses over a few minutes. These descriptions suggest an allergic or hypersensitive reaction to heroin or its adulterants. A vasculopathy similar to polyarteritis nodosa has been described in patients dying after combined use of heroin and metamphetamine [5].

IATROGENIC AND MEDICINAL TOXINS

Severe respiratory depression is a hallmark of heroin intoxication and the pathophysiology of this picture in the case of overdosage appears similar to that seen with morphine. High central nervous system levels of heroin suppress respiratory functions by direct brain stem depression as well as by depressed chemosensitivity to changes in pCO_2. Additionally, however, the acute toxic reaction seen with heroin addiction is accompanied by a profound degree of pulmonary edema. The minimal respiratory efforts that continue to exist are often enough to whip the pulmonary fluid into an obstructive froth that exudes from the mouth and nose. Hemoptysis may be present and severe.

Several hypotheses have been proposed to explain the pulmonary edema. Abnormal stimulation of autonomic or limbic system structures in the brain can induce pulmonary edema and, because of the other known neurologic effects of heroin, centrally mediated pulmonary edema has been suggested. Hypoxia, acute allergic reactions, or direct toxic effects at the alveolar membrane have also been proposed. The pulmonary edema may be a species-specific reaction in man, since intravenous injection of "street" heroin in several species of animals including primates induces predictable coma and hypoventilation but never pulmonary edema [20].

Treatment of the acute toxic syndrome involves judicious oxygenation, control of the pulmonary edema, and naloxone 0.4 mg (1 cc) given intravenously to reverse the respiratory and central nervous system depression. Naloxone may also be given intramuscularly or subcutaneously. The peak effect of intravenous naloxone occurs within two minutes and the drug may be given every five minutes until the patient awakens. If there is no response after several doses, the overdose is likely due to nonopiate depressant drugs like barbiturate medications or methaqualone. Since naloxone activity is short-lived, any patient with opiate overdose must be watched for at least 24 hours for recurrence of central nervous system depression or apnea. Narcotic antagonists can precipitate an acute withdrawal syndrome in an addicted person; restitution of low-dose opiate drugs may be necessary for a short withdrawal time. Importantly, pulmonary edema may occur as much as 24 hours after the overdose; the patient should be observed carefully for fluid overload. Since patients are often debilitated or exposed to contaminated needles, cellulitis, osteomyelitis, endocarditis, and pneumonias are to be anticipated and treated when there is evidence. However, prophylactic antibiotics are not necessary. Seizures may also occur and are treated usually with phenytoin. Once the acute toxic syndrome has resolved, seizures usually do not occur.

Transverse Myelitis

An acute transverse myelitis can occur in opiate addicts presenting with sudden onset of weakness, a band level of diminished sensation, and unusual bladder and bowel incontinence. Myelograms on such patients have been normal when performed and at autopsy, extensive necrosis of the spinal cord is seen. In many of these cases, no underlying medical disease other than narcotic addiction was present. In survivors, a moderate to severe paraparesis with a thoracic sensory level is the typical picture. The involvement of both pain and temperature as well as vibratory sense suggest that this is not a vascular lesion involving the anterior spinal artery, but instead a diffuse necrotic process [18].

Seizures and Myoclonus

Meperidine is used extensively in the treatment of cancer patients and their pain syndromes. Recently, the neuroexcitatory effects of this drug have become appreciated and both seizures and myoclonus have occurred in patients taking large doses of meperidine. Case histories include patients ingesting up to 10 grams per week of meperidine who develop coincident seizures and myoclonus. The neurologic complications occur while the patient receives the drug and not as a withdrawal phenomenon. The neuroexcitatory toxic effect appears to relate to normeperidine, which accumulates, especially in patients with chronic renal failure. In the latter population, the half-life of normeperidine increases from 14.2 to 34.4 hours [13].

Endogenous and exogenous opioids may play a role in epilepsy, as suggested by recent animal studies, where methionine-enkephalin, morphine, or beta-endorphine produced a prolonged immobile stuporous state with intermittent sudden twitches and abnormal electroencephalographic seizure activity. Such behavioral changes and EEG patterns were immediately reversed by naloxone, an opiate antagonist [4].

Myopathies

Two types of muscle abnormalities are seen in heroin abusers. The first is an acute rhabdomyolysis occurring within a few hours after the intravenous injection of drug. Severe muscle pain and tenderness, swelling, and progressive weakness follow. Myoglobinuria precipitates renal failure in many patients. Rarely, additional cardiac myolysis may occur. Histologically, devastating necrosis of muscle fibers with edema and focal hemorrhage may occur.

A chronic fibrosing myopathy also occurs in "skin poppers" who use the drug by intramuscular or subcutaneous/intramuscular injection. Again, it is unknown whether this myopathy relates to the opiate itself or to the additives. The myopathy may be associated with a brawny edema when the patient's veins are eventually obliterated superficially.

IATROGENIC AND MEDICINAL TOXINS

Neuropathy

Numerous peripheral nerve lesions have been seen in opiate addicts. Mononeuritis may occur following a drug injection (usually in an anatomic area distant from the injection site) or may occur with no temporal relation to drug administration. The motor and sensory signs usually do not appear upon awakening and therefore do not seem to relate directly to pressure neuropathy.

A mild, predominantly distal and symmetric polyneuropathy may occur in these patients and appears to relate to the general poor nutrition of many opiate abusers. In addition, a fulminating ascending neuropathy typical of Guillain-Barré Syndrome can also be seen. In such cases, segmental demyelination can be prominent. A third type of neuropathy is that involving the brachial or lumbosacral plexies. Severe burning causalgia can accompany the usual weakness and hyperreflexia in the involved limb. In most cases some degree of recovery occurs. Treatment of the neuropathy involves good nutrition and vitamin supplementation. No specific therapy is otherwise available.

Ts AND BLUES

A recent report characterizes patients who self-administered intravenous "Ts and Blues" (pentazocine and tripelennamine: Talwin and Pyribenzamine) [3]. This combination of drugs is mainly used as a substitute for heroin. Seizures following the injection occurred frequently and status epilepticus also was seen. Seizures were usually generalized. Cerebrovascular accidents occurred in three of thirteen patients—two with deep cerebral infarctions. Infection in the form of mycotic aneurysms, nocardial abscess, cerebrogranulomatosis, or cerebral aspergillosis also occurred.

As with heroin and morphine, it is difficult to separate those neurologic syndromes directly related to the drugs from those related to the addict's lifestyle. Infection most likely relates directly to the nonsterile technique of self-injection, although seizures and cerebrovascular accidents could relate to primary drug activity on parenchyma or blood vessels.

MPTP

In the early 1980s, an illicit chemist researched the scientific literature and identified a narcotic derivative which the government had failed to control, 1-methyl-4-phenyl-4-propionoxy-meperidine, or MPPP. A byproduct of this drug, 1-methyl-phenyl-1,2,3,6-tetrahydropyridine (MPTP), has now been identified by Langston et al. [15] as a highly potent neurotoxin that produces clinical parkinsonism and marked depletion of pigmented cells in the substantia nigra. In animals given the agent, the same nigral depletion occurs as well as a behavior that includes hypokinesia and mild tremor. Acutely the drug may induce toxic hallucinations, generalized tremors and irregular myoclonus; however, within days or weeks after one or more doses, bradykinesia, rigidity, resting tremor and gait abnormalities develop in these often very young subjects. In man, the condition is permanent and nonextrapyramidal signs are lacking. The patient shows a dramatic response to levodopa and agonist therapy initially and hence, behaviorally, pharmacologically and histologically, the syndrome resembles quite closely idiopathic Parkinson's disease.

The neurotoxic effect at the cellular level is unknown. It has been suggested that it is converted into a charged quaternary amine, which may become trapped intraneuronally. There is no explanation for its selectivity to nigral dopaminergic cells.

Most remarkable is the pattern of drug response in affected patients. Although they respond dramatically to initiation of dopaminergic therapy with abatement of their parkinsonian signs, they develop the spectrum of drug toxicity seen typically in patients with idiopathic Parkinson's disease, at a dramatically fast rate. Hence, drug-induced chorea, hallucination, on-off, loss of efficacy (see Chapter 11), are all seen but begin within weeks or months of therapy. The entire clinical picture of Parkinson's disease from onset, through response, and finally through toxicity is distilled into a disturbingly short time frame. Other toxins can induce parkinsonian signs, but such a picture without other complicating clinical features has never been seen. The selectivity of the toxin to substantia nigral cells may relate to melanin concentrations in this nucleus.

■ HYPNOSEDATIVE AGENTS

Hypnosedative agents are prescribed and marketed to calm patients and facilitate sleep. In high doses they can usually induce general anesthesia. They act diffusely on the central nervous system and are often used additionally as anticonvulsants, muscle relaxants, or antianxiety agents. Generally, neurotoxicity syndromes associated with hypnosedatives relate to oversedation and diffuse encephalopathy, and hence are the extreme extension of the desired clinical effect.

BARBITURATES

Many variations of barbituric acid have been chemically synthesized to alter lipid solubility and thereby change their duration of action, latency to onset of activity, and metabolic degradation (see Table 13.1). Pharmacologically, barbiturates depress the activity of all excitable tissue, although the CNS is far

TABLE 13.1 Barbiturates

Official name	Trade name	Classification	Duration (hr) of action in therapeutic dose	Serum levels associated with toxicity	Significant dialysis of drugs
Barbital	Veronal	Long-acting	12-24	8 mg/dl or more	H (yes)
Phenobarbital	Luminal	Long-acting	12-24	40 mg/dl or more	P (yes)
Amobarbital	Amytal		8-10		H (minimally effective)
Butabarbital	Butisol	Intermediate acting	8-10	5 mg/dl or more	
Allobarbital	Diadol		8-10		P (no)
Secobarbital	Seconal		4-10	3 mg/dl or more	H (no)
Pentobarbital	Nembutal	Short-acting	6-8		P (no)
Hexobarbital	Evipal	Ultra-short-acting	3-4	1.5 mg/dl or more	H (no)
Thiopenal	Pentothal		3-4		P (no)

H = hemodialysis
P = peritoneal dialysis

more sensitive than skeletal, cardiac, or smooth muscle. Reticular activating system activity is depressed with all barbiturates; those containing a 5-phenyl substitute elevate the threshold for cortical after-discharges and suppress seizure foci.

Barbiturate toxicity is a frequent and hazardous complication of drug ingestion, and is associated with death in 0.5% to 12% of all toxic cases. Most of these cases are the result of deliberate attempts at suicide, but many are accidental poisonings in children or in drug abusers, especially those using more than one drug.

Clinical Features

Phenobarbital and its derivatives represent the oldest class of modern antiseizure drugs and are relatively devoid of serious neurotoxicity when kept within the therapeutic plasma level range of 15–40 µg/cc. Drowsiness is undoubtedly the most common complaint, especially when the drug is introduced. The intense sedation side effect of phenobarbital usually lasts only weeks, although patients may continue to complain for months and even years until the drug is switched or discontinued. The tolerance that develops is not related to decreased blood levels of the drug; there may be both an adaptive central mechanism and a shortened half-life of phenobarbital after continued use.

Even after long-term habituation to the therapeutic dose of phenobarbital, patients will become sedated and ataxic (often without nystagmus) when the plasma level rises above 50 µg/cc. Since the phenobarbital is metabolized hepatically (50%) and also excreted unchanged (50%), patients with either liver or renal disease are subject to unexpected intoxication at seemingly therapeutic doses.

When phenobarbital levels rise above 80 µg/cc, severe ataxia, nausea, vomiting, and nystagmus predominate. The patient may be so disabled by the somnolence, ataxia and nausea that he cannot sit up. Above 120 µg/cc, coma and respiratory depression occur. These enormously high levels are seen occasionally in chronically treated patients without the presence of dramatic toxic sedation; this paradox may relate to enzyme induction with a resultant diminished half-life of the drug. Both the sedative encephalopathy and cerebellar dysfunction resolve with the cessation of the drug.

A second encephalopathic syndrome occurs in children on phenobarbital and is highly distinctive. Instead of somnolence, these children develop remarkable agitation and hyperactivity. Sleep rhythms are often disrupted and there is prolonged nocturnal awakening. Inattentiveness, poor memory, and decline in school performance may suggest attentional deficit disorder (ADD) or childhood hyperactivity. Since epileptic children as well as those with a past history of febrile convulsions are frequently treated with phenobarbital, this syndrome is not rare; components of the problem have been reported in up to 40% of children receiving phenobarbital for febrile seizures [6]. When this syndrome occurs another drug must be substituted. Curiously, when Mebaral (mephobarbital) is used, the hyperactivity often abates, even though Mebaral is converted to phenobarbital systemically.

A peculiar third toxic encephalopahy, which may relate to the high incidence of lethal toxicity, has been termed "drug automatism." The patient fails to sleep after ingesting one or two doses of barbiturates, but becomes confused and unknowingly overdoses himself. In presumed cases of attempted suicide where patients deny intentional overdosage, some investigators feel this denial is of psychogenic origin. Jansson, however, investigated almost 500 cases of barbiturate intoxication and estimated that one-quarter could be explained as drug automatism [14]. Barbiturates are the most commonly used drugs in suicide by overdose; in the United States, an estimated 3,000 suicide deaths per year are attributed to barbiturates.

A variety of other neurologic signs and symptoms are seen in patients with moderate barbiturate overdose. These often resemble alcoholic inebriation. Early agitation followed by somnolence and difficulty walking and slurred speech are characteristic. In severe intoxication, patients are comatose and their pupils may be constricted. If the patient becomes hypoxic, however, pupillary dilatation will be seen. In barbiturate coma the EEG may show a characteristic burst suppression pattern with brief episodes of electrical silence. Because of barbiturate effects on the brain-stem respiratory system, breathing abnormalities are seen early [10]. Severe hypothermia may be induced and may be associated transiently with an electrically flat EEG.

Chronic forms of barbiturate intoxication may result from cumulative effects. The resulting signs and symptoms depend upon the amount administered as well as upon individual sensitivity to the drug and the variation in the rate of drug metabolism.

Patients with chronic toxic exposure to barbiturates show ataxic gait and slurred speech with periods of intermittent agitation, but generally depressed effect. Tremors and confusion are also characteristic. Ocular symptoms, including diplopia and blindness along with signs such as ptosis and nystagmus have also been reported.

The wide variety of short-, medium-, and long-acting barbiturates are all associated with the above neurologic syndromes. The onset of action and duration of toxicity differs according to the half-life of each drug (see Table 13.1).

Although the sedative and anticonvulsant activity of barbiturates is believed to relate to both pre- and postsynaptic effects on neurotransmitter systems and ions, as well as nonsynaptic effects reducing sodium and potassium conductance, the neurotoxic effects of barbiturates at the subcellular level are unknown [16]. The half-life is long (days), therefore acute withdrawal does not occur. However 4-5 days after abrupt cessation, withdrawal seizures may ensue; therefore propitious discontinuation of phenobarbital usually takes 3-4 weeks of slow tapering. Even with slow withdrawal, transient neurologic signs may develop, especially postural tremor and internal agitation, accompanied by irritability and sleeplessness. Neonates born of mothers ingesting phenobarbital are hypotonic, irritable, and vomit over the first five days of extrauterine life [2]. Phenobarbital participates in important drug-drug interactions with other anticonvulsants, which can result in additional systemic and neurologic problems (see Table 13.1).

Practical Management

Supportive care with attention to respiration is the primary mode of treating phenobarbital overdose. Activated charcoal, which probably absorbs gastrointestinal phenobarbital, which is subsequently excreted in the stool, has been shown in volunteers to reduce the serum half-life by more than 50% [1]. In comatose patients, the coma resolved with this treatment more rapidly than would have been expected with traditional supportive care alone.

In the past, patients in barbiturate coma were treated with stimulant drugs, but the increased metabolic demands provoked additional toxicity and therefore these added drugs are no longer recommended. Currently, the management of acute toxicity focuses on: (1) correction of life-threatening symptoms, hypoxia, cardiac arrhythmias; (2) prevention of further absorption of the drug by lavage and activated charcoal (1 gram of charcoal can bind 300-350 mg barbiturate). The recommended dose is 1 gram/kg. Saline cathartic will hasten intestinal transit and further reduce absorption; (3) facilitation of drug inactivation by forced diuresis, alkalinization of the urine and dialysis if necessary. The aim of diuresis is to produce a urine output of 300-400 ml/hr through fluids and diuretics until the drug levels decline. Since the barbiturates are weak acids, alkalinization will maximally maintain the drugs in ionized (nonabsorbable) form. Sodium bicarbonate can be used to maintain urine pH at least at 8. The alkalinization of the blood stream further enhances the diffusion of barbiturate out of cells. If the patient has ingested short-acting or intermediate-acting barbiturate, alkalinization is less useful.

Every patient recovering from acute barbiturate overdose must be observed for possible withdrawal symptoms. Excitement, sleeplessness, delirium and psychosis, or even seizures may occur. If such problems develop, the proper management is to reinstitute a barbiturate, phenobarbital 30 mg for every 100 mg of intermediate-acting or short-acting preparation formerly used, divided in four daily doses. Gradual reduction will then be effected over 3-4 weeks [21].

Hemodialysis and hemoperfusion may be more effective for the occasional patient in whom rapid removal of the drug is necessary [11]. The phenobarbital excretion must not be too rapid or withdrawal seizures may occur, complicating the treatment and threatening the patient's prognosis.

ETHCHLORVYNOL (PLACIDYL)

This agent is a hypnosedative with a rapid onset and short duration of action. In addition, it has anticonvulsant and muscle relaxant properties. As with the barbiturates, the hypnotic effect of this agent is greatly amplified by concomitant alcohol ingestion [7]. The most common side effects associated with ethychlorvynol use is a strange mintlike aftertaste, dizziness, nausea, vomiting, and facial paresthesias. These latter effects may be associated with hyperventilation. Some patients complain of mild mental confusion or "hangover" effects after consuming the drug. Profound hypnosis, weakness, and syncope unrelated to hypotension have been reported. Idiosyncratic reactions, characterized by marked excitement and histrionic behavior, have been seen when the drug was ingested and a delirium may result when the drug is ingested along with antidepressants. The drug is clearly contraindicated in patients with acute intermittend porphyria. Severe intoxication induces deep coma, respiratory depression, bradycardia and hypotension. Death has occurred with a blood concentration of 4 mg/dl.

Chronic abuse of the drug results in both tolerance and physical dependence. Such chronic patients may appear similar to chronic barbiturate patients and may be uncoordinated, ataxic, and have slurred speech, confusion, and have nystagmus or other visual complaints that include scotomas, amblyopia or diplopia. Withdrawal symptoms mostly resemble those seen with delirium tremens and may be especially severe in elderly patients. In treating the acutely intoxicated patient, exhaustive attention must be paid to respiratory and cardiac function. Unlike barbiturate poisoning, with ethchlorvynol use forced diuresis can be extremely dangerous, forcing patients into shock and severe hypovolemia. Since the decline of serum levels is biphasic for this drug, careful monitoring is needed for several days; the first half-life distribution phase is 5-6 hours and the second is over 100 hours with acute intoxication. In obese patients, there is further sequestration in fat, making clearance even slower potentially.

Withdrawal symptoms are treated with restitution of the ethchlorvynol with gradual tapering, or by substitution with phenobarbital 100-200 mg/2 hours until the patient is quiet; the 6-hour cumulative phenobarbital dose may then be administered four times daily with gradual tapering over one week. Babies born to ethchlorvynol-medicated mothers have undergone withdrawal and should be treated with 3 mg/kg phenobarbital for several days.

METHAQUALONE

While all 2,3-disubstituted quinazolines possess hypnotic activity, only methaqualone is available legally. The drug has antitussive activity comparable to that of codeine, although it lacks independent analgesic properties. The drug may possess tranquilizing properties distinct from its sedative effects, but this has not been fully established. In hypnotic doses, numerous neurologic side effects have been reported. There are reports of transient or persisting paresthesias and other signs of peripheral neuropathy that may last months to years after the cessation of drug ingestion, although in such patients multiple drugs were usually ingested [17]. Paradoxical restlessness and anxiety instead of sedation and sleep are also reported with this drug. Excessive dreaming and somnabulism may also occur. As with many of the drugs already mentioned, there is an additive sedating effect of methaqualone with alcohol. Other drug interactions include an enhanced effect of MAO inhibitors and tricyclic antidepressants, and when methaqualone is ingested along with phenothiazines or tricyclics, epistaxis and menstrual irregularities have been reported in a higher frequency. Unlike many of the drugs already discussed, methaqualone has been used without difficulty in patients with intermittent porphyria. In overdosage, restlessness and excitement occur followed by delirium and marked myoclonus. Most lethal cases have been in patients who have ingested multiple drugs or methaqualone with alcohol.

Treatment is primarily supportive. Convulsions can be treated with phenytoin. Forced diuresis should be avoided since patients are often already hypotensive and only 2% of absorbed methaqualone is excreted in the urine. Furthermore, some patients have pulmonary edema, making added fluids hazardous. Although hemodialysis and peritoneal dialysis have been used with some success, general care and support is the most important focus. As withdrawal syndromes are well described, the development of agitation and tremors after the acute phase should lead the physician to reintroduce low doses of the methaqualone or phenobarbital.

Methaqualone has become a widely abused substance, presumably based on the popular view that it has aphrodiasic activity. Drug culturists have reported that it induces a "high" without the drowsiness seen with barbiturates. Chronic abusers may employ doses ranging to 2 grams per day. Severe generalized seizures have been seen upon abrupt withdrawal from such high doses. The use of methaqualone by high-school students rose sharply from 1976 to 1981. The increase has been suggested to relate to the dramatic increase in cocaine use, since methaqualone is often used to "bring down" a cocaine "high." Illicit tablets produced clandestinely or in foreign laboratories supply most methaqualone subjects.

IATROGENIC AND MEDICINAL TOXINS

CHLORAL HYDRATE

Following oral ingestion, chloral hydrate is rapidly absorbed from the intestinal tract. It is detoxified in the liver, but part is excreted in the urine. Chloral hydrate has been combined with alcohol to produce the well-known "Mickey Finn." There is a wide variation in individual response to chloral hydrate. It is estimated that 10 grams or more is generally needed to produce acute intoxication, but death may result with as little as 4 grams. Some degree of tolerance may develop, and habitual users have consumed as much as 92 grams without fatal outcome [10].

The initial toxic symptoms are nausea and vomiting, followed by ataxia and stupor. The medullary centers are often depressed, with a resultant drop in blood pressure, slowing of respiration, and cyanosis. General vasodilatation is frequently marked, causing a slight diminution in body temperature. There may be conjunctivitis and lacrimation with swelling of the eyelids. Pupillary constriction suggestive of morphine poisoning and diplopia may be seen. Aberrations of vision and partial blindness may result from congestion of the optic nerve. In fatal cases death usually occurs within 5 to 10 hours. In some instances, fatal relapse may occur after apparent recovery. Respiratory paralysis is the most frequent cause of death, but cardiac deaths have been reported.

Chronic chloral hydrate intoxication is rare in the United States, but in India, where chloral hydrate addiction is common, chronic toxicity is frequent. In chronic poisoning the face becomes deep red to purple in color. The icteric skin and sclerae are evidence of hepatic damage. Dermatoses of erythematous, urticarial, or purpuric types are frequent. Gastrointestinal disorders are common and, together with hepatic damage and poor nutrition, contribute to the emaciation usually seen in chloral hydrate addicts. Fatigue and sensations of intense cold and faintness are usual. Loss of libido and urinary and menstrual disorders also occur, as well as joint pains, increased sensitivity to cutaneous stimuli, weakness of the legs, and facial palsies.

Treatment of the intoxicated patient involves general supportive measures and frequent monitoring for cardiac arrhythmias, especially in children and adolescents. Chloral hydrate depresses the contractility of the myocardium and shortens the refractory period as do other hydrocarbon drugs. Forced diuresis is useful using mannitol (2 grams/kg for children or 100 grams for adults) or furosemide (1 mg/kg for children or 40-80 mg in adults). Hemodialysis has also been used. A withdrawal syndrome may occur; in that case, chloral hydrate may have to be reinstituted, or phenobarbital added in small doses. After 48 hours, a gradual withdrawal of the sustaining drugs may be instituted, although the withdrawal period should last 7-10 days.

GLUTETHIMIDE

Although claimed to be a nonbarbiturate hypnotic, glutethimide (Doriden) is closely related to phenobarbital in structure. Since its introduction in 1964, it has become a remarkably popular prescription sedative. As a result, acute poisoning is not unusual. Clinically, the symptoms resemble those of barbiturate overdosage; treatment involves the same supportive measures. Glutethimide has additional strong anticholinergic properties; as a result, in the case of overdosage, pupillary and other anticholinergic effects are evident. The drug may remain in the gastrointestinal tract for extensive periods of time; therefore, gastric lavage may be particularly efficacious in preventing more extensive toxicity.

Acidosis is a particular problem in patients with glutethimide toxicity. Sodium bicarbonate should be administered and fluids will help to maintain the blood pressure. Since this drug induces anticholinergic effects, one might consider physostigmine to reverse such toxic symptoms. However, the dangers associated with this drug appear to outweigh the potential benefits; therefore physostigmine is not recommended for use in glutethimide toxicity. In those patients who do not respond to the general supportive measures, charcoal and resin hemoprofusion have been used with success. The withdrawal syndrome associated with glutethimide addiction should be treated with resubstitution of glutethimide at a decreased dose, or with small doses of phenobarbital that are then tapered over a two-week period.

▪ STUDY QUESTIONS

A known morphine addict is hospitalized after a car accident with fractures of the clavicle and multiple ribs. He is in severe pain, and an analgesic is prescribed. Symptoms of apparent morphine withdrawal develop soon afterwards. Which was the most likely analgesic given?

1. Codeine
2. Meperidine (Demerol)
3. Aspirin
4. Nalorphine (Nalline)

Answer: 4

Nalorphine is an opiate antagonist and a potent analgesic. It competitively antagonizes mu receptors, and is a partial agonist at kappa receptors. As such, it is associated with the precipitation of morphine withdrawal in subjects dependent on high levels of a strong opiate (morphine), but can be used as an analgesic in patients with lower levels of dependency. The analgesia induced by nalorphine is distinct from that seen with morphine itself, in that the former interferes primarily with nocioceptive input to the spinal cord, whereas morphine also acts on superspinal loci.

Children are often the victims of inadvertent barbiturate overdose because they receive these drugs for:

1. Migraine
2. Febrile convulsions
3. Chronic cough
4. Hyperactivity and poor attention span

Answers: 1, 2, 4

Children often receive barbiturates regularly for the prevention of febrile convulsions and the control of hyperactivity. Those with severe headaches may receive these drugs intermittently as well. Sometimes when children have flu or gastrointestinal upset and become irritable and cranky, their parents may give them barbiturate suppositories. Importantly, phenobarbital may be associated with either increased somnolence and lethargy or paradoxical hyperactivity; thus, a clinical picture of unexplained nervousness and irritability is within the realm of phenobarbital toxicity in the pediatric group.

The acute toxic narcotic syndrome has the following important features:

1. Hyperventilation
2. Coma
3. Constricted pupils
4. Transverse myelopathy

Answers: 2, 3

Although the pathophysiology of the acute toxic narcotic syndrome is obscure, the clinical hallmarks are hypoventilation, pulmonary edema, depressed level of consciousness, and constricted pupils. It has been suggested that the response is a hypersensitive allergic reaction, although this is not confirmed. The massive pulmonary edema is associated with a froth in the mouth and nose, which leads to further ventilatory compromise.

The combination of pentazocine and tripelennamine (Talwin and Pyribenzamine, or "Ts and Blues") is associated with a clinical syndrome, including:

1. Seizures and cerebrovascular accidents
2. Myasthenia gravis
3. Pseudotumor cerebri or increased intracranial pressure
4. Myoclonus and dementia

Answer: 1

Generalized seizures and focal cataclysmic cerebrovascular events were hallmarks of a recent report on "Ts and Blues." Whether this reaction is due to the toxic products themselves or to underlying infection or aneurysm is unclear. The syndrome is seen when the drugs are combined and administered intravenously, and is not associated with oral ingestion of Talwin.

When a patient admitted to the hospital is a known addict of a sedative agent, which of the following general guidelines can be used in avoiding the withdrawal state:

1. A short-acting barbiturate is best.
2. A dose equivalent of phenobarbital at 30-50% of the suspected chronic dose may be used, with increases or decreases depending on the patient's clinical state.
3. Phenobarbital should in all instances be avoided because of its liver toxicity and masking effect of withdrawal.
4. Withdrawal can be effectively managed with a long-acting barbiturate preparation, with the exception of chloral hydrate addiction, where true withdrawal does not occur.

Answer: 2

The treating physician can never know with certainty what the patient's chronic addictive dose has been. This is because patients are often unreliable and, if they are ingesting street medications, the amount of adulteration is variable. Therefore, the basic adage is that the equivalent sedative dose of phenobarbital at a 30-50 percent reduction can be started. This dose may have to be increased or decreased depending on whether the patient is overly sedated or whether he is in fact used to a higher dose of medication. After a week to 10 days, the dose established can be gradually decreased, and the patient withdrawn safely.

■ REFERENCES

1. Berg MJ, Berlinger WG, Goldberg MJ, Spector R, Johnson GF: Acceleration of the body clearance of phenobarbital by oral activated charcoal. N. Engl. J. Med. 307:642-644, 1982.
2. Bleyer WA, Marshall RE: Barbiturate withdrawal syndrome in a passively addicted infant. JAMA, 221:185-186, 1972.
3. Caplan LR, Thomas C, Banks G: Central nervous system complications of addiction to "T's and Blues." Neurology 32:623-628, 1982.
4. Chugani HT, Ackermann RF, Chugani TC, Engel J: Opioid-induced epileptogenic phemomena: anatomical, behavioral, and electroencephalographic features. Ann. Neurol. 15:361-368, 1984.
5. Citron BP, Halpern M, McCarron M, Lundberg GD, McCormick R, Pincus J, Tatter D, Haverback BJ: Necrotizing angiitis associated with drug abuse. N. Eng. J. Med. 283:1003-1011, 1970.
6. Consensus Statement: Febrile seizures: Long-term management of children with fever-associated seizures. Pediatrics 66:1009-1012, 1980.
7. Cummings LM, Martin YC, Scherfling EE: Serum and urine levels of ethchlorvynol in man. J. Pharmacol. 60:261-263, 1971.

8. Fultz JM, Senay EC: Guidelines for the management of hospitalized narcotic addicts. Ann Intern. Med. 82:815-818, 1975.
9. Goetz CG: Neurotoxins and respiratory dysfunction. In WJ Weiner: Respiratory Dysfunction in Neurologic Disease, pp. 197-211. Futura Press, Mount Kisco, NY, 1980.
10. Goetz CG, Klawans HL, Cohen MM: Neurotoxic agents. In AB Baker, EL eds.: Clinical Neurology, pp. 1-84. Hagerstown, Md., Harper and Row, 1981.
11. Goldberg MJ, Berlinger WG: Treatment of phenobarbital overdose with activated charcoal. JAMA 247:2400-1, 1982.
12. Hiller JM, Pearson J, Simon EJ: Distribution of stereospecific binding of the potent narcotic analgesic etorphine. Res. Commun. Chem. Pathol. Pharmacol. 6:1052-1057, 1973.
13. Hochman MS: Meperidine-associated myoclonus and seizures in long-term hemodialysis patients. Ann. Neurol. 14:593, 1983.
14. Jansson B: Drug automatism as a cause of pseudosuicide. Postgrad. Med. J. 30:A34-A40, 1961.
15. Langston JW, Ballard P, Tetrud JW, Irwin I: Chronic parkinsonism in humans due to a product of meperidine-analog synthesis. Science 219:979-980, 1983.
16. Macdonald RL, McLean MJ: Cellular bases of barbiturate and phenytoin anticonvulsant drug action. Epilepsia 23(Suppl. 1):S7-S18, 1982.
17. Marriott PF: Methaqualone with psychotrophic drugs: Adverse interaction. Med. J. Aust. 1:412-418, 1976.
18. Pearson J, Richter RW: Neurologic aspects of addiction opiates. In PJ Vinken and GW Bruyn, eds.: Handbook of Clinical Neurology, Vol. 37, pp. 365–400. Amsterdam, North-Holland Press, 1979.
19. Pentiah P, Reilly F, Borison HL: Interaction of morphine sulfate and sodium salicylate on respiration in cats. J. Pharmacol. Exp. Ther. 154:110-118, 1966.
20. Reichman LB, Shim CS, Baden MM, Richter RW: Development of tolerance to street heroin in addicted and non-addicted primates. Am. J. Pub. Health 63:801-803, 1973.
21. Skoutakis VA, Acchiardo SR: Barbiturates. In VA Skoutakis, Clinical Toxicology of Drugs, pp. 61-76. Lea & Febiger, Philadelphia, 1982.

CHAPTER 14

Stimulants and Hallucinogens

STIMULANT drugs and hallucinogens are two classes that significantly overlap. Central stimulants are defined as those drugs that diminish the need for sleep, reverse the effects of fatigue, and enhance performance tasks. Hallucinogens are those agents that provoke visual, auditory, or tactile perceptual hallucinations as their primary clinical effect. Although amphetamine and its congeners are the prototypes of central stimulants, they can in fact induce hallucinations. Other agents with a structural basis rather closely related to amphetamine are considered hallucinogens, not stimulants, since their prominent hallucinogenic effects clinically outweigh their stimulatory activity. The classification of a drug therefore relates to the agent's predominant effect rather than its absolute qualities. The following categories may be established, all of which are summarized in Table 14.1: (a) stimulants related to catechols, usually with a phenylethylamine structure, including amphetamine, methylphenidate, and pemoline; (b) stimulant drugs without a catecholamine base, including cocaine and caffeine; (c) anorectic agents that at high doses cause central stimulation, in contrast with (d) phenylethylamine derivatives that are anorectic, but even at high doses lack significant stimulatory effects; (e) hallucinogens with amphetamine-like structures, the prototype being mescaline; (f) derivatives of tryptamine; and (g) derivatives of LSD. Finally, miscellaneous psychoactive agents like phencyclidine, which combine stimulatory, depressive, and hallucinogenic properties should be considered in another class. There are yet other agents with multiple neurologic effects, including stimulation and hallucinations, which are discussed in other sections of this volume.

TABLE 14.1 Psychoactive Drugs, Classified by Predominant Clinical Effect

Stimulants		Anorectic drugs		Hallucinogens			Mixed psychoactive drugs
With catechol structure	Without catechol structure	Catechol derivatives without stimulant effects at high dose	Catechol derivatives without significant stimulatory effect	With catechol structure	With tryptamine structure	With lysergic acid diethylamine structure	
Prolintane		Menfenorex	Amphecloral	Mescaline			
Dextrofemine	Cocaine	Levamphetamine	Chlorphenetime	DOM (STP)	N,N, Dimethyltryptamine (DMI)	LSD	
Methylphenidate		Norpseudoephedrine	Formetorex	DOET			Phencyclidine
Methamphetamine		l-Methamphentamine	Fludorex	MDA	Diethyltryptamine		
Phenmetrazine		Phendimetrazine	Amfepentorex	TMA			
Phenmetrazine		Furfenorex	Cloforex	TMA-2			Marijuana
Pipradrol	Caffeine	Ethylamphetamine	Fenfluramine	TMA-3	Dipropyltryptamine		
Dimethamphetamine		Metamfepramone	Fluminorex	DMA			
	Nicotine	Diphemethoxidine	Ortetamine	MMDA			
Fencamfamine		Fenbutrazate	Clominorex	DMMDA	Psilocybin		
Pemoline		Ephedrine	Fenmetramide				
Alfetamine		Phentermine	Trifluorex		Psilocin		
Zylofuramine		Benzphetamine					
Xylopropamine		Diethylpropion					
Cypenamine		Pentorex					
Facetoperan		Aminorex					
Dexamphetamine							

STIMULANTS WITH CATECHOL STRUCTURE

AMPHETAMINE

Amphetamine, or phenylisopropylamine, is the prototype of central nervous system stimulants. It is a specific compound, so that the commonly used word "amphetamines" is technically inappropriate. Amphetamine derivatives are most commonly used in promoting weight loss, although the treatment of narcolepsy and attentional deficit disorder in children are two well-recognized indications for the clinical use of amphetamine compounds.

Amphetamine appears to act predominantly as a dopaminergic agonist. It acts indirectly to induce release of presynaptic dopamine into the synaptic cleft. Amphetamine does not appear to promote exocytotoxic release of catecholamines, but induces calcium independent release. There is some evidence that amphetamines may also block the uptake of dopamine so that more active neurotransmitter remains in the synaptic cleft to stimulate receptors. Amphetamine also causes activation of norepinephrine systems, and the noradrenergic pathway from the locus coeruleus to cerebellar Purkinje neurons has been shown to be very sensitive to amphetamine [8].

Abusive amphetamine use has become a significant clinical and social problem. In the past, stimulants were used by the military and even advocated for school children to improve their attention span and to reduce fatigue. In a 1978 report it was estimated that eight percent of the United States population had used stimulants for nonmedical purposes and that one percent were current users, which was defined as having used a stimulant drug within the last month. The age group most likely to use stimulants are the 25-year-olds with 21% having used a stimulant at least once and 3% reported as current users [22]. Accidental ingestion by small children is a significant source of stimulant morbidity.

Clinical Features

The clinical picture of a patient intoxicated with amphetamine may range from mild restlessness to coma and death. Espelin and Done have established a rating severity score of 1-4 for amphetamine intoxication [7]:

1. Irritability, insomnia, tremor, and sweating;
2. Hyperactivity, confusion, excessive sweating, and mild fever;
3. Delirium, often with hallucinations, manic behavior, and hyperpyrexia;
4. Convulsions and death.

The determination of a toxic dose of amphetamine is difficult, since there is a wide range of individual susceptibility. Furthermore, tolerance develops with chronic exposure; the toxic dose will change in each individual with experience. In adults, the acute lethal dose is estimated to be between 20-25 mg/kg, whereas in children 5 mg/kg may be fatal [25].

Tremor is one of the prominent neurologic effects of amphetamine compounds. The tremor is postural and most marked when the patient holds his hands out in front of him; it tends to abate when the patient relaxes his hands on his lap. The tremor resembles that seen in patients with hyperthyroidism, high states of anxiety, or those who ingest high doses of caffeine. Pathophysiologically, the tremor appears to relate to increased activity of the noradrenergic system, with possible activation of both central and peripheral nervous system mechanisms [23].

Hyperthermia is also frequently encountered after amphetamine ingestion. Temperatures as high as 43° C (109.4°F) have been reported. The central or peripheral nervous system may be involved in the generation of this high body temperature. Stimulation of dopaminergic neurons usually produces hypothermia, whereas stimulation of peripheral noradrenergic systems usually produces hyperthermia. Body temperature and plasma amphetamine levels tend to follow a similar time course, both peaking approximately 1½ hours after the ingestion of a single dose. Likewise, the pupils tend to be widely dilated and sluggishly reactive to light at this time. The pupillary response appears to be related to the alpha adrenergic stimulation of the radial muscle of the iris. Hypertension, with increase in both diastolic and systolic blood pressure, and tachycardia relate to the activation of both alpha and beta adrenergic systems [25].

The hallucinations and psychotic behavior that are seen with amphetamine are not usually acute effects, but occur after chronic abuse of amphetamine compounds. Psychosis, however, does occur after a single acute dose when the patient has previously experienced a chronic amphetamine psychosis. Hallucinations are usually auditory, although tactile and visual hallucinations may be seen. The observation that amphetamine-induced psychosis is a chronic effect suggests that chronic drug exposure in some way alters receptor site populations in the brain. These changes may not be fully reversible since even after the patient has recovered from a hallucinatory state, a subsequent single exposure to amphetamine may reactivate the psychosis acutely [24].

Chorea is also associated with the use or abuse of amphetamine products, and is seen in three different clinical settings, the first two rarer than the third. In patients with already present Huntington's chorea, amphetamine will acutely exacerbate the abnormal movements of this disease. Since amphetamine is a dopaminergic agonist, and the chorea of Huntington's disease is felt to relate to a degenerative overactivity of striatal dopaminergic systems, this exacerbation by amphetamine may well relate to an amplification of the already heightened striatal dopaminergic function. In patients without chorea but with a history of prior abnormal movements related to Sydenham's chorea or chorea due to systemic lupus erythematosus, amphetamine may acutely precipitate new transient chorea that will disappear after the drug is withdrawn. Normal volunteers receiving an identical acute dose of amphetamine demonstrate no adverse effect. The induction of chorea in response to such an acute dosage of a central stimulant would suggest that an underlying structural abnormality of the basal ganglia renders these neurons supersensitive to exogenous dopaminergic stimulation. Similarly, some children who are treated with amphetamine compounds or other stimulants for hyperkinesis or attentional deficit disorder develop irregular choreic movements after an acute exposure to the drug. This phenomenon is rare (1.3% in a large series), but again suggests that an underlying striatal abnormality is already present in these few children [4,23].

By far the most common and therapeutically most troublesome form of amphetamine-induced chorea is the late-onset form, seen after long-term drug exposure [12]. Because amphetamine compounds are so often abused, the dose and duration of exposure are rarely documented. Some authors have tended to discuss chorea as a part of the broader category of chronic stimulant-induced stereotypy [30]. Although discrimination between the two phenomena may be difficult, various clinical experimental observations suggest that the choreiform movements are distinct from behavioral stereotypy. The similarity of amphetamine-induced lingual-facial-buccal movements to those observed in classic tardive dyskinesia and levodopa-induced dyskinesias suggest that they represent a distinct drug-mediated phenomenon. Since the movements in the above two categories are felt to relate to chronic increased activation of striatal dopaminergic receptors, the same biochemical alteration may underlie the movements seen after chronic amphetamine exposure. Laboratory work in animals has demonstrated that after chronic exposure to amphetamine, animals demonstrate increased sensitivity to amphetamine and alterations in both the affinity and the number of dopaminergic receptor sites in the striatum [33]. Amphetamine when used on a chronic basis may induce similar structural alterations at the level of the striatum in man, rendering the subject supersensitive to stimulation by dopaminergic agents, either endogenous or exogenous. An analogous change at other nonstriatal receptor populations may underlie the chronic psychosis seen with amphetamine. Tics have also been precipitated with amphetamine.

Another movement complication of amphetamine exposure is behavioral stereotypy. Some authors state that stereotypy is not seen in the absence of psychosis, although this is a controversial point [6]. Complex stereotypy, referred to as "punding," may assume diverse forms. These small behavioral fragments, which might easily be seen as part of the normal daily behavior, become, under the influence of central stimulants, nongoal-directed, socially meaningless, and continuously repeated rituals. Repetitive assembly and disassembly of small machines, repetitive copying of numbers or lists, and continuous cleaning of objects are all within the repertoire of punding. The anatomic basis of such behavior is unclear, although animal studies of amphetamine-induced stereotypic behavior suggest that stereotypic gnawing relates to the striatal dopaminergic system. Such behavior in animals, however, is an acute phenomenon seen within minutes after amphetamine exposure, whereas the stereotypes in man are seen after chronic exposure only. The similarity of such stereotypy to automatisms observed in temporal lobe epilepsy suggests that limbic pathways may be more involved than striatal.

A significant neurovascular complication of amphetamine congeners is cerebrovasculitis. Usually this syndrome is seen after chronic intravenous use of metamphetamine, but has recently been described also after the use of oral agents. Small vessels less than 1 millimeter in diameter become occluded and large and medium vessels may also be involved. These observations may relate to embolic or thrombotic disease caused by the drug or to impurities. Beading of the vessels is one of the characteristic angiographic features observed.

Related to the above vasculitic disease may be subarachnoid or intracerebral hemorrhage. Some cases of intracerebral hemorrhage may relate to amphetamine-induced hypertension as well. The intracerebral hemorrhage is seen after oral or intravenous use of the amphetamine drugs. Vasculitic changes are not seen on all angiograms in such patients, suggesting that there may be multiple mechanisms underlying intracranial extravasation of blood [14].

Practical Management

The various toxic syndromes seen with amphetamine are handled differently, although the unifying treatment is that of amphetamine withdrawal [25]. In the acute setting, the first step is to evaluate the severity of the intoxication. Since amphetamine toxicity can be life-threatening, immediate emergency attention to life support systems is essential. Convulsions, hyperpyrexia, hypertensive crisis, and cardiovascular collapse are the immediate dangers of the intoxicated patient. Prior to the development of convulsions, agitation and combative delirium are seen; phenothiazine drugs that effectively quiet the patient act quickly after intramuscular injection, and will have a later effect on hypertension as well [7]. Neuroleptic drugs block dopaminergic receptor sites. It has been recommended that if chlorpromazine is selected, 1 mg/kg may be used and repeated at 30-minute intervals as needed. Because so often a patient takes amphetamine with other drugs, if there is any question of combination medication, especially sedative, half the recommended dose of chlorpromazine should be used. Butyrophenones like haloperidol may in fact be superior to chlorpromazine, since less respiratory depression and less sustained hypotension with reflex tachycardia has been reported with them. The values of a neuroleptic must be weighed against the risk that they may lower seizure threshold. In a mildly affected patient (severity rating 1, as described above on

Epelin's and Done's scale, diazepam can be used, since in patients with a rating of other systemic effects requiring dopaminergic blocking agents are not present. In these mild cases, diazepam orally or intravenously at a dose of 10 mg for an adult or 0.1-0.3 mg/kg in a child may be used [25].

To lower body temperature, the patient should be placed in a cooled room, under a hypothermic blanket, and neuroleptic medications may help to control shivering. Temperature should be monitored every 15 minutes until stabilized at a temperature below 39°C (102.2°F).

Hypertension often is controlled sufficiently by the administration of neuroleptic drugs. If, however, the blood pressure is severely elevated, an alpha blocking agent, such as phenoxybenzamine or even sodium nitroprusside may be needed.

Once these emergency measures are taken, steps to minimize absorption of the drug from the GI tract may be instituted. Emesis and lavage cannot be performed if the patient is undergoing a seizure and in some instances, such procedures have been associated with the precipitation of amphetamine seizures. If the patient has received medication to control agitation, emesis can be dangerous because of aspiration complications. If the patient has ingested amphetamines within the past four hours, evacuation of the stomach is usually recommended. If the patient is alert, syrup of ipecac may be administered. If, on the other hand, the patient is lethargic or comatose, lavage should be performed. When ingestion has occurred longer than four hours before the patient is encountered, activated charcoal and saline should be administered, since at this point, emesis and lavage are probably not beneficial.

Once absorbed, amphetamine drugs are widely distributed in the body and easily cross the blood-brain barrier. Amphetamine compounds are metabolized by several pathways, with deamination the predominant one in man. Forced acidic diuresis is indicated to enhance the renal elimination of amphetamine compounds, but forced fluid administration can be hazardous if there is hypertension. The goal is a urine flow of 3-6 ml/kg/hr in children and 2-4 ml/kg/hr in adults, with a urine pH of 5.5 or lower.

Peritoneal dialysis or hemodialysis may also be employed, especially if the patient does not improve with more conservative means of therapy as outlined above. Hemoperfusion has not been extensively investigated.

Amphetamine-induced psychosis may be controlled by the use of dopaminergic-blocking neuroleptic drugs. Of course, withdrawal of amphetamine is the major form of therapy. Likewise, the chronic amphetamine-induced chorea will be controlled by cessation of the drug, although severe chorea can temporarily be managed with a neuroleptic drug. In cases where the chorea involves the respiratory apparatus, patients may be significantly more comfortable with low doses of neuroleptics for several days. In the case of the drug-induced vasculopathy, traditional management for the cerebrovascular accident is used and steroids have been used empirically with reports of benefit [31].

Other Catechols

Besides amphetamine, numerous other drugs have been developed that share many clinical properties. The most widely used is methylphenidate (Ritalin). This drug differs from amphetamine in its mode of action, in that it acts predominantly to inhibit the reuptake of dopamine and norepinephrine [10]. The drug may also have some releasing effect on presynaptic dopamine and may even have a direct synaptic stimulatory effect. The paranoid psychosis described with amphetamine can also be seen with methylphenidate, as well as the development of a chronic choreic state, stereotypies, and alterations in effect. Pemoline (Cylert) also acts to increase dopaminergic activity centrally. Used predominantly to treat attentional deficit disorder in young children, this drug is more recently available than either amphetamine or methylphenidate. Significant neurotoxic side effects are less commonly reported with this drug, although this may well reflect its more recent release rather than its lower absolute potential for chronic toxicity. The neurotoxic effects described above for amphetamine and similar compounds should be considered as potential hazards of methylphenidate and pemoline [25].

■ STIMULANTS WITHOUT CATECHOL STRUCTURE

COCAINE

Cocaine is a naturally occurring central nervous system stimulant extracted from the leaves of the coca plant. Chronic exposure creates a psychological dependence with a strong craving sensation. Intranasal and intravenous usage are progressively common. The drug has vasoconstrictive effects peripherally and induces a mild febrile state with dilated pupils, increased heart rate, and increased blood pressure. There is an immediate feeling of euphoria, confidence and energy, which apparently underlies its popularity. Approximately ten million Americans have used cocaine, and it is estimated that cocaine is second only to marijuana in its popularity. A 1982 report indicated that approximately 16% of U.S. high school graduates of 1981 had tried cocaine [26].

Because a feeling of depression or "letdown" occurs rapidly (often within 15 minutes after an intranasal dose), the user is often compelled to repeat the dose to recapture the fleeting exhilaration. After repeated administration of the drug at short intervals, users often complain of formications on the skin, anxiety, and often terrifying visual and auditory hallucinations. Paranoid delusions may also occur, with subjects suddenly becoming fearful and hypersensitive to even the most mild stimuli.

Most cocaine-dependent subjects use about 0.4 g of cocaine daily, but may intermittently take as much as 4 g [36]. Hypertension, tremor, muscle twitches and sometimes convulsions may accompany the behavioral toxic changes seen with cocaine abuse. Cocaine is often taken along with other agents, including alcohol (this combination is called a "liquid-lady"). New combinations, may have more complicated and more diverse clinical effects than those described in this section, with both marked stimulation and depression occurring. Pure oral use is uncommon, and most oral cases described have been subjects swallowing large amounts to escape police detection during smuggling.

Chemically pure cocaine is exquisitely rare and adulterated products are more commonly available; hence the estimate of a toxic dose is always crude. With twenty-four subjects who died after oral ingestion, the amount released into the gastrointestinal tract appeared to be 1 g or more [35]. By other routes, 1.2 g is usually considered fatal [26].

Clinical Features

Clinically, the toxic effects of cocaine can be divided into CNS alterations, autonomic nervous system activation or depression, and cardiovascular and/or respiratory changes. The CNS effects are both stimulatory and depressive. Descending inhibitory pathways are blocked, causing excitation. With low doses, such stimulation is primarily cortical, inducing the desired effects of euphoria and exhilaration. These may be replaced by less pleasant confusion and apprehension if intoxication persists. As stimulation involves brain stem and spinal cord regions, tremors like those seen with amphetamine may develop. Convulsions that may relate directly to CNS excitation or to complications of cardiovascular and respiratory systems may occur and are life-threatening if further systemic complications develop.

Cocaine produces both central and peripheral sympathetic nervous effects. Vasoconstriction, pupillary dilatation, and fever occur with acute intoxication. Cocaine produces an initial increase in the respiratory rate and depth of inspiration. With large doses, this is followed by rapid and shallow breathing and progressive respiratory depression resulting in apnea. These effects appear to relate to the stimulation and depression of the medullary center in the brain stem. Small doses of cocaine slow the heart secondary to central vagal stimulation, whereas with moderate doses, cocaine produces tachycardia and hypertension. Arrhythmias have been reported with cocaine used in a control setting for medical purposes, as well as with cocaine abuse and overdose. Sinus tachycardia is the most common abnormality, although ventricular arrhythmias are well documented [26].

Cocaine exerts central and sympathomimetic actions through potentiation of the actions of catecholamines. The drugs block reuptake of dopamine and norepinephrine from the sympathic cleft. It does not release catecholamines and, as with methylphenidate, the reuptake inhibition of dopamine in vitro is not altered by reserpine pretreatment [15]. Such changes in catecholamine are actively important to central as well as peripheral nervous system alterations and may also directly affect the cardiovascular changes. An effect of cocaine on serotonin activity has also been suggested.

Patients who abuse cocaine on a chronic basis are subject to hallucinations. Siegel examined altered perceptions in a group of cocaine users in which 37 of 85 subjects experienced altered images [32]. Many had chronic mydriasis and complained of hypersensitivity to light and halos around bright lights. Approximately 18% of the group had hallucinatory experiences, which were first noticed after six months of cocaine use. Initially, these were predominantly visual, but were followed by tactile hallucinations, often olfactory, auditory, and even gustatory hallucinations eventually occurred. Tactile hallucinations or "cocaine bugs" present the sensation of crawling under the skin, although when the subjects look at their skin they see no movement. Although hallucinations are usually associated with chronic use, they can be seen when an acute large dose is administered. The chronic cocaine user may be prone to violence, irrational thinking, and delusions of persecution and grandeur [32].

The concept of pharmacologic kindling was established with research using cocaine. The concept is based on electrical studies showing that very low intensity stimulation in certain brain regions eventually provoked major motor seizures when administered chronically and intermittently. Similarly, cocaine, when administered intermittently and chronically in subhallucinogenic doses, may later mimic system function and eventually induce full hallucinations [28].

Practical Management

When a patient is acutely intoxicated with cocaine, attention to the respiratory and cardiovascular systems is essential. If the patient has seizures and is intubated, intravenous or intramuscular phenobarbital may be administered and titrated to control the fit. To control the cardiovascular changes, Rappolt and associates have recommended the intravenous use of propranolol at a dose of 1 mg/min as needed, up to a total of 8 mg [29]. Usually, heart rate and blood pressure will return to normal within three minutes. This protocol has been somewhat controversial, however, since such cardiac effects are usually short-lived, occurring only during the high stimulatory phase of intoxication.

Since most cocaine exposures occur with intravenous or intranasal route, prevention of absorption is not indicated. If, however, cocaine is ingested orally, the stomach may be emptied as long as the patient has ingested the drug within four hours. If the CNS depressive phase has developed, an emetic is dangerous and lavage should be performed. In the event that a patient has swallowed condoms filled with cocaine, removal by endoscopy may rupture the packet; therefore, surgical removal is recommended.

Only a small percentage of cocaine is excreted unchanged in the urine; thus, altering the pH does not significantly affect cocaine excretion. Metabolic pathways for cocaine degradation are multiple and the byproducts include norcocaine, benzoylecgonine, and ecgonine. These products may be slightly altered by pH changes, but the net effect does not appear to be major.

CAFFEINE AND NICOTINE

Although there is little data to compare the relative stimulatory effects of caffeine or nicotine to amphetamine, caffeine and nicotine also appear to interact with dopaminergic systems. Caffeine potentiates amphetamine-induced behaviors in experimental animals and the stimulatory effect of nicotine is blocked by co-administration of an antagonist drug to dopamine synthesis [18]. There has also been the suggestion that an inverse relationship exists between smoking and the development of Parkinson's disease in humans. The precise mechanism of caffeine's stimulatory effect may relate to antagonism of adenosine receptors [11]. Since adenosine has been reported to inhibit the amphetamine-induced release from synaptosomes, it is reasonable that caffeine might exert its stimulant effect through antagonism of such inhibition [8]. Nicotine stimulates the release of striatal dopamine, as well as hypothalamic norepinephrine. In contrast to caffeine, nicotine might exert stimulant effects through specific nicotinic receptors, whose activation may facilitate dopaminergic transmission centrally. These cholinergic receptors would be in distinct contrast to the traditional muscarinic cholinergic receptors that are usually antagonistic to dopaminergic function, at least in the striatum.

Caffeine and other xanthine derivatives, including aminophylline, are central nervous system stimulants that may excite all levels of the CNS—the cortex being the most sensitive. An increased awareness of the environment or hyperesthesia may be an unpleasant experience to some patients upon ingestion of xanthine. Motor activity tends to increase and recently acquired or delicately coordinated skills may be adversely affected [13]. The patient becomes loquacious and restless and often complains of ringing in the ears and giddiness. Whether these manifestations relate to direct cerebral effects of xanthines or secondary results of vascular change is uncertain. In contrast to their dilating effect on systemic blood vessels, xanthines increase cerebrovascular resistance, with a resultant decrease in total cerebral blood flow [20]. Caffeine also stimulates the medullary respiratory, vasomotor, and vagal centers, with resultant increased rate and depth of breathing. This effect can be therapeutic, but it can also induce respiratory metabolic imbalance, which may manifest as a mild diffuse encephalopathy. In high doses, xanthines affect the spinal cord, which responds to stimulation with increased reflex excitability, tremulous extremities, and tense muscles.

Caffeine clearly alters sleep patterns. If taken within one hour of attempted sleep, caffeine increases sleep latency, decreases total sleep time, and worsens the subject's estimate of sleep quality. Less time is spent in stage 3 and 4 and more in stage 2. The popular concept that caffeine interferes with sleep is in fact well justified [3].

Xanthine seizures are seen as a complication of aminophylline therapy, especially when the drug is administered intravenously. Usually generalized, these seizures may be focal. The EEG pattern of periodic lateralized epileptiform discharges (PLED) is characteristic but not universal for these seizures. It has been suggested that the physiology of xanthine-induced epilepsy may relate to increased levels of cyclic adenosine monophosphate (cAMP), or to relative hypoxia due to the vasoconstrictor effect of the drug.

Numerous over-the-counter preparations have recently gained publicity because of their neurotoxic effects. These medications usually include high doses of caffeine with lesser amounts of phenylpropenolamine, plus an occasional third drug. Such agents are often manufactured to look like prescription medication and in the community are often referred to as over-the-counter amphetamines or "look-alikes." Such pills are also sold as street drugs and stimulants. Associated side effects have included headache, tremor, and agitation, but more importantly seizures and cerebrovascular accidents. The severe neurologic consequences may relate to the vasoactive properties of phenylpropenolamine, especially when combined with pseudoephedrine [21].

Nicotine is also a powerful stimulant and has no major therapeutic application. Its high toxicity and presence in tobacco smoke give nicotine a considerable medical importance, however. The drug alters both the peripheral and central nervous system. Clinically, tremors and convulsions are major neurologic signs of nicotine intoxication. Respiration is stimulated by medullary activation and also by chemoreceptor stimulation in the carotid aortic bodies. Vomiting results both from peripheral and central stimulation and the marked antidiuretic action of the drug results from hypothalamic stimulation. If acutely ingested, nicotine can be fatal at approximately 60 mg of the base product. Smoking tobacco usually contains 1-2 percent nicotine and it is estimated that each cigarette delivers 0.05-2.5 mg of nicotine. Gastric absorption of nicotine from tobacco taken by mouth is delayed because of slow gastric emptying, and nicotinic induced vomiting will remove much of the inadvertently taken toxin. If the patient has not vomited, vomiting should be induced with syrup of ipecac, and alkaline solutions should be avoided.

Autonomic overactivity with dilated pupils, irregular pulse, sweating, and twitching of the muscles are characteristic signs of nicotine toxicity. Coma may rapidly supervene, although convulsions are usually not present. If death occurs, it is due to the paralysis of respiratory muscles; artificial respiration is uniformly successful in preventing death in experimental animals. Cardiac arrhythmias are significant and are other potential sources for demise. Both suicidal and homicidal cases of nicotine poisoning have occurred. The famous 1843 case of Conte de Bocarme, whose wealthy brother-in-law was suspiciously found dead, brought nicotine poisoning to notoriety. When a fatal dose is ingested, death usually occurs within minutes to a few hours.

Chronic intoxication due to nicotine also occurs. Green tobacco pickers or "croppers" develop nausea, vomiting, dizziness, and prostration. The illness lasts intermittently between 12 and 24 hours and clears, only to recur when workers return to work. There are no mortalities or long-term sequelae, however. During the 1973 harvesting season, an estimated 9% of the 60,000 tobacco growers in North Carolina reported illnesses. Unusual manifestations of nicotine intoxication have included eighth nerve toxicity in a chronically exposed tobacco worker, and polyneuritis in an acutely intoxicated individual, although the significance of these features is difficult to ascertain since they are so rare.

■ HALLUCINOGENS

As described in the introduction to this chapter, the class of hallucinogens includes those drugs that effect hallucinations as their prominent attribute [36]. With these agents, there is no state of confusion or delirium as seen with agents like anticholinergic drugs that may cause hallucinosis amidst a more global encephalopathy. Phencyclidine is discussed separately, as it often has a confusional state accompanying the hallucination.

Biochemistry

Mescaline was the first hallucinogen to be discovered; it is a naturally occurring compound found in certain Mexican cacti. The chemical has been analyzed in detail with numerous substitutions made to test the relative activity of each grouping. Any substitute at the beta carbon or the terminal nitrogen abolishes activity, except if a methyl group is added at the alpha carbon, whereby activity of mescaline will double. With this alpha alteration, the molecule backbone structure becomes that of amphetamine. Methoxy substitution in the 2,4,5 and 3,4,5 positions appears to produce the most potent hallucinogens [2]. Unlike LSD, mescaline does not appear to alter serotonergic systems significantly. It has mild curarelike blocking effects at the neuromuscular cholinergic junction, which may be explained in part by its structural similarity to tubocurarine. This peripheral anticholinergic activity suggests the possibility that mescaline may also alter central nicotinic cholinergic receptors.

Mescaline itself can produce a wide range of psychotomimetic effects, including distortion of visual perception, illusions, visual as well as auditory hallucinations, and feelings of depersonalization. Alternatively, an intense feeling of personal significance for external and internal stimuli has been described. Aberle commented on a prayer meeting of the Navajo Indians where he wrote, "the user is prompted to ask of everything, what does this mean for me" [1]? The patient is not confused and the clear sensorium prompts the patient to be often more perplexed and awed by the situation than might be expected in a more confusional delirium.

The abuse of nutmeg, the seed of *Myristica fragrans,* as a hallucinogen relates to a naturally occurring amphetaminelike derivative in the nut oil. Neither mescaline nor phenylethylamine relatives occurs naturally in human or mammalian body fluids. The closest compound is 3,4-dimethoxyphenyl-ethylamine (pink spot compound), which may be a dietary product of ingested tea. In former studies, it was suggested that this product might relate to the pathophysiology of schizophrenia.

Hallucinogens related to tryptamine were first extracted from seeds of plants used as snuff in South American native ceremonies. The active component appears to be NN-dimethyl-tryptamine (DMT) and variations that include diethyltryptamine and dipropyltryptamine are both hallucinogenic and longer lasting than DMT. 5-Methoxydimethyltryptamine, also a natural ingredient in pergrina seeds of South America, is an even more potent hallucinogen. The mushroom *Psilocybe mexicana,* used by the Aztecs, has been shown to contain psilocybin (4-O-phosphoryl-DMT) and psilocin (4-OH-DNT). All these products bear a close structural relationship to serotonin, suggesting that the serotonergic system either through excessive agonism by the drugs, or partial antagonism by the drugs, relates to the pathophysiology of hallucinations. Amine hallucinations are typically exotic and elaborate with a clear sensorium [2]. Mushroom hallucinogens are discussed in Chapter 10.

The most potent known hallucinogen, active at doses as low as 25–100 micrograms by mouth, is lysergic acid diethylamide (LSD). It is a synthetic compound and is not found in nature, although it is structurally related to naturally occurring ergot preparations. Some of these compounds are discussed with botanical toxins and induce gangrenous and convulsive disorders. Naturally occurring ergot hallucinogens include lysergamide, lysergic acid, methylcarbonolamide, and lysergic acid propanolamide. Such lysergates which predate more modern chemical distillations may well have played a role in certain Aztec ceremonies and other ancient rituals. 250 micrograms of LSD will produce overwhelming voyages of fantasia, superimposed on a clear sensorium.

Stimulants and Hallucinogens

The pharmacology of LSD is perplexing. Its structural similarity to serotonin suggests an interaction with this neurotransmitter system and its effects appear rather selective to the S2 receptor site population. The primary source of brain serotonin is the raphe, located in the region of the midbrain and pons. The raphe projects axons to the cortex, including the frontal lobe, hippocampus, and visual area, as well as to the spinal cord. Serotonergic receptors have been identified in each of these three regions: S1, which are postsynaptic receptors in the cortex; S2, which are presynaptic (autoreceptors) in the raphe itself, and S3, which are receptors in the spinal cord. Serotonin of course is active in all three, but LSD may have preferential effects at the raphe. Since the usual activity of a presynaptic receptor is to provide inhibition, and the raphe is basically inhibitory to the visual cortex serotonergic system, selective activation of S2 receptors leads to "inhibited-inhibition," or facilitation. This electrical facilitation would activate the visual cortex and reasonably be associated with spontaneous visual illusions (hallucinations). LSD appears to have little effect on S1 receptors. LSD cannot be viewed as a global serotonergic agonist, since it has little effect peripherally. Other classic serotonergic blocking agents, like methysergide and cyproheptadine, appear to have much more peripheral serotonergic blocking activity than central effects.

The "presynaptic" theory of LSD activity has significant flaws and obviously is not a completely satisfactory explanation of the drug's hallucinogenic activity. In the cat, where much behavioral research with LSD is performed, destruction of the raphe does not induce LSD-like behavior. Furthermore, even when the raphe is lesioned, LSD can induce behavioral changes, demonstrating its activity inside the raphe region. Attempts to study the binding of ^{3}H-LSD and ^{3}H-5HT in brain membranes have demonstrated that 5-HT and LSD sites are quite similar, although there are some important differences. 5-HT showed one-hundred times more affinity for serotonin itself than for the LSD binding site, while the classical serotonin antagonist had more affinity for the LSD site. These studies suggest that LSD may bind to the 5-HT receptor in both its agonist and antagonist state. Mescaline does not fit to this serotonin model nearly so well, partly because of the curarelike effects that are described above.

LSD dramatically alters adrenergic mechanisms in the periphery and also acts as a partial agonist in the dopaminergic system. Small changes in the structure of the compound will change its hallucinogenic properties, so that studies only with pure LSD give definitive information. Clearly, the 9, 10 double bond in the LSD structure appears to be an essential component for hallucinogenic activity. Any variation in the structure appears to reduce hallucinogenic potency.

IATROGENIC AND MEDICINAL TOXINS

Clinical Features

Much has been written about the hallucinatory patterns seen with LSD. The subjects describe multiple feelings that may coexist, although usually euphoric effects predominate in the midst of the hallucination. Perceptual changes, such as micropsia or macropsia may occur, and the hallucinations may be overpowering in its magnificence or in its exquisite detail. Auditory hallucinations are rare with LSD, but Baudelairian synesthesias may occur, with colors being heard and sounds seen. During the hallucinatory experience, thoughts and memories can vividly emerge, often unexpectedly to the user's distress. Elation may suddenly shift to fear and tension may reach panic proportions. Although the half-life of LSD in man is approximately three hours, the entire "trip" begins to clear after about twelve hours. Although the user may be personally impressed with his apparent new sensitivity for art, human feelings, and the harmony of the world, there is little evidence for changes in beliefs or values after the LSD experience.

In addition to the hallucinogenic effects of LSD, the compound produces somatic effects that are largely sympathomimetic in nature, including pupillary dilatation, hypertension, tachycardia, postural tremor, nausea, pyeloerection and hyperthermia. Mydriasis and hyperreflexia may also occur [2].

The clinical description of LSD hallucinations is probably no different from that induced by the other hallucinogens. The dose and duration of action and administration route differ among agents. For instance, DMT is inactive by mouth, and must be injected, sniffed, or smoked [16]. LSD is longer acting, a hundred times more potent than psilocybin and psilocin, and four thousand times more potent than mescaline in producing altered states of consciousness. With LSD, the somatic effects are typically linked to the hallucinogenic effects, which are in contrast to DOET, where euphoria and self-awareness are produced without perceptual distortions in the lower dosage ranges.

A high degree of tolerance to the behavioral effects of LSD develops after three or four daily doses, although sensitivity returns after a drug-free period of approximately the same duration. There is significant cross-tolerance among LSD, mescaline, and psilocybin, but none between LSd and amphetamines. Withdrawal after LSD does not seem to occur. Suicides in the midst of an LSD intoxication have occurred, although deaths attributable to the direct effects of LSD are poorly established. In animals, death can occur from respiratory failure and hyperthermia.

The evidence for significant long-term psychological damage due to hallucinogens is not established. Surely, subjects complain of recurrence of the drug effects without ingesting the drug; these are called "flashbacks." The pharmacology of such events is puzzling, although they are effectively treated with reassurance. Subjects who expose themselves to hallucinogens often have a long-term history of depression, paranoid behavior, and prolonged psychotic episodes. Whether such episodes would have occurred without the drug has not been established [9]. Because of the phenomenon of kindling with cocaine and possibly amphetamine, there is concern that LSD used chronically could in fact induce a chronic hallucinatory state. Complaints that subtle abstract thinking may be altered after the chronic repeated use of LSD have been minimized by some authors [19].

The patient with hallucinogen intoxication should be protected from harming himself or others in the midst of his encephalopathy. Calming verbal contact is often enough to keep the patient manageable. Sedatives and phenothiazines have been used in patients who are excessively agitated or hyperactive, although low doses should be tried (chlorpromazine 50 mg; haloperidol 1 mg) to avoid drug interactions. Forced restraints can be emotionally harrowing for all concerned. No antidotes are available. A drug screen should be obtained from blood or urine samples to assess the possibility of multiple drug intoxication.

■ MISCELLANEOUS PSYCHOTROPIC AGENTS

MARIJUANA (CANNABINOIDS)

The active product in marijuana is derived primarily from the flowering top of hemp plants, although all parts of both the male and female plant contain psychoactive compounds. Most commonly, the plant is cut, dried, chopped and then incorporated into cigarettes.

Among the cannabinoids are cannabinol, cannabidiol, cannabinolic acid, and several other congeners. The isomer believed responsible for most of the psychological effects of marijuana is delta-9-THC or tetrahydrocannibinol. In man, this compound exerts its most prominent effects on the central nervous system and the cardiovascular system. The nervous system effects differ depending on the dose, route of administration, and the experience and expectation of the subject. It is estimated that in the United States, hemp plant content of delta-9-THC ranges from 0.5–6 percent.

Oral doses of 20 mg or a cigarette containing two percent delta-9-THC induces alterations in mood, memory, motor coordination, and self-perception. There is usually a sense of mild euphoria and well being, as well as relaxation. In an isolated environment, sleepiness may be a prominent feature, which contrasts significantly with the effects of LSD and hallucinogens, which induce heightened arousal. After several cigarettes, short-term memory is impaired and there is objective evidence of difficulty carrying out tasks requiring multiple mental steps [16]. Balance and stability of stance may be affected and driving and tasks requiring complex integration of perception and attention are impaired with as little as one or two cigarettes. Impairment produced by alcohol is additive to that of marijuana.

Higher doses of marijuana can produce frank hallucinations, delusions, and paranoid feelings. Thinking generally becomes confused and disorganized and subjects complain of depersonalization. Anxiety may be mild or can reach panic proportions, changing suddenly from the prior euphoria. Because the delta-9-THC content of marijuana in the United States is low, most users are able to regulate their dose in order to avoid the excessive dosage that produces these unpleasant effects. Importantly, however, schizophrenics appear to be particularly sensitive to the acute exacerbation of their symptomatology by marijuana [16].

Cardiac alterations include tachycardia, and an increase in systolic blood pressure. The heart rate appears to be dose-related with its onset and duration correlating rather well with the concentrations of delta-9-THC. Tremor, respiratory stimulation, and increases in deep tendon reflexes, so common with the other drugs discussed in the chapter, are not usually seen with marijuana. There is also a slight tendency toward hypothermia.

The pharmacologic mechanism of action of delta-9-THC is unknown. When subjects are pretreated with alphamethylparatyrosine, which reduces brain concentrations of dopamine and norepinephrine, the psychological effects are unaltered. This finding suggests that dopamine and norepinephrine activity is not directly related to the compounds' mental properties.

The long-term neurotoxicity of marijuana has been controversial. There have been reports of male sexual dysfunction, including decreased sperm motility and depressed testosterone levels in many users, although other studies failed to reveal any noticeable decreases in sexual potency or fertility. Subtle changes in personality, decreased interest in achievement and pursuit of conventional goals (amotivation) have been reported, although substantial evidence of personality change due to irreversible brain damage is lacking.

Abrupt discontinuation of cannabinoids after chronic use of high dosages is followed by irritability, nervousness, decreased appetite and weight loss, and there may be rebound increase in REM sleep.

Management of the intoxicated patient focuses mainly on protecting the individual from imprudent actions of self-injury during the time when the drug is active. Reassurance is essential, since the hallucinations may change from magnificent to intensively horrible very rapidly. Depending on the dose of medication ingested, the hallucinations may last several hours. Using sedatives is particularly dangerous as patients have often ingested multiple medications or adulterated street drugs.

PHENCYCLIDINE

Phencyclidine (PCP) has become an epidemic drug of abuse in urban North America. In particular, adolescents and young adults smoke the agent or ingest it in capsule or tablet form. The agent has mixed activity and alters many neurotransmitter systems; its clinical effects are dramatically variable. People with prior psychiatric illness appear to be exceptionally vulnerable, however, to PCP-induced psychosis. It is estimated that PCP is now the most common and most dangerous drug of significant abuse [17].

The drug is taken in order to produce a state of calm or "nothingness." Overdose with serum levels above 100 ng/ml renders the patient comatose with hypertension and generalized seizure activity. Chronic users may be ambulatory with the same high PCP blood levels, demonstrating only slurred speech and dulled sensorium.

From clinical studies, it appears that people who inhale 1-10 mg PCP have no significant psychiatric or physiologic impairment. Chronic exposure, however, may be associated with alterations in the threshold.

A major presenting problem with PCP toxicity is acute hallucinations and psychosis with schizophreniform or manic symptomatology. There may or may not be a clouded sensorium accompanying the psychosis. When the patient is confused, agitated, and delirious, he resembles a patient with acute anticholinergic toxicity more than one who has digested any of the hallucinogens already discussed. Some patients are withdrawn and catatonic, while others are euphoric and hyperkinetic. In the same patient, waxing and waning alterations in affect and motor activity may occur.

Prominent nystagmus is seen when this drug is ingested, and vomiting and hypersalivation may also be seen. There is no mydriasis. Opisthotonic posturing, especially in children, has been described, as well as seizure activity.

The curious complex of symptoms seen with PCP makes it imperative that it be kept in the differential diagnosis of suspected hallucinogen overdose, suspected hypnosedative overdose, and suspected stimulant or anticholinergic overdose. Importantly, when fluids are sent for analysis, gas chromatography with nitrogen detection ($GC-N_2$) is essential, since gas chromatography with flame ionization detection methods are often negative in spite of significantly toxic levels found by the former method [27].

PCP perturbs all neurotransmitter systems studied to date with prominent effects on cholinergic and adrenergic systems. There is a mild dopaminergic effect, as evidenced by animal studies, and PCP also increases serotonin concentrations in whole brain. It appears to have mixed effects on the cholinergic system in that it antagonizes the acetylcholine receptor and simultaneously has potent anticholinesterase activity. The overall effect, however, is one of predominant anticholinergic activity. Since the drug is so highly lipophilic, PCP is found in high concentrations in brain.

The specific management of the PCP-intoxicated patient depends on the clinical presentation. In all patients, a reduction in sensory stimulation is usually beneficial and a quiet room is recommended. When the patient is merely agitated, diazepam in divided doses may be given in order to keep the patient calm. Acidifying the urine by intravenous means or by oral intake of cranberry juice, ascorbic acid, or ammonium chloride will promote the excretion of PCP. When hypertension accompanies agitation, propranolol (40–80 mg, PO initially and 20–40 mg' TID) usually reduces sympathomimetic symptoms. Since these patients may be psychologically sensitive and agitated, extensive testing and manipulation with wires and tubing is to be avoided.

When the patient is confused and agitated or hallucinating, an anticholinesterase agent like physostigmine may be used. This will rapidly reverse the anticholinergic effect of PCP. Importantly, if there is any question that the patient may have ingested multiple drugs, the use of phenothiazines must be used with extreme caution. Seizures are usually managed with phenytoin; if the patient is intubated, then barbiturates can also be used.

In patients dying from phencyclidine overdose, the usual cause of death is respiratory depression. Hypertensive crisis followed by intracerebral hemorrhage and death have been reported [5]. An observation used by clinicians to suggest that an intoxicated patient has taken PCP is the bland nonchalance during venapuncture. Since this agent is an anesthetic, patients do not feel the needle and in spite of altered behavior and even violence, show little response to blood drawing.

■ STUDY QUESTIONS

An obese, chronic schizophrenic bank teller with a history of intermittent alcohol abuse last week stopped taking his maintenance neuroleptic drugs and 5 hours ago took a single dose of amphetamine for a new weight-reduction program. He presents to the emergency room hallucinating and combative and demonstrates upon examination severe irregular and involuntary lingual-facial-buccal movements as well as choreic movements of the extremities. Which are reasonable statements?

1. The alcohol, chronic neuroleptic exposure and schizophrenia probably have no direct impact on the patient's acute presentation since acute psychotic behavior and chorea are typical acute side-effects of amphetamine.
2. Since this patient recently stopped his neuroleptic, his dopaminergic receptor sites are heavily blocked and the amphetamine probably caused further blockade.

3. Amphetamine would precipitate the same type of choreic reaction with a prior history of Sydenham's chorea.
4. Methylphenidate should have been prescribed for a weight-conscious schizophrenic, since it has no dopaminergic activity centrally.

Answer: 3 only.

Essential parts of this patient's history include his past schizophrenic behavior and chronic exposure to neuroleptic drugs. Neuroleptic drugs block dopamine receptor sites and after chronic use it has been proposed that these receptor sites become hypersensitive to ambient dopamine. When the neuroleptics were stopped, the lingual-facial-buccal movements that appeared were termed tardive dyskinesia and theoretically related to the hypersensitive dopamine receptors no longer blocked by the neuroleptic. The exposure of dopaminergic receptors to an acute dose of amphetamine (a dopaminergic agonist) could precipitate new psychotic behavior and an exacerbation of the lingual-facial-buccal movements. Similarly, a patient with prior striatal damage in the form of Sydenham's chorea or occasionally in systemic lupus erythematosis could demonstrate the same unusual choreic response to a single dose of amphetamine. Ordinarily, chorea and psychosis are only seen in patients who ingest centrally active dopaminergic agonists over a chronic period of time. This could occur with amphetamines but could also occur with methylphenidate.

A patient is admitted to an acute emergency medical unit in great agitation. She is hallucinating and screaming that bugs are crawling under her skin and disfiguring her face. After 10 minutes in a quiet room, she calms down but is confused about the date and city. She sees the uniformed doctors and nurses and says that they are bakers "about to pop her into the flaming oven." Her skin is dry and hot although she is not perspiring. Serum and urine drug screens are sent but what drugs are significant possibilities for acute toxicity in this patient?

1. Amphetamine
2. Mescaline
3. LSD
4. Phencyclidine
5. Anticholinergic overdose
6. Cocaine

Answers: 4 and 5

The patient's presentation is that of a confusional delirium with hallucinosis. The presence of dry skin without dehydration is suggestive of anticholinergic toxicity. Phencyclidine also has anticholinergic properties and can present with a similar picture. Amphetamine, mescaline, LSD, and cocaine classically present with a clear sensorium and the very prominent confusional state of this patient would not be expected. Of course, often patients will ingest more than one agent, so this presentation does not obviate the physician from sending for an extensive serum and urine drug screen.

Amphetamine acts primarily to:

1. Block reuptake of dopamine.
2. Force release of dopamine.
3. Antagonize serotonergic receptors.
4. Antagonize dopamine and acetylcholine receptors.
5. Both 3 and 4

Answer: 2

Amphetamine is known as an indirect agonist in that it has little activity at the dopamine receptor itself but causes activation of the presynaptic stores of the neurotransmitter. As such, if the dopaminergic neurons are depleted of their dopamine, the administration of amphetamine has little impact. Drugs that classically block the reuptake of dopamine include amantadine and some tricyclic antidepressants. Drugs that stimulate directly the dopaminergic receptor site include apomorphine, bromocriptine, and newer experimental antiparkinsonian agents. Amphetamine has no known direct effect on the serotonergic system, although it does have agonist effects on the noradrenergic system.

A patient ingested phencyclidine (PCP) 3 hours ago and is now fluctuating between severe agitation and somnolence. Which of the following measures are indicated?

1. Prophylactic nitroprusside for the control of potential hypertension crisis.
2. Acidification of urine.
3. Atropine or another anticholinergic.
4. Phenothiazines.

Answer: 2

Acidifying the urine promotes the excretion of PCP and is an important aspect of treatment. Additionally, a quiet environment will often calm the patient. If hypertension is present, propranolol may be used, although the increased blood pressure is usually quite temporary. In those cases where agitation and confusion are prominent, physostigmine, an anticholinesterase agent, can quickly reverse the anticholinergic effect.

■ REFERENCES

1. Aberle DF: The Peyote Religion Among the Navaho. Wenner-Gren Foundation for Anthropological Research, Inc., New York, 1966.
2. Bradley RJ, Morley BJ, Barker SA, Smythies JR: Hallucinogens. In Handbook of Clinical Neurology, PJ Vinken and GW Bruyn, eds. Vol. 37, pp. 329-346, North-Holland Publishing Co., Amsterdam, 1979.
3. Curatolo PW, Robertson D: Health consequences of caffeine. Ann. Intern. Med. 98:641-653, 1983.
4. Denckla MB, Bemporad JR, Mackay MC: Tics following methylphenidate: 70 cases. JAMA 235:1349-1351, 1976.

5. Eastman JW, Cohen SN: Hypertensive crisis and death associated with phencyclidine poisoning. JAMA 231:1270-1271, 1975.
6. Ellinwood EH, Sudilovsky A, Nelson LM: Evolving behavior in the clinical and experimental amphetamine (model) psychosis. Am. J. Psychiatry 130: 1089-1093, 1973.
7. Espelin DE, Done AK: Amphetamine poisoning. N. Engl. J. Med. 278:1361-1365, 1968.
8. Fink JS, Smith GP: Mesolimbicocortical dopamine terminal fields are necessary for normal locomotor and investigatory exploration of rats. Brain Res. 199:359-384, 1980.
9. Freedman DX: The psychipharmacology of hallucinogenic agents. Ann. Rev. Med. 20:409-418, 1969.
10. Gerhards HJ, Carenzi A, Costa E: Effect of nomifensine on motor activity, dopamine turnover rate and 3'5'-adenosine monophosphate concentrations of rat striatum. Naunyn-Schmeidebergs Arch. Pharmacol. 286:49-59, 1974.
11. Giorguiett-Chesselet MF, Kemel ML, Wandscheer D, Glowinski J: Regulation of dopamine release by presynaptic nicotinic receptors in rat striatal slices: Effect of nicotine in a low concentration. Life Sci. 25:1257-1262, 1979.
12. Goetz CG, Klawans HL: Stimulant-induced chorea: Clinical studies and animal models: IN I. Creese, ed., Stimulants: Neurochemical Behavioral and Clinical Perspectives. Raven Press, New York, 1983.
13. Goldstein A, Kaizer S, Warren R: Psychotropic effects of caffeine. J. Pharmacol. Exp. Ther. 150:146-151, 1965.
14. Goodman S, Becker DP: Intracranial hemorrhage associated amphetamine abuse. JAMA 212:480-481, 1970.
15. Groves PM, Wilson CJ: Monoaminergic presynaptic axons and dendrites in rat locus coeruleus seen in reconstructions of serial sections. J. Comp. Neurol. 193:853-862, 1980.
16. Jaffe JH: Drug addiction and drug abuse. In AG Goodman, LS Gilman, A Gilman, eds., Pharmacologic Basis of Therapeutics, pp. 535-584. Macmillan, New York, 1980.
17. Johnson KM: Neurochemical pharmacology of phencyclidine. In RC Peterson and RC Stillman, eds., Phencyclidine (PCP) Abuse: An Appraisal, pp. 48-49. NIDA Research Monograph 21, 1978.
18. Kuczenski R: Biochemical actions of amphetamine and other stimulants. In I. Creese, ed., Stimulants: Neurochemical, Behavioral and Clinical Perspectives, pp. 31-61. Raven Press, New York, 1983.
19. McWilliams SA, Tuttle RJ: Long term psychological effects of LSD. Psychol. Bull. 79:341-351, 1973.
20. Moyer JH, Tashnek AB, Miller SI, Snyder H, Bowman RO: Effect of theophylline on cerebral hemodynamics. J. Clin. Invest. 31:267-272, 1952.
21. Mueller SM, Solow EB: Seizures associated with a new combination "pick-me-up" pill. Ann. Neurol. 11(3):322, 1982.
22. National Inst. Drug Abuse Capsule, March 17, 1978.

23. Nausieda PA: Central stimulant toxicity. In PJ Vinken and GW Bruyn, eds., Handbook of Clinical Neurology, Vol. 37, pp. 223-298. North-Holland Publishing Co., Amsterdam, 1979.
24. Ney PG: Psychosis in a child associated with amphetamine administration. Can. Med. Assoc. J. 97:1026-1029, 1967.
25. Oderda GM, Klein-Schwartz W: Central nervous stimulants. In VA Skoutakis, ed., Clinical Toxicology of Drugs, pp. 183-199. Lea & Febiger, Philadelphia, 1982.
26. Oderda GM, Klein-Schwartz W: Cocaine. IN VA Skoutakis, ed., Clinical Toxicology of Drugs, pp. 201-215. Lea & Febiger, Philadelphia, 1982.
27. Pitts FN, Yago LS, Aniline O, Pitts AF: Capillary GC-nitrogen detector measurement of phencyclidine (PCP), ketamine and other arylcycloalkylamines in the picogram range. J. Chromatogr. 193:157-160, 1980.
28. Post RM, Kopanda RT: Cocaine, kindling, and psychosis. Am. J. Psychiatry 133:627-634, 1976.
29. Rappolt RT, et al., Propranolol in cocaine toxicity. Lancet 2:640-641, 1976.
30. Schiorring E: Changes in individual and social behavior induced by amphetamine and related compounds in monkeys and man. In E. Ellinwood and M. Kilbey, eds., Cocaine and Other Stimulants. Plenum, New York-London, 1977.
31. Shukla D: Intracranial hemorrhage associated with amphetamine use. Neurology 32:917-918, 1982.
32. Siegel RK: Cocaine hallucinations. Am. J. Psych. 135:309-314, 1978.
33. Stefanis C, Dornbush R, Fink M, eds.: Hashish: Studies of Long-Term Use. Raven Press, New York, 1977.
34. Weiner WJ, Goetz CG, Nausieda PA, Klawans HL: Amphetamine induced hypersensitivity in guinea pigs. Neurology 29:1054-1057, 1979.
35. Wetli CV, Wright RK: Death caused by recreational cocaine use. JAMA 241:2519-2522, 1979.
36. Wikler A: Drug dependence. In AB Baker and LH Baker, eds., Clinical Neurology, pp. 1-73. Harper & Row, Philadelphia, 1980.

CHAPTER 15

Antibiotics

ANTIMICROBIAL drugs account for 20%-30% of all reported adverse drug reactions. Although most of these are not specifically neurologic, a number of well established neurologic syndromes have been associated with the use of these agents (see Table 15.1).

▪ ANTIBACTERIAL AGENTS

PENICILLINS

Despite wide use of penicillin agents, neurotoxic reactions are infrequent and cerebral reactions extremely uncommon. Historically, radiculitis, paraplegia, hemiplegia, and convulsions occurred after penicillin was administered into the cerebral spinal fluid either intrathecally, intraventricularly, or into the cisterna magnae. Since these modes of administration have been abandoned, such reactions are exceedingly rare, although seizures and myoclonic jerks have been reported after high intravenous doses of penicillin agents [2]. Penicillin G appears to be the most epileptogenic form of penicillin on a weight basis and has been responsible for the largest number of cases. Neurotoxic signs usually appear within 24-72 hours after beginning penicillin therapy and terminate within 48 hours after cessation of drug. In those with renal compromise, a longer clearance period is to be anticipated. Seizures usually do not respond to traditional anticonvulsant therapy, although paraldehyde has been used with some success. The incidence of seizures correlates with the concentration of penicillin in the cerebrospinal fluid. The EEG pattern usually is that of focal or generalized epileptiform activity.

IATROGENIC AND MEDICINAL TOXINS

TABLE 15.1 Neurotoxicity of Antibiotics

Antibiotic	Associated neurologic syndrome
Penicillins	Seizures, myoclonus, myopathy, (hypokalemia), sensory neuropathy
Aminoglycosides	Cranial nerve neuropathy, neuromuscular blockade, polyradiculitis
Polymyxin	8th cranial nerve neuropathy, neuromuscular blockade, peripheral neuropathy, seizures
Amphotericin B	Peripheral neuropathy, myelopathy, radiculopathy
Miconazole	Behavioral alterations
Isoniazid	Peripheral neuropathy, seizures, optic neuropathy, ataxia, meningitis, myalgia
Ethambutol	Peripheral neuropathy, optic neuropathy
Cycloserine	Behavioral changes with hallucinations, seizures, tremors, myoclonus
Ethionamide	Mental alterations, seizures, tremor
Sulfonamide	Peripheral neuropathy, behavioral alterations, cerebrovascular accidents, myelopathy
Chloroquine	Myopathy, dystonia, peripheral neruopathy, cranial nerve neuropathy (bilateral abducens nerves)
Metronidazole	Peripheral neuropathy, behavioral alterations
Nitrofurantoin	Peripheral neuropathy (similar to Guillain-Barré Syndrome), optic neuritis
Chloramphenicol	Peripheral neuropathy, behavioral alterations, 8th cranial nerve neuropathy, optic neuropathy
Tetracyclines	Neuromuscular blockade, pseudotumor cerebri, 8th cranial nerve neuropathy
Erythromycin	8th cranial nerve neuropathy
Lincomycin and Clindamycin	Neuromuscular blockade
Nalidixic acid	Seizures, behavioral alterations, pseudomotor cerebri

Myoclonus seen with penicillin may be isolated eye twitching or extensive continuous body jerks without loss of consciousness. Asterixis, a focal form of myoclonus, may also be seen. Myoclonus may occur in the absence of any EEG abnormality.

Neurotoxic effects appear more commonly in elderly patients with compromised renal function. The incidence of renal insufficiency (BUN greater than 25) in penicillin seizure patients ranges from 77% to 84%. The toxicity relates to the following: acidic drugs are bound poorly in uremic serum so that free penicillin circulates; poor renal clearance causes higher absolute blood and CSF levels [19]; the blood-brain barrier functions less efficiently in the uremic state. Menigitic inflammation may enhance neurotoxic effects by promoting the penetration of these drugs into the CSF and decreasing their egress. This is not, however, well established since seizures are characteristic of meningoencephalitis and in practice, it would be difficult to distinguish whether the disease or the treatment is more responsible.

An additional risk factor that may be associated with increased blood-brain barrier penetration of penicillin is the underlying disease state for which penicillin is prescribed. It is known from laboratory studies that multiple microemboli can disrupt blood-barrier function. Since patients with vasculopathies, cardiovalvular disease, and cardiopulmonary bypass surgery are often exposed to penicillin, and are often at high risk for embolic disease, they may be victims of penicillin-related toxic signs. The mechanism of neurotoxicity of penicillin is as yet unestablished, although alteration in electrolytic flux at the cellular level of cortical tissue has been demonstrated in vitro after penicillin administration [26].

A final risk factor appears to be the mode of administration. Continuous infusion of penicillin, currently relatively obsolete, was found to account for the highest incidence of penicillin-related toxic signs [6]. Two other toxic signs are associated with penicillin drugs, although they are more related to the vehicle rather than the penicillin moiety. A wide variety of neurologic symptoms have been associated with procaine penicillin G, but appear to relate to procaine toxicity. These include altered behavior states ranging from anxiety and unexplained apprehension to wild and bizarre violent behavior. Generalized muscle weakness related to hypokalemia may also be seen when the sodium salts of penicillin are used. Potassium levels must be carefully monitored during penicillin therapy, since this form of toxicity is fully reversible by cation supplementation.

A curious acute sensory neuropathy associated with penicillin or penicillin analogs has been reported in three patients. A profound sensory ataxia with widespread sensory loss in the face and body and no motor impairment developed during antibiotic therapy and did not significantly improve even after withdrawal of antibiotic drugs. The clinical picture resembles the sensory neuronopathy associated with malignancy and has features distinctive from demyelinating or axonal neuropathies. The investigators suggest that the likely pathologic basis is in the dorsal roots and ganglia as well as the gasserian ganglia to explain the selective sensory features in the body and face [24].

AMINOGLYCOSIDES

The toxicity of all aminoglycoside antibiotics—neomycin, kanamycin, streptomycin, gentamycin, tobramycin, and amikacin—is similar. There are two major adverse affects of aminoglycosides: first, damage to the eighth cranial nerve and hearing apparatus and second, a potentiation of neuromuscular blockade. Cochlear and vestibular damage are the result of direct toxicity of these drugs. The exact incidence of such toxicity depends on the definition of hearing loss or vestibulopathy, since different studies have used different measurement instruments and criteria for definitions. The Boston Collaborative Drug Surveillance group demonstrated that aminoglycoside antibiotics are the most frequent cause of drug-induced deafness in the hospital setting, 1.3 cases per hundred exposed patients, markedly in excess of those cases reported for aspirin and quinidine [1]. Other studies indicate the incidence of clinical ototoxicity ranges from 5%-25% depending on whether audiometry or other measures were used to detect the hearing deficit [16]. Aminoglycosides differ in their ability to cause auditory or vestibular toxicity. Whereas streptomycin and gentamycin induce predominantly vestibular damage, amikacin, kanamycin and neomycin provoke predominantly auditory damage. Tobramycin produces equal vestibular and auditory toxic signs.

Early detection of hearing losses is felt to be essential, since dead hair cells are not replaced. The earliest detectable sign is usually loss of high-frequency reception, which cannot be detected as conversational hearing difficulties. Since these early signs are often reversible, apparently such abnormalities are not linearly related to hair death. Once extensive hair death has been induced, one would anticipate poor resolution even after withdrawal of the antibiotic. In over 80% of abnormal audiograms, the damage is bilateral.

Vestibular toxicity is manifested by the patient with complaints of vertigo or dizziness and in the laboratory by electonystagmographic caloric changes. Vestibular damage may occur insidiously or be cataclysmic, mimicking Menière's disease. The causation can be confusing because in up to 15% of cases vestibular signs occur 10-14 days after stopping the antibiotic.

The risk factors for the development of ototoxicity have been studied in a variety of ways. A recent prospective study indicated that the significant risk factors included: the patient developing a high temperature during therapy, the total dose of antibiotic received, a high creatinine clearance for cochlear toxicity, a poor medical condition or critically ill state, and a duration of therapy greater than ten days [5]. Nonsignificant variables included the dose rate per day, absolute serum levels, age, prior noise exposure, prior aminoglycoside exposure and prior ear infections. Importantly, in this study the serum levels never exceeded the recommended maximum blood levels of drug. Since increased risk of ototoxicity is seen when trough or peak levels are excessive, recommendations for three typical aminoglycosides are given in Table 15.2.

Age greater than 60 years may be an additional risk factor due primarily to the altered creatinine clearance. Although significant ototoxic signs have

TABLE 15.2 Aminoglycosides and Ototoxicity

Drug	Peak level (mcg/cc) should not exceed	Trough level (mcg/cc) should not exceed
Gentamycin	8	2-3
Tobramycin	10	2
Amikacin	32	10

From: MF Parry, Antibiotic neurotoxicity. In A. Silverstein, Neurologic Complications of Therapy. Futuro Publishing, Mount Kisco, New York, 1982.

not been seen in most newborns exposed to aminoglycosides, individual cases of drug-associated deafness in babies have been reported.

Drug level and renal function must be assessed frequently and dosage adjusted accordingly. Fee suggests the important addition of the baseline audiogram as soon as the patient's medical condition will allow it to be practically obtained. Following this baseline test, follow-up testing should be performed. There is animal data suggesting that aminoglycoside toxicity is more pronounced in a noisy environment. Since many patients who receive aminoglycosides are temporarily housed in an intensive care unit or in close proximity to noisy medical equipment, Fee suggests an attempt to diminish noise around the patient and especially to avoid noisy environments after hospitalization [5].

Interestingly, intraventricular and intrathecal administration of aminoglycoside antibiotics have not been associated with high incidences of ototoxicity. This finding suggests that such toxic signs relate more to serum than to CSF concentrations. These data, however, are not firm since patients receiving CSF aminoglycosides are often exceedingly ill and vestibular or audiologic testing may not be feasible.

Intrathecal kanamycin and gentamycin may induce polyradiculitis, with paresthesias, paralysis, and loss of tendon reflexes. Whether this effect relates to the aminoglycoside itself or to its vehicle is unknown.

A potentially fatal neurotoxic effect of all aminoglycosides is neuromuscular blockade. Rapid absorption from a large epithelial surface or rapid intravenous infusion may result in respiratory paralysis. Neuromuscular blockade is believed to be the result of curarelike effects of the aminoglycosides and possibly competition with calcium by these antibiotics [16]. The result is a nondepolarizing, flaccid paralysis. The effects are enhanced by anesthesia, and other neuromuscular blocking agents such as tubocurarine and pancuronium bromide and magnesium ions. Aminoglycosides may further potentiate ether and other drugs used to induce muscular relaxation during anesthesia. The aminoglycoside activity can be effectively antagonized by calcium ions, but only slightly by neostigmine. Electromyographic studies of the patient under neuromuscular blockade are similar to those seen with curare. In addition to the curarelike effect, there is additional depression of acetylcholine release after stimulation. The combined pre- and postsynaptic effects help to explain the activity of the aminoglycoside antibiotics.

The aminoglycosides may induce neuromuscular blockade when used alone, but the usual report is that of a marked neuromuscular blockade in association with anesthesia. Importantly, there is potentiation of neuromuscular dysfunction in patients with botulism, myasthenia gravis, and Guillain-Barré when they receive aminoglycosides. For this reason, such drugs should be used with extreme caution and best avoided in such situations. With such neuromuscular blockade there is significant compromise of respiratory function and a high risk of aspiration pneumonia and respiratory arrest. There is depression of the gag reflex, decrease in diaphragmatic movements, and a poor tidal volume. Hence, patients with nonneuromuscular diseases or with poor pulmonary reserve, such as those with chronic obstructive lung disease, should also avoid aminoglycosides whenever possible.

The practical management of neuromuscular blockage, once present, involves the prompt discontinuation of the causative aminoglycoside. Calcium and neostigmine have been associated with reversal, although this is not a predictable effect in humans. Other less common nervous system symptoms associated with aminoglycoside therapy consist of transient diplopia, scotomas, blurring of vision, dysesthesias in the distribution of the fifth cranial nerve or perioral paresthesias, paralysis of the vocal cords, toxic psychosis, and convulsive movements [11]. Intrathecal injection may cause pain and spasm of the erector spinae muscles accompanied by radicular pain, meningismus, twitching of the leg muscles, and finally, convulsions and stupor.

SULFONAMIDES

Sulfonamides, pyrimethamine, and trimethoprim inhibit the synthesis of tetrahydrofolinic acid, the one-carbon donor needed for the synthesis of methionine, serine, and purines. Mainly used in the treatment of urinary tract infections, these drugs are associated with a low incidence of neurotoxicity. A variety of uncommon adverse reactions, however, occur during therapy, the pathogenesis of which is not understood. Included among these are headache, fatigue, tinnitus and acute psychosis [13]. These may be accompanied by stiff neck and fever, simulating the symptoms of a meningitis [15]. Euphoria, nausea, vomiting, and somnolence may be observed on the second or third day of therapy, with the patient complaining of difficulty in concentration and some impairment of judgment. In some instances, generalized convulsions may occur. A wide variety of scattered focal symptoms have been reported, such as agraphia, aphasia, stammering, altered distance perception, teleopsia, and macropsia. Polyneuritis occurs in a small number of cases and myelitic symptoms with weakness of the lower extremities or paraplegia are seen occasionally [7].

Pathologically, a variety of lesions have been reported in fatal cases of sulfonamide intoxication, including focal necrosis and demyelination of the cerebral white matter, hypothalamus, and pons, as well as hemorrhages in the fourth ventricle, brain stem, cerebral gray matter, and nuclear structures. The vascular endothelium is swollen and necrotic, often with occlusion of the vessel lumen. The spinal cord may show neuronal changes with fragmentation of the myelin.

The pathophysiology of the neurotoxic signs may relate to a drug-induced hypersensitivity reaction, since they often occur in the context of a larger serum sickness or drug-induced vasculitis. In cases of neurotoxicity seen with combination sulfamethoxazole-trimethoprim (Bactrim, Septra), neurotoxicity is felt to relate to the sulfonamide moiety; this conclusion is based on the observation that the signs seen resemble those described with sulfonamides alone and that trimethoprim has no well-established neurotoxicity of its own.

NITROFURANTOIN

Nitrofurantoin is a commonly used drug in the treatment of chronic or recurrent urinary tract infections. Neurologic toxicity occurs in approximately 0.2% of all patients receiving the drug. A single significant neurological syndrome has been associated with nitrofurantoin, a progressive and often disabling polyneuropathy. This neuropathy is usually seen in patients who have been receiving the drug for several days (80% developing symptoms after less than 45 days of treatment). Similar to the Guillain-Barré syndrome, this neuropathy is usually subacute, and begins in the distal extremities, often with sensory complaints of paresthesias or numbness. Vibratory and position sense may be more affected than pain or temperature sensation at this early point. The neuropathy ascends and involves the motor system with progressive weakness and areflexia. When recognized, drug discontinuation is essential, although 10%-15% of patients will not improve and 15% will have only partial recovery. The prognosis appears to relate most significantly to the extent of the neuropathy at the time of drug withdrawal, but not to the total dose exposure, the duration of therapy, or to the age or sex of the patient. If the drug is continued, neuropathy progresses and respiratory changes have also been described in unusual cases [19].

The peripheral neuropathy associated with nitrofurantoin does not appear to be an allergic phenomenon as is pulmonary toxicity, since eosinophilia is not present. The spinal fluid in such patients is usually normal, although in 25% of patients there is a slight increase in protein, which in no way approaches the high levels seen in typical Guillain-Barré syndrome. There is no pleocytosis. Pathologic changes include demyelination, axonal swelling, and Wallerian degeneration of the peripheral nerve. Such changes may extend into the root, and even anterior horn cells may show chromatolysis. Importantly, there is no local information.

CHLORAMPHENICOL

Chloramphenicol, although associated with one of the most feared and notorious adverse effects of any medication—aplastic anemia—causes few other undesirable reactions. Toxic encephalopathy with symptoms of confusion and delirium has been reported after use of more than 8 grams of chloramphenicol daily. Underlying neoplastic disease, liver and renal dysfunction may predispose to excessive drug accumulations and hence to toxic encephalopathy. Prolonged therapy with high doses ($>$ 2 grams/kg) of chloramphenicol has been associated with the production of reversible optic neuritis. Most patients who develop decreased visual acuity while receiving chloramphenicol have had cystic fibrosis, and the direct relationship of the drug or disease to the visual compromise is unclear [10].

The optic neuropathy is sudden in onset and associated with decreased visual acuity and ocular pain. The optic discs are hyperemic and edematous. Pathologically, ganglian cells in the macular and perimacular region are degenerated. Early edema is followed by atrophy of the papillomacular bundle. The degree of these findings dose not correlate well with the visual compromise, since the clinical syndrome is relatively reversible. There may be some residual constriction of visual fields and mildly diminished acuity.

Ototoxicity has been reported after chloramphenicol installation into the middle ear. In most of the cases reported, the patients had multiple drug therapy or an underlying condition that could have left residual hearing deficits. Thus, a causal relationship has not been firmly established in man. In animals, however, installation of chloramphenicol into the middle ear does induce sensorineural hearing loss [21].

Finally, a peripheral neuropathy may occur in association with chloramphenicol therapy and often accompanies the optic neuropathy. The neuropathy is predominantly sensory, so that patients complain of numbness and paresthesias predominantly in a distal distribution over the feet.

Chloramphenicol inhibits the metabolism of phenytoin and phenobarbital, and there will be a marked elevation in anticonvulsant blood levels of patients receiving the antibiotic and anticonvulsant. This effect occurs quickly, and therefore immediate adjustment of anticonvulsant dose must be effected to avoid toxicity. The practical management of seizure patients who require chloramphenicol must include careful monitoring of the blood level of the anticonvulsants. Once the chloramphenicol is stopped, the blood levels of anticonvulsants will quickly plummet, and thus augmentation of phenytoin or phenobarbital must be initiated when chloramphenicol is stopped.

OTHER ANTIBACTERIAL AGENTS

Tetracyclines

The neurotoxicity of tetracycline drugs is uncommon, although the syndrome of pseudotumor cerebri or "benign" intracranial hypertension occurs rarely in children and infants taking tetracycline. The syndrome is characterized by headache, papilledema, elevated cerebral spinal fluid pressure and, in the babies, bulging fontanels. Visual disturbances may also occur as well as sixth nerve paresis. Signs and symptoms disappear within a few days after drug discontinuation, although papilledema may persist for weeks.

Significant vestibular toxicity has been associated with a tetracycline derivative, minocycline, in approximately 50% of patients; it is more common, however, in females, where toxicity is estimated at 70% [4]. The vestibular toxic reaction is seen within three days of therapy. The patient will complain of lightheadedness, unsteady gait, nausea and extreme vertigo. Such complaints may precede any electronystagmogram abnormality. The toxicity correlates well with achievement of a threshold blood level and this correlation may explain the higher toxicity in women, who have a smaller blood volume and hence higher blood levels of tetracycline on a fixed-dose schedule. Although vestibular toxicity is more likely in patients with pre-existing vestibular disease or a past history of vestibular abnormalities, many patients have no prior history of balance or inner ear difficulties and yet exhibit vestibular toxicity with tetracycline. The reaction is transient, and even in the most severe cases, usually resolves within five days.

Erythromycin

Erythromycin is probably the least toxic of the commonly used antibiotics [9]. An uncommon side effect of this agent is temporary hearing loss [12]. This reaction has occurred during treatment with 4 grams or more of the lactonate derivate of oral erythromycin and is reversible with dosage reduction or discontinuation. The patient's complaints are usually those of tinnitus rather than of distinct difficulty hearing. Since the erythromycin is metabolized by the liver, those patients with hepatic abnormalities may be at higher risk for this ototoxic reaction.

Erythromycin interacts with carbamazepine, and carbamazepine levels rapidly increase when erythromycin is introduced. Careful monitoring of the carbamazepine blood level should be performed on all patients who receive erythromycin; the clinical symptoms of carbamazepine toxicity (slurred speech, ataxia, mental changes) must be closely evaluated for such patients.

IATROGENIC AND MEDICINAL TOXINS

Lincomycin and Clindamycin

Lincomycin and clindamycin are remarkably free from adverse reactions other than the well-known gastrointestinal disorders of pseudomembranous colitis and diarrhea. Potentiation of neuromuscular blockade has rarely complicated therapy with these antibiotics, but since this effect is potentially threatening, it must be rapidly identified [20]. Lincomycin or clindamycin should be considered possible causes of prolonged postoperative respiratory depression in patients receiving curarelike neuromuscular blocking agents. Respiratory depression, however, is only one-tenth as common as that seen with aminoglycoside antibiotics [28]. Although the clinical syndrome resembles that seen with aminoglycosides, clindamycin induces muscle relaxation by an effect on the contractility and not by effecting neuromuscular transmission directly. Hence, unlike the aminoglycoside-induced paralysis, calcium and neostigmine may have no effect. Lincomycin, in addition, induces both neuromuscular blockade and direct muscle relaxation. Practical management of lincomycin-induced paralysis could include calcium supplementation. A final possibly neurotoxic effect of lincomycin has been gustatory dysfunction.

Nalidixic Acid

Nalidixic acid is an antiseptic product used predominantly in the treatment of urinary tract infections. Visual disturbances occur in up to 20% of patients receiving nalidixic acid. Patients complain of halo vision, changes in color perception, and visual hallucinations. The visual disturbances are rapidly reversible with discontinuation of the drug. Altered behavioral states may accompany such visual problems and may range from mild agitation and anxiety to severe delirium and psychotic behavior. These mental symptoms usually occur when the drug is at its peak level and disappear rapidly when the medication is stopped. Convulsions have occurred in patients who have received nalidixic acid; they are estimated to be more frequent in patients who have renal failure, since this drug is cleared by the kidney. Such seizures may be accompanied by hyperglycemia, the cause of which is unknown. Finally, the syndrome of "pseudotumor cerebri" or "benign" intracranial hypertension has been rarely described. This occurs usually in young children or infants and is similar to the syndrome described under tetracyclines. The syndrome quickly resolves with cessation of the medication, although the papilledema may remain for weeks.

Antibiotics

■ ANTITUBERCULOUS DRUGS

ISONIAZID (INH)

INH is associated with two types of neurotoxic effects: those related to acute, high-dose intoxication and those related to chronic exposure. In both instances, the toxicity relates at least in part to an interaction between INH and pyridoxine. In the case of acute toxicity, direct toxic effects of INH may also be responsible for neurologic symptoms [23]. INH inhibits the phosphorylation of pyridoxine and chelates whatever pyridoxal phosphate remains. The latter effect is more significant in acute intoxication and probably relates to the induction of convulsions. In chronic toxicity, INH predominantly inhibits the phosphorylation of pyridoxine to induce a peripheral neuropathy.

Acute INH intoxication due to intentional of inadvertent overdosage is associated with severe ataxia, generalized seizures, altered behavior including psychosis, and coma. Metabolic acidosis, hyperglycemia, and aceturia may accompany the acute neurologic syndrome. Pyridoxine should be administered immediately, along with standard anticonvulsants and supportive measures needed to restore metabolic homeostasis. The acute toxic syndrome usually occurs when a subject ingests more than 6 grams in a single dose, or with less in the presence of renal insufficiency, malnutrition, alcoholism, or a co-existing seizure disorder. Since pyridoxal phosphate is a cofactor important to the GABA system, it has been hypothesized that the diminished GABA activity centrally may relate to the pathophysiology of INH-induced seizures. Clearly, however, the direct involvement of the GABA system has not been demonstrated, and pyridoxine is a cofactor for numerous decarboxylation reactions.

A prominent polyneuropathy is associated with chronic INH administration, presenting with paresthesias and diminished temperature discrimination, position sense loss, and eventual weakness. This neurotoxic syndrome is dose-related and most common in "slow inactivators," alcoholics, and patients with malnutrition. INH is predominantly metabolized by the liver and in those patients with bilirubin levels greater than 2.0 mg/dl, significant dosage adjustment may be required. It has been estimated that 40% of patients receiving more than 15 mg/kg/day and 10% receiving 6–15 mg/kg/day will develop neuropathy [19]. An additional form of neuropathy, also preventable by concurrent treatment with pyridoxine, is optic neuropathy.

More unusual INH-related neurotoxic syndromes include a drug-induced systemic lupus erythematosis picture with meningitis. Patients present with meningeal signs, CSF pleocytosis, and elevated protein but normal glucose.

Seizures may occur in such patients and the treatment is withdrawal of the causative drug and administration of adrenal corticosteroids. Myalgias and ataxia may also occur with or without the peripheral neuropathy described above. Again the treatment is withdrawal of the INH. Since seizures are a complication of INH therapy, this drug is not recommended for patients with preexisting seizure disorders if another drug can be chosen. When INH is required in patients already receiving anticonvulsant therapy, the dosage of the latter drugs may have to be adjusted, since INH decreases the clearance of such agents as phenytoin. Careful monitoring of drug serum levels during the treatment phase with INH is essential.

OTHER ANTITUBERCULOSIS DRUGS

Ethambutol

With ethambutol, reversible optic neuritis may occur at a dose of 25 mg/kg/day. At the currently recommended dose $\leq$ 15 mg/kg/day, the incidence of optic neuritis is less than 0.1%. Bilateral visual acuity deficits have been reported in patients on prolonged low-dose ethambutol therapy. The drug should be stopped after the first sign of visual change; recovery can be anticipated although it may require weeks to months. The baseline visual acuity test prior to ethambutol therapy with follow-up visual acuity testing at periodic levels may detect visual change at the earliest point. Rarely, blindness has been associated with this drug, although the doses were always above 15 mg/kg/day and the drug was continued when the patient was demonstrating declining visual acuity. The optic neuropathy appears to be a demyelinating process, and the reason for the optic nerve's sensitivity to this drug is unknown. Other side effects include a metallic taste in the oral cavity, which is frequently associated with ethambutol, and which may be due to impairment of receptor activity, alteration of sensory cellular function, or a defect in impulse transmission [22]. A mild peripheral neuropathy may also occur, but is not a common finding.

Cycloserine

Cycloserine is a severely neurotoxic product and is currently used only in the treatment of drug-resistant tuberculosis. Significant neurotoxic signs occur in 10% of patients receiving 1 gram cycloserine/day. Usually these are behavioral changes that may range from mild depression or anxiety to severe psychotic reactions with hallucinations and confused bizarre behavior. Additionally, myoclonus, unusual tremors, and even seizures may occur. Such problems are dose-related and reverse when the drug is stopped. Patients who have a co-existing seizure disorder are probably at a greater risk for the cycloserine epileptic toxicity. Even when the dose of cycloserine is reduced to less than 500 mg/day, significant neurotoxicity occurs in 3%-5% of patients [19]. Whether the neurotoxicity of this drug relates to a direct effect on the central nervous system or is an indirect result of calcium, magnesium, and pyridoxine alterations is undetermined. Pyridoxine has been administered in those patients suffering with neurotoxic signs; electrolytes and calcium must be carefully monitored in such patients.

Ethionamide

Ethionamide, also used in the treatment of drug-resistant tuberculosis, may induce an unusual mental aberration. Depression, anxiety and psychotic changes may occur but are significantly rarer than those seen with cycloserine. Also tremor, visual disturbances, and seizures have been reported. Pyridoxine administration has been associated with improvement. After ethionamide is stopped, recovery may take several days.

Rifamycin, para-aminosalicylic acid, and pyrazinamide are not associated with established neurotoxic syndromes, although asymptomatic xanthochromia of the cerebrospinal fluid has been seen in some patients receiving rifamycin.

■ ANTIFUNGAL AGENTS

Polymyxins are closely related to the aminoglycosides in structure and in neurotoxicity. The incidence of neurotoxic reactions to the polymyxins has been estimated at 7%. Most of the reactions are transient and completely reversible with discontinuation of therapy. The various unusual adverse effects of polymyxins include paresthesias, peripheral neuropathy, diplopia, dysphagia, muscle weakness, dizziness, seizures, confusion, and psychosis. However, with aminoglycoside therapy, respiratory paralysis is the most serious neurotoxic reaction to polymyxin administration. Underlying renal dysfunction predisposes to neuromuscular blockade induced by this drug group, and as many as 2% of treated patients have been observed to develop respiratory insufficiency [17]. Prodromal symptoms of dyspnea, restlessness, diplopia and weakness may precede respiratory paralysis. Because the mechanism of this drug-induced respiratory depression is unknown, treatment lies with ventilatory support and drug withdrawal upon recognition of the prodromal symptoms. Like the aminoglycosides, polymyxins may increase the effect of neuromuscular blocking agents used in anesthesia.

Ototoxicity is the final adverse neurotoxic syndrome, but this is seen with topical therapy and is less well-documented after a parenteral administration. Hearing deficits have been seen after drug installation in the ear canal and polymyxin in otitis is to be cautioned, especially if the tympanic membrane is perforated. With parenteral administration, ataxia and vertigo with staggering gait have been reported, but whether these effects relate directly to eighth nerve or ear damage is not known. Such signs disappear with cessation of polymyxin treatment.

Amphotericin B is an effective agent against systemic fungal infection. Neurotoxic effects are associated primarily with its intrathecal use, although seizures have been reported on a presumed anaphylactic basis [8]. Intrathecal use of the drug has been associated with pain along lumbar nerves, mononeuropathies including foot drop, chemical meningitis, difficulty with micturition, and paresthesias [27]. Headache and impaired vision have also been reported. Myelopathy may relate to direct spinal cord damage or to vascular compromise. Although the amphotericin B molecule binds to sterols in cell membranes of fungi and thereby promotes its antifungal effect, it may be cross-reactivity at the host cell membrane that underlies the neurotoxic signs.

Miconazole is a broad-spectrum antifungal drug that has been associated with various behavioral changes like euphoria and lightheadedness when administered intravenously. Rarely, a toxic psychosis may accompany miconazole therapy; The drug also may induce inappropriate ADH secretion and thereby provoke various electrolyte imbalances that can precipitate mental alterations and diffuse weakness [25].

■ ANTIMALARIAL AGENTS AND PROTOZOACIDES

Chloroquine is an antimalarial agent associated with uncommon and mild neurotoxicity. Headache, visual disturbances, nausea, and tinnitus with progressive hearing loss may occur. Optic nerve dysfunction may appear as scotomatous field defects, decreased acuity or, rarely, optic atrophy. Abnormal involuntary movements including torticollis, blepharospasm, and dystonic tongue protrusion have occurred during chloroquine therapy, especially in patients under 30 years of age. As with other drug-induced dystonias, intravenous anticholinergic agents usually reverse the abnormality [3].

Chloroquine has also been advocated for the treatment of rheumatoid arthritis. Peripheral neuropathy, cranial nerve palsies, and myopathy have been described in these chronically treated patients. The peripheral neuropathy is a distal, sensorimotor polyneuropathy that is reversible after drug withdrawal [18]. Bilateral abducens nerve paralysis, also reversible with cessation of chloroquine therapy, has been described.

The neuropathy associated with prolonged high-dose chloroquine administration is often characterized by proximal weakness with less severe bulbar compromise that develops over several weeks.

Antibiotics

Metronidazole, a 5-nitroimidazole compound, is a well-established protozoacide used in the treatment of trichomoniasis, giardiasis, and amebiasis, and has been used to control Crohn's disease. With conventional oral doses of the drug, a peripheral neuropathy may develop that is predominantly distal and sensory. Although full recovery usually occurs after withdrawal of the drug, it is important to identify the cause early, since pathologic investigation has shown a major degree of nerve degeneration in affected patients. Confusion, irritability, depression, and headache as well as a peculiar metallic phantoguesia have been reported as additional drug complications [14]. High doses of metronidazole (total dose exceeding 50 gr over a 21-day period) have recently been introduced as a radiosensitizing dose in patients with advanced malignancies. In these cases, generalized convulsions and a profound sensory neuropathy temporally coincident with the introduction of the drug have been reported. Since only 7% of the drug is excreted unmetabolized in the urine, renal insufficiency does not appear to be associated with an increased incidence of neurotoxicity.

▪ STUDY QUESTIONS

A patient without neurologic disability receives procaine penicillin treatment and develops wild, belligerent behavior. The neurologic exam reveals a delirious state, but no focal findings. Blood gases are normal. Which statements are true?

1. The patient deserves a spinal tap to evaluate for possible meningitis.
2. Spinal taps are contraindicated for patients with suspected penicillin encephalopathy because of fear of likely herniation.
3. The clinical picture could be caused by the procaine or the penicillin.
4. The patient has the picture of a chemically induced myasthenia gravis.

Answer: 1 and 3

A patient with systemic infection and a change in mental status must receive a lumbar puncture to evaluate for the possibility of infectious spread to the meninges. Penicillin itself is not associated with frequent neurologic syndromes, and the encephalopathy in the above case would be due to either the drug or the procaine. If penicillin is a needed antibiotic, a switch-over to another form could be reasonable. Penicillin is not associated with a myasthenic syndrome and furthermore mental changes in the absence of hypoxia are not seen in myasthenia gravis.

Aminoglycosides should be avoided in all patients with the following disorders:

1. Diphtheria
2. Botulism
3. Myasthenia gravis
4. Seizure disorder

Answers: 2 and 3

Aminoglycosides block neuromuscular transmission and hence are dangerous in any patient with already underactive neuromuscular junctions. Such patients would include those with botulism, since botulinum toxin decreases release of presynaptic/prejunctional acetylcholine. Also, patients with myasthenia gravis should not receive aminoglycosides, since in myasthenia, there is a blockade by antibodies to muscle acetylcholine receptors at the neuromuscular junction. Polymyxins, clindamycin, and lincomycin also provoke neuromuscular blockade and should be avoided. Diphtheria and seizures are not specifically affected by such drugs.

As a class, antibiotics are not associated with high neurotoxic risks. Which of the following, however, are exceptions to this rule and are associated with a high incidence of neurotoxicity?

1. Penicillin
2. Cycloserine
3. Trimethoprim
4. Chlorophenol
5. Minocycline
6. Erythromycin

Answers: 2 and 5

With cycloserine, mental alterations, myoclonus and seizures are frequent and even when the dose is decreased to the range of 500 mg/day, neurotoxicity occurs in up to 5% of patients. Minocycline provokes ototoxicity in 50%–70% of cases, with higher incidence in females.

Pyridoxine is useful in which of the following instances:

1. Acute management of neurotoxicity related to INH overdose.
2. Chronic prevention of INH-induced peripheral neuropathy.
3. Both
4. None.

Answer: 3

INH neurotoxicity relates to its effects on pyridoxine and possible GABA function so that pyridoxine supplementation is important to both acute and chronic toxic cases. The marked INH chelation of pyridoxyl phosphate that occurs with acute overdose should be counteracted with pyridoxine therapy. Regular pyridoxine supplementation along with INH is felt to inhibit the likelihood of optic neuritis and peripheral neuritis. The situation is complicated in such cases as tuberculosis, where peripheral neuropathy can develop in association with INH treatment.

REFERENCES

1. Boston Collaborative Drug Surveillance Program: Drug induced deafness. JAMA 224:515-516, 1973.
2. Cohen MM: Fatality following the use of intrathecal penicillin. J Neuropath. Exp. Neurol. 11:335-338, 1952.
3. Eronini EA, Umez-Eronini EM: Chloroquine induced involuntary movements. Br. Med. J. 1:945-946, 1977.
4. Fanning WL, Gump DW, Sofferman KA: Side effects of minocycline. A double blind study. Antimicrob. Agents Chemother. 11:712-717, 1977.
5. Fee WE: Aminoglycoside ototoxicity in the human. Laryngoscope 90:1-19, 1980.
6. Fossieck B, Parker RH: Neurotoxicity during intravenous infusion of penicillin. A review. J. Clin. Pharmacol. 14:504-512, 1974.
7. Gammon GD, Schoenbach EB: Neural toxicity from the sulfonamides. Arch. Neural. Psychiatry 63:1010, 1950.
8. Gilman AG, Goodman LS, Gilman A: Pharmacologic Basis of Therapeutics. Macmillan, New York, 1980.
9. Harrell WE: Hazards of antibiotic therapy. JAMA 168:1975-1878.
10. Huang NM, Harley RD, Promadhattavedi V, et al.: Visual disturbances in cystic fibrosis following chloramphenicol administration. J. Pediatr. 68: 32-34, 1966.
11. Hunnicutt T, Graf WJ, Hamburger M, Ferris B, Scheinker IM: Fatal toxic encephalopathy apparently caused by streptomycin. JAMA 137:599-601, 1948.
12. Karmody CS, Weinstein L: Reversible sensorineural hearing loss associated with intravenous erythromycin lactobionate. Ann. Otolaryngol. 86:9-10, 1977.
13. Koch-Wesser J, Sidel VW, Dexter M, et al: Adverse reactions to sulfisoxazole, sulfamethoxazole and nitrofurantoin. Arch. Intern. Med. 128:399-403, 1971.
14. Karamer J, Klawans HL: Iatrogenic neurology: Neurologic complication of non-neuropsychiatric agents. In HL Klawans, ed., Clinical Neuropharmacology, Vol. 4, 175-198, 1979.
15. Lawrence JS: The Sulphonamides in Theory and Practice. London, H. K. Lewis & Co., Ltd., 1946.
16. Lerner SA, Seligsohn R, Matz GJ: Comparative clinical studies of ototoxicity and nephrotoxicity of amikacin and gentamicin. Am. J. Med. 62:1919-1924, 1977.
17. Lindesmith LA, Baines RD, Bigelow B, et al.: Reversible respiratory paralysis associated with polymyxin therapy. Ann. Intern. Med. 68:318-320, 1968.

18. Loftus CR: Peripheral neuropathy following chloroquine therapy. Cand. Med. Ass. J. 89:917-920, 1963.
19. Parry MF: Antibiotic neurotoxicity. In A Silverstein, Neurological Complications of Therapy. Futura Publishing, Mount Kisco, New York, 1982.
20. Pittinger C, Adamson R: Antibiotic blockade of neuromuscular function. Ann. Rev. Pharmacol. 12:169-178, 1972.
21. Proud GO, Mittelman H, Seiden GD: Ototoxicity of topically applied chloramphenicol. Arch. Otolaryngol. 87:34-41, 1968.
22. Rollin H: Drug-related gustatory disorders. Am. Otolaryngol. 87:37-43, 1978.
23. Schwietzer CH: Pilzgifte und Pilzvergiftungen. Munch. Med. Wschr. 112: 1085-1086, 1970.
24. Stesman AB, Schaumburg HH, Asbury AK: Acute sensory neuropathy syndrome. Ann. Neurol. 7:354-358, 1980.
25. Stevens DA: Miconazole in the treatment of systemic fungal infections. Am. Rev. Respir. Dis. 116:801-806, 1977.
26. Swanson PD: Penicillin induced metabolic alterations in isolated cerebral cortex. Arch. Neurol. 26:169-172, 1972.
27. Utz JP: Amphotericin B toxicity. Ann. Intern. Med. 61:340-343, 1964.
28. Wright JM, Collier B: Characterization of the neuromuscular block produced by clindamycin and lincomycin. Can. J. Physiol. Pharmacol. 54: 937-944, 1976.

CHAPTER 16

Antineoplastic Agents

ANTICANCER drugs destroy tumor cells, but induce a variety of cytotoxic effects elsewhere as well. Rapidly growing tissues like bone marrow and gastrointestinal mucosa are highly vulnerable, while the nervous system is rather resistant to such incidental toxicity. Nevertheless, significant morbidity and rarely mortality relate directly to drug-induced toxic damage to the nervous system, either peripheral or central. Additionally, indirect or secondary nervous dysfunction in the form of drug-induced hepatic or renal damage can lead to a metabolic encephalopathy, and drug-induced immune suppression can similarly lead to a secondary opportunistic encephalitis or meningitis. These indirect consequences of chemotherapy are not discussed in this chapter, which instead focuses on direct established drug-induced neurotoxic syndromes. Also mentioned is drug-radiation interaction leading to neurologic dysfunction, since combination therapy is currently used extensively. In most cases, once the toxic signs are recognized and the diagnosis of drug-induced neurotoxicity is established, the treatment is withdrawal of the etiologic agent. In some cases, certain antidotes can be administered to help prevent the side effect or at least hasten maximal recovery once induced.

It is important to understand that drug-induced side effects can clearly mimic and in fact be indistinguishable from cancer. Hence, neuropathy can result from various dugs, but can also be seen in nontreated tumor patients and drug-induced cerebellar ataxia can be indistinguishable from a cerebellar metastatic lesion. Drug effect must always be considered in a patient receiving chemotherapy, but no assumption should be made; a thorough metastatic, metabolic and nutritional evaluation is essential in all cancer patients developing new neurologic syndromes.

Chemotherapy often involves more than one drug and the combinations are said to be based on a logical consideration of cell kinetics [31]. Some drugs are "cell cycle specific," primarily affecting S-phase, when DNA is replicated, or cell division (M-phase). Examples include methotrexate and cytarabine for S-phase and Vinca alkaloids for M-phase. Other agents work throughout the replication cycle and are termed non-cycle-specific, such as alkylating agents. Combining information related to drug kinetics, drug penetration, and tumor growth rates allows the therapist to estimate treatment doses for cancer at various stages. While one dose may be recommended at the induction of therapy, another may be more reasonable for consolidation or use during remission. Table 16.1 summarizes the drugs and syndromes discussed.

■ ALKYLATING AGENTS

The alkylating agents are cell cycle nonspecific drugs, which alkylate purine and pyrimidine moieties of DNA, thereby altering synthesis of nucleotides. Nitrogen mustard is the prototype of this class, although other drugs have been developed to improve therapeutic efficacy and reduce toxicity. At present, cyclophosphamide is the most widely used alkylating agent; thiotepa, melphalan, chlorambucil and busulfan are the other important drugs of this class. The major toxicity of this group is bone marrow suppression, and in general, neurotoxicity is not a major feature.

A variety of other drugs have similar actions to the alkylating agents and are grouped by some authors under that same general heading. These would include the nitrosoureas, cis-platinum, and some antibiotics that act as neoplastic agents. These, however, will be discussed separately.

NITROGEN MUSTARD (NM) MECHLORETHAMINE

Nitrogen mustard, although having largely been replaced by newer drugs, is often used in Hodgkin's disease and other lymphomas as well as in solid tumors of the lung and ovary.

This drug is occasionally used in combination with other antitumor drugs as MOPP: mechlorethamine, oncovin (vincristine), procarbazine, and prednisone in the treatment of lymphoma. NM administered intravenously in a dose of 0.4 mg/kg is ordinarily without neurotoxicity. Hemiplegia and coma, however, were reported in one patient seven days after the second of two intravenous doses of NM at the recommended dose schedule [4]. Increased intracranial pressure and cerebrospinal fluid pleocytosis were also found. Post-mortem examination revealed areas of focal gliosis and neuronal loss within the brain with no evidence of intracranial tumor. This episode was felt to be an idiosyncratic response by the CNS to nitrogen mustard.

Antineoplastic Agents

TABLE 16.1. Anticancer Drugs and Neurotoxicity

Alkylating agents:
 Eighth cranial nerve neuropathy
 Seizures
 Hemiplegia (stroke syndrome)
 Myelopathy
 Encephalopathy
 Peripheral neuropathy

Methotrexate:
 Intrathecal
  Aseptic meningitis
  Myelopathy
  Seizures
  Leukoencephalopathy
  Cortical atrophy
  Possible:
   Cerebellar dysfunction
   Optic atrophy
 Intravenous
  Leukoencephalopathy
  Cerebral vascular accidents

5-FU:
 Cerebellar dysfunction
 Encephalopathy
 Parkinsonism

Cytosine arabinoside:
 Asceptic meningitis after intrathecal use
 Cerebellar dysfunction with ataxia
 Possible optic atrophy

5-Azacytidine:
 Myopathy
 Mental changes

Vincristine, vinblastine, and vindesine:
 Peripheral neuropathy
 Autonomic neuropathy
 Cranial neuropathies
 Myopathy
 Mental changes (may be secondary to inappropriate ADH secretion)
 Seizure

Nitrosoureas:
 Encephalopathy (by itself in high doses intra-arterially)
 Additive brain damage with radiation therapy

Cis-platinum:
 Eighth cranial nerve neuropathy
 Peripheral neuropathy

Hexamethylmelamine:
 Encephalopathy with hallucinations
 Peripheral neuropathy
 Cerebellar ataxia
 Tremor: parkinsonism or postural

L-asparaginase:
 Encephalopathy
 Seizures

Massive intravenous injections of NM have caused hearing loss, vestibular dysfunction and tinnitus, presumably from damage to the eighth cranial nerve. Intracarotid NM injection has been associated with hemiplegia, seizures, coma, and death. One pathological study showed diffuse cerebral edema, greater on the side of the injection [12]. Extensive gliosis and demyelination were also present in that cerebral hemisphere, presumably from a previous injection. Clinical evidence of lower motor neuron damage has been observed following high-dose intra-arterial perfusion of NM to treat pelvic or limb tumors.

Experimental evidence suggesting potential neurological toxicity of NM has shown that high concentrations of labeled NM are found in the eighth nerve after intravenous administration [22]. In addition, demyelination, axonotmesis, epineurial and endoneurial thickening as well as hemorrhagic foci were noted in the sciatic nerve after exposure to high doses of NM. Conduction velocities distal to the injury were significantly prolonged.

CYCLOPHOSPHAMIDE (CYTOXAN)

Cyclophosphamide (Cytoxan), currently one of the most widely used alkylating agents, is associated with very little neurologic toxicity. It is used to treat Hodgkin's disease, non-Hodgkin's lymphoma, adult leukemia, and numerous solid tumors, including breast carcinoma and oat cell carcinoma of the lung.

Rapid intravenous infusion of cyclophosphamide has occasionally caused dizziness, a posterior pharyngeal tingling sensation, and a feeling of euphoria [2]. These symptoms are brief, lasting only seconds to minutes, and are completely reversible. Inappropriate diuretic hormone secretion has also occurred rarely and is exacerbated by the high fluid loading required in high-dose Cytoxan therapy to prevent renal toxicity. The remarkable safety of this drug may well relate to the fact that only tiny quantities of the drug or its metabolites can be detected in the cerebrospinal fluid.

CHLORAMBUCIL (LEUKERAN)

Chlorambucil is a drug used often in the treatment of chronic lymphocytic leukemia and certain non-Hodgkin's lymphomas. Although generally regarded to be non-neurotoxic, acute severe CNS abnormalities consisting of lethargy, ataxia, seizures, and coma developed in two children inadvertently injected with massive overdoses of chlorambucil [14]. Recovery within one week occurred without any neurological sequelae.

Seizures have rarely been reported to be a complication of chlorambucil. Such seizures have been described in children with nephrotic syndrome, occurring in 7 of 91 patients and ceasing when the drug was stopped. Chlorambucil has also provoked focal motor fits in an adult, which resolved with cessation of the medication [23].

THIOTEPA

Thiotepa is an intravenously administered alkylating agent commonly used in the treatment of bladder cancer. Due to its low neurotoxicity, it is one of the few anticancer drugs that can be injected into the CSF [28]. In one series of ten patients with meningeal leukemia and carcinomatosis treated with multiple courses of intrathecal thiotepa, clinical neurotoxicity developed in only two

Antineoplastic Agents

[15]. The toxicity consisted of progressive lower extremity weakness, back and leg pain, areflexia, and a progressive myelopathy. Electromyography in one patient revealed diffuse lower motor neuron abnormalities. Gliosis and demyelination in the posterior columns of the spinal cord and the nerve roots of the cauda equina were present at post-mortem study. No evidence of meningeal leukemia or arachnoiditis was found. In animal studies, doses of 12 mg/m^2 injected intracisternally provoked opisthotonic posturing and hyperextension of the limbs.

OTHER ALKYLATING AGENTS

Melphalan used predominantly to treat multiple myeloma, is without established neurotoxicity. Busulfan (Myleran), also considered neurologically safe, was associated with the development of myasthenia gravis in one case of a patient with chronic myelogenous leukemia. The relationship between the myasthenia, the Myleran, and the leukemia was not clarified.

■ ANTIMETABOLITES

METHOTREXATE (MTX)

Methotrexate is an alkylating agent but acts primarily during DNA synthesis (S-phase) as an antifolate antineoplastic drug. It prevents the conversion of folic acid to tetrahydrofolic acid, as well as preventing the conversion of tetrahydrofolic acid to folinic acid. The synthesis of proteins is thereby diminished. As an oral or intravenous drug in the usual described doses, MTX has long been regarded as a neurologically safe agent. MTX has only limited abilities to cross blood–brain barriers; CSF concentration is less than 10% of that in plasma after oral or usual parenteral doses.

When given by alternate routes or in higher doses, however, MTX is associated with a number of neurologic syndromes. The majority of MTX neurotoxicity is known to occur in association with intrathecal drug administration, and may be acute or chronic. The acute effects include a mild to moderate transient meningoencephalitis, usually beginning within hours of intrathecal administration and characterized by headache, nausea, vomiting, nuchal rigidity, lethargy, and fever. The illness usually lasts 1-3 days, but may persist for two weeks. CSF examination frequently reveals a moderately severe pleocytosis initially, although this reaction does not usually recur with subsequent therapy. The cause of the syndrome is presently unknown, but impurities in the drug or its mixture have been implicated, since the syndrome has occurred sporadically with different lots of drug penetration. The reaction occurs in patients with active CNS or meningeal tumor as well as in those patients given methotrexate prophylactically.

Another acute complication occurring within hours of intrathecal MTX is an acute transverse myelopathy with paraplegia which may be permanent [13]. An ascending myelopathy after treatment with multiple doses of combined intrathecal methotrexate and Ara-C for meningeal leukemia has also been described.

Transient radiculopathies, possibly related to epidural or subdural injection, have also been described. Intrathecal injection of MTX can also cause secondary spinal subdural hemotomas resulting in either myelopathy or radiculopathy, and since these complications are treatable, they should be considered in a patient who develops neurologic complications after methotrexate therapy.

Finally, intraventricular injections of MTX may induce nausea and vomiting, although gradual injection of this drug prevents the problem. High intrathecal doses of methotrexate in dogs can provoke seizures, and epileptic fits have occasionally been attributed to intrathecal methotrexate in man [25].

Delayed neurotoxic reactions to intrathecal MTX are more frequent than the above-mentioned acute effects. Of these, encephalopathy is the most important and usually follows repeated doses of MTX into the lateral ventricle or lumbar subarachnoid space. The clinical syndrome is characterized by slowly progressive confusion, dementia, somnolence, tremor, ataxia and seizures or, less commonly, sudden onset of hemiplegia and coma eventuating in death [27]. Pathologically, the lesion is usually a leukoencephalopathy, with areas of coagulative necrosis and demyelination similar to the changes seen in radiation damage to the CNS. These alterations may occur throughout the white matter after intrathecal administration, but have a predilection for the periventricular areas when given intraventricularly.

The pathophysiologic basis of the methotrexate encephalopathy is controversial. Shapiro et al. [27] suggested that ventricular obstruction was a critical factor to methotrexate encephalopathy in that the hydrocephalus associated with obstruction allowed an increased transependymal absorption of methotrexate into the periventricular white matter. Although the encephalopathy is seen when methotrexate is administered alone, a combination of drug therapy plus radiation appears to enhance the neurologic syndrome. Nevertheless, cases have been well described where the periventricular distribution of encephalopathic lesions are well outside the port of brain radiation.

Radiologic investigations of methotrexate encephalopathy with CT scanning shows extensive patchy white attenuation, mostly in the periventricular area. These changes may be diffuse or multifocal and they may occur in patients who have no neurologic dysfunction on clinical examination. In a study by Arnold et al. [3], the incidence of these CT changes range as high as 50%. Autopsy material has shown variable changes in the cerebral white matter including gliosis, spongy changes, and altered neuronal structure. Optic atrophy with blindness and cerebellar dysfunction have been described in patients treated with multiple therapeutic regimens including intrathecal MTX [14].

Although the leukoencephalopathy has been predominantly noted after intrathecal methotrexate, a similar clinical and pathologic syndrome has been seen with high-dose intravenous MTX. In seven patients treated over a period of 4-5 months (doses ranging from 8-20 grams/m^2), an encephalopathy developed during the second or third month after initiation of treatment. The syndrome included a gradual dementia, pseudobulbar palsy, and spastic quadraparesis. In four, episodes of delirium and agitation occurred and six of the patients became stuporous. With cessation of the drug, neurologic improvement occurred, although sequelae were present throughout the patients' remaining life. In CT scans obtained, there was cerebral atrophy and attenuation of the white matter, and in one, there was a focal contrast-enhancing lesion. This complication is estimated to occur in less than 2% of patients receiving high-dose methotrexate. It has been suggested by Bleyer that those patients who demonstrate prolonged elevations of CSF methotrexate levels are most likely to develop the encephalopathic syndrome. In the cases cited above, all seven patients had detectable levels of methotrexate at least three and often nine days after their last treatment [5].

The treatment of methotrexate-induced leukoencephalopathy is withdrawal of the provocative agent. In spite of this, however, many patients will progress from moderate personality changes to stupor, coma, and death and others may maintain a persistent altered mental state. Fortunately, most patients improve, although often with significant sequelae. The use of citrovorum factor has been advised by some investigators [20], since this agent given systemically can circumvent the actions of folic acid antagonists on some normal tissues, specifically bone marrow. The usefulness of this agent in regard to the neurologic system is not established. If intrathecal therapy is still required, an alternative agent could be cytarabine.

The risk factors involved in methotrexate-induced leukoencephalopathy may be multiple. Clearly, radiation therapy to the whole brain enhances the risk. A general correlation exists between total cumulative dose of MTX and the development of encephalopathy, although clear exceptions can be found. In patients with active meningeal disease, leukoencephalopathy is quite frequent and the hydrocephalus associated with meningeal disease may be a provoking factor. Any mechanism that enhances methotrexate exposure to brain cells appears to enhance the potential risk of this agent. Interestingly, methotrexate acts on dividing cells, and neurons, of course, are not in active reproduction. The white matter changes seen at autopsy and on CT scan suggest that the damage may relate to oligodendroglial or vascular cells, but it is possible that other actions are in fact in play.

Other long-term but less common side effects associated with methotrexate have included cerebellar dysfunction a patient given combined MTX-therapy; and progressive brain stem dysfunction marked by quadraparesis and pseudobulbar palsy in patients who received X-ray therapy as well as MTX (and in one case, methyl-CCNU). More significant are concerns over mild changes that might be induced in large numbers of children who do not demonstrate such pronounced neurologic impairment. Of 23 leukemic children treated with prophylactic radiation and intrathecal MTX, 50% showed some evidence of gait and motor abnormalities, seizures, and incoordination 10-18 months after treatment. Other studies following patients up to five years have shown normal neurologic and psychometric development, although CT scans have demonstrated cerebral atrophy in as high as 25% of children. These long-term developmental studies must be continued to assess the effects on both children and adults whose tumors are successfully treated, but who may in fact be at risk for new neurologic disease secondary to the antitumor treatment [30].

A final syndrome altogether distinct from the chronic encephalopathy described above is a sudden, cataclysmic cerebral dysfunction that resembles a cerebral vascular accident. Such patients may suddenly develop a hemiplegia, speech disturbance, or focal epilepsy. The signs may be focal or multifocal, static or fluctuating. Generally, recovery is quite complete, although a mild residual might be detected. The origin and pathologic substrate of these sudden neurologic apoplexies are unknown, but it has been suggested to occur in 1-2% of patients treated with repetitive doses of high-dose methotrexate, specifically those young children with osteogenic or other sarcomas.

5-FLUOROURACIL

5-fluorouracil is a chemotherapeutic drug given orally or intravenously for treatment of breast, ovarian, and gastrointestinal cancer. An antipyrimidine drug, 5-fluorouracil (5-FU) is associated with a characteristic cerebellar syndrome in 1% of patients. When doses of 5-FU exceed the usual recommendations, the incidence of this cerebellar syndrome may be as high as 3%-7%. Ataxia of the extremities, dysmetria, hypotonia, and coarse nystagmus are the clinical hallmarks. The symptoms are generally subacute in onset, and once identified, they are controlled by a reduction of 5-FU dose or an increase in intervals between treatments [30]. The syndrome is reversible, although cases of its re-emergence after a subsequent treatment have been reported [31].

Other neurotoxic reactions reportedly associated with 5-FU include memory loss and mild to moderate encephalopathy, as well as a parkinsonian syndrome. The encephalopathy may occur in as many as 40% of treated patients and, interestingly, cerebellar symptoms are not typical of this encephalopathic group. Reduction of medication is followed by improvement over approximately one month. Likewise, the parkinsonian syndrome is generally reversible, although in one instance long-term residual was seen. Blurring of vision and diplopia have also been reported with this agent; both clear upon cessation of therapy.

The origin of the cerebellar syndrome and other neurotoxic effects related to 5-FU is unknown. When intracarotid or intrathecal 5-FU was administered to cats, cerebellar damage was induced, and was believed to relate to the high production by these routes of 5-FU metabolites, including fluoroacetate and fluorocitrate. A further metabolite, 5-fluoro-2-deoxyuridine-5-monophosphate, concentrates in mouse cerebellum. When thymidine was added to 5-FU as a trial combination in therapy, cerebellar dysfunction was rapidly increased.

CYTARABINE (CYTOSINE ARABINOSIDE; ARA-C)

Ara-C acts by competing for natural cytidine nucleotides and subsequently interfers with the synthesis of DNA. It is primarily used in the treatment of acute myelogenous leukemia as part of combination therapy. It diffuses quite well into the CSF when given intravenously and once in the CSF is eliminated very slowly. It can also be given directly intrathecally when there is meningeal leukemia or lymphoma. As part of combination therapy, methotrexate and ara-C are given intrathecally to treat various solid tumors.

Aseptic meningitis can occur with intrathecal ara-C, although this is less common than the meningitis seen with methotrexate [1]. In one case where there was a permanent paraplegia following ara-C intrathecal therapy, extensive white matter demyelination and axonal swelling were seen in the spinal cord. Two cases of optic atrophy and blindness were seen while patients were receiving ara-C, although in both patients whole-brain radiation and several systemic drugs, as well as prior ara-C and methotrexate, had been delivered. Such cases make it impossible to relate the optic damage specifically to ara-C. In fact, when the optic nerve was biopsied, the changes were those typically seen in relation to radiation damage. Ataxia may begin 6-8 days after starting ara-C and may become so severe that the patient is unable to eat. In those cases that have progressed to death, autopsy examinations have shown loss of Purkinje cells [32].

OTHER ANTIMETABOLITES

5-Azacytidine is an unusual drug that has significant neurotoxicity and is restricted by and large to treating acute myelogenous leukemia. In one series of patients, 17 of 18 developed generalized muscle tenderness, difficulty rising from a chair, and abnormal gait after receiving the drug for 5 days. Additionally, in over half, there were significant mental changes and confusion. The symptoms were completely reversible within one week, and an associated hypophosphatemia appears to correlate with the development of these symptoms [18].

Antipurine agents include 6-mercaptopurine (6-MT), 6-thioquanine (6-TG), and 8-azaguane (8-AZ). 6-MT and 6-TG are commonly used in the treatment of leukemic states and are not associated with significant toxicity. 8-AZ, however, may become a drug used in the treatment of brain tumors in the future, since such tumors lack the degradating enzyme for this product, in contrast to normal brain tissue. Such enzymatic differences suggest that direct tumor bed administration of this drug could offer potential efficacy, although preliminary studies have in fact not yielded therapeutic benefit [30].

■ NATURAL PRODUCTS

PLANT ALKALOIDS

Vincristine (VCR) and vinblastine (VBL) are alkaloid derivatives of the periwinkle plant, and are toxic to both the central and peripheral nervous systems. Vincristine is the more widely used drug and is effective against several neoplasms, including breast cancer and leukemia. The major limiting factor in its use in cancer therapy is its neurotoxicity. The average required dose of VCR results in a predictable sensorimotor peripheral neuropathy. In addition, VCR affects the central nervous system, the cranial nerves, and the autonomic nervous system. Vincristine neuropathy often occurs after only one or two weekly treatments and often has as its first sign depression of ankle tendon reflexes. Paresthesias in the fingers and toes are followed by distal sensory loss and eventually distal weakness. Deep tendon reflexes diminish maximally approximately two weeks after a single dose and may return to normal in one to three months after drug cessation. Weekly doses appear to have a cumulative effect and as additional doses are given, depression of all reflexes occurs, with complete areflexia being quite common [7]. Weakness is usually minimal in the routine dose schedules, but when it does occur, the feet are most affected, mainly the dorsiflexors and evertors. If more severe, the extensors of the fingers and wrists may become involved. Motor signs may occur in 5%-36% of patients [30]. Sensory and motor complaints are usually reversible with the cessation of vincristine therapy, although permanent changes have been seen.

Nerve conduction studies reveal some reduction in motor nerve conduction as well as sensory nerve velocities. Progressive decreases in conduction velocities occur during VCR therapy, but may remain in the normal range despite obvious clinical neuropathy [6]. Needle electromyography demonstrates denervation in distal musculature. Reduction in amplitude of sensory evoked potentials and prolonged distal motor latencies are often found in these patients, suggesting that the pathology is one of axonal degeneration with a component of "dying back" phenomena. Studies of the sural nerve confirm this hypothesis, demonstrating axonal degeneration without segmental demyelination.

VCR is also associated with an autonomic neuropathy, with constipation the most common problem, occurring in almost one-third of patients in one large series [19]. Mild abdominal pain is common, and may be neurogenic in origin. It usually starts 4-70 hours after the dose of VCR and therefore precedes the loss of deep tendon reflexes. Autonomic side effects appear to be dose-related, and patients may present with the clinical picture of bladder dysfunction, impotence, and orthostatic hypotension or an acute abdominal crisis due to a paralytic ileus [19].

Cranial nerve dysfunction is rare. When there is significant peripheral weakness, bilateral seventh nerve paresis occasionally occurs, especially in children. The facial weakness is usually symmetric, a feature that helps to differentiate this VCR reaction from meningeal seeding of tumor, which usually presents asymmetrically. Ocular motor paresis, usually presenting as ptosis, has also been reported and in one series occurred in 10% of patients receiving VCR [26]. Laryngeal paresis, hoarseness, and dysphagia associated with paralysis of the vocal cord and optic atrophy have been documented as well [10]. Finally, jaw or throat pain occurring early in the course of therapy, often within hours of a dose and subsiding after a few days, is a well-accepted side effect of VCR therapy and may be neurologic in origin. Myopathy, usually with tenderness and pain, frequently develops in children after 1-2 weeks of VCR therapy. Focal muscle necrosis with myofibrillary disruption has been seen histologically in electron microscopic studies.

Abnormalities of the brain and spinal cord are rare when VCR is given intravenously because of the drug's poor permeability across the blood-brain barrier. Seizures have, however, been reported, but are usually in association with the syndrome of inappropriate ADH. Not all vincristine-associated seizures can be explained by ADH abnormalities, however, since up to 4% of patients show no underlying metabolic abnormalities. Confusion, mental changes, and hallucinations have also been reported in a few patients.

A number of factors appear to enhance the toxicity of vincristine in some individuals. Preexisting neuropathy appears to predispose patients to greater risk of vincristine-induced damage. As an example of such a patient with a mild form of Charcot-Marie-Tooth disease developed a severe paraplegia with bulbar paresis that resulted in death after two weekly doses of vincristine. Patients with underlying neuropathy or muscle disease should be given vincristine with extreme caution. Other drugs may enhance vincristine neuropathy. Severe neuropathic syndromes have been seen in combination VCR, L-asparaginase, and isoniazid therapy. Furthermore, when L-asparaginase was given before or simultaneously with VCR to patients with acute leukemia, the incidence of neuropathy was greater than if VCR was given first. Malnutrition may also enhance VCR neuropathy, although vitamin supplementation does not appear to reverse the syndrome.

Vinblastine has similar neurotoxic reactions, but only at doses that are usually not prescribed because of concomitant severe hematologic reactions. Paresthesias, distal sensory loss with weakness, jaw pain, urinary dysfunction, vocal cord paralysis and hypotension have been described as side effects of VBL.

Vindesine (DVA), a newer agent used for non-small-cell carcinoma of the lungs and other relatively resistent tumors, has a similar neurotoxic profile to that of vincristine. Unlike the usual vincristine neuropathy, however, weakness often appears more significant than the sensory complaints. The weakness may be distal, suggestive of neuropathy, or proximal, suggestive of a myopathic process. On EMG studies, even the proximal weakness appears to relate predominantly to a neuropathy.

ANTIBIOTIC ANTINEOPLASTIC AGENTS

Various antibiotics that are effective antimicrobial agents are not used for such purposes because of cytotoxic properties. However, these drugs have been used in the treatment of various cancers, often with excellent effects. Several of these agents appear to act as alkylating agents, although the mechanism of action of some antibiotic-antineoplastic agents is not clear.

Bleomycin

Bleomycin is chiefly used to treat tumors of the head and neck, testis, and lung. Because the drug is ordinarily used with other chemotherapeutic agents, pure bleomycin-related neurotoxicity is uncertain. Mental status abnormalities and peripheral neuropathy have been associated with bleomycin therapy, although no pathological changes have been reported in brain or peripheral nerves in such patients [14]. Although bleomycin-related cochlear damage has been demonstrated in animals, there is no comparable clinical evidence in man. The most significant toxic effect of bleomycin is pulmonary fibrosis, which does not appear to be directly dose-related.

Adriamycin and Actinomycin D

Adriamycin and Actinomycin D, in the usual prescribed doses, produce no neurologic side effects in man. Neurotoxicity, however, has been produced in experimental animals with both drugs. Adriamycin can produce an initial severe posterior limb ataxia and later a mild forelimb ataxia, with associated pathological change in the dorsal root ganglia [9].

Actinomycin D causes tremors, myoclonus, seizure, ascending myelopathy, and encephalopathy when injected into the CSF in animal models. Demyelination and necrosis have been found in the brain on pathological studies. When these drugs are administered systemically, there is virtually no entrance into the CSF.

L-ASPARAGINASE

L-asparaginase is an enzyme that hydrolyzes asparagine to aspartic acid and ammonia. Hence, in those tumor cells that require this essential amino acid and cannot manufacture it on their own, L-asparaginase is effectively cytotoxic. Systemic side effects are often dose-limiting and include nausea, vomiting, and bone marrow suppression. Central nervous system neurotoxicity, however, may also be dose-limiting in that there may be an acute alteration in mental function associated with this agent. In doses greater than 1,000 IU/kg/day lethargy and confusion occurred in as many as 60% of patients [21]. Encephalopathy is less frequent in the usual currently prescribed doses (200-1,000 IU/kg/day), although 15% of cases may need to discontinue the drug because of the encephalopathic syndrome. Although the fully developed encephalopathy may be preceded by more subtle but detectable changes, the early encephalopathy may go unnoticed; the mental changes are usually reversible, but in high doses, progression to coma and even death have occurred during treatment regimes with L-asparaginase. Although the encephalopathy relates to dosage, significant mental changes have been seen in some patients on very low doses. Seizures are not a usual accompaniment of this syndrome. Curiously, the enzyme is too large to cross the blood–brain barrier and so the origin of central nervous system toxicity remains unexplained. The changes may relate to the elevation of L-asparaginase, L-glutamate, and ammonia, or to the systemic hepatic dysfunction. However, while some encephalopathies result from secondary metabolic derangements, many patients with L-asparaginase-related encephalopathy have acceptable liver function tests. Drug-induced hypofibrinogenemia and hypoantithrombin III can lead to sagittal sinus thrombosis with strokes. In these cases, fresh frozen plasma, steroids, and heparin, are used to treat this drug-related complication.

■ OTHER CHEMOTHERAPEUTIC AGENTS

NITROSOUREAS

The nitrosoureas are a group of cancer chemotherapeutic agents which have alkylating properties but probably also inhibit protein and DNA synthesis. The most common agents used in this group are BCNU and CCNU, which readily cross the blood-brain barrier following systemic administration. These two agents are commercially available, although a wide variety of other nitrosureas are currently being used in investigational institutions (methyl-CCNU, streptozotocin, PCNU, ACNU, and DCNU).

BCNU and CCNU show minimal neurologic toxicity in the dose regimens used, and in fact have been used extensively in the management of CNS malignancies. However, BCNU and CCNU are clearly neurotoxic when used in unconventional manners and may, even in usual doses, act synergistically with other forms of therapy to induce chronic neurotoxic effects. An example of the former condition is the experimental treatment of primary and metastatic brain tumors with carotid injections of BCNU. Although therapeutic efficacy was demonstrated in such cases, orbital, eye and neck pain at the time of injection, focal seizures, and transient encephalopathy were complications in this small group. During vertebral artery injection, a transient ischemic episode was reported [30].

When BCNU has been used in very high doses (1500–3000 mg/m^2/dose instead of the usual 200–240 mg/m^2) multifocal abnormalities developed within three months of treatment [31]. The changes seen at autopsy included coagulative necrosis, fibrinoid necrosis, and no evidence of inflammation; these changes were remarkably similar to those seen with radiation necrosis of the brain. (These patients, however, had received no prior brain radiation.) Significantly, there was no evidence of brain metastatic disease in such cases.

Examples of synergistic activity of the nitrosoureas with other antineoplastic therapy is the synergism with radiation therapy demonstrated with BCNU. In a small percentage of patients treated with BCNU and radiation for malignant glioma, an insidious dementia associated with cerebral atrophy develops. Similarly, systemic methyl-CCNU has been reported to be associated with multifocal demyelinative lesions in a patient who also received radiation therapy. Such lesions were remarkably similar to those seen with radiation methotrexate treatment.

Antineoplastic Agents

CIS-PLATINUM

Cis-platinum is a recently available chemotherapeutic agent with the significant neurotoxic effect of ototoxicity. Deafness often begins within three to four days of the initial treatment, slowly improving over succeeding weeks after treatment is stopped. In most cases, deafness is reversible, but when profound, it may be permanent [24]. Direct toxicity of cis-platinum on the organ of Corti appears to be the cause of the induced deafness, since nystagmus and vertigo have only rarely been reported. The predominant hearing loss is for high frequencies of 4,000-8,000 Hz. Such ototoxic effects are more prominent in elderly patients and the combination of slow infusion of the drug and widespread use of pretreatment with intravenous hydration and often mannitol to enhance renal excretion has significantly reduced the problem of ototoxicity [16].

An additional side effect of cis-platinum is peripheral neuropathy, mainly sensory in nature and characterized by distal paresthesias and diminished proprioceptive sense. Usually such neuropathies occur after several courses of cis-platinum. While most patients show a diffuse loss of sensory discrimination, some patients demonstrate profound posterior column dysfunction without temperature and pain involvement. Such predominant involvement of posterior and vibratory senses can help to differentiate this neuropathy from vincristine-induced peripheral damage, where all modalities are much more consistently involved [30]. Cis-platinum neuropathy is not altogether reversible and in such cases meningeal seeding of cancer as well as the remote effect of carcinoma must be considered in the differential diagnosis. Whether this neuropathy is predominantly demyelinative or axonal is controversial.

Central nervous system involvement with cis-platinum has also been reported. An acute reversible encephalopathy and occasional seizures have been documented in patients who have significant metabolic abnormalities, including hypomagnesemia or hypocalcemia [17]. Optic nerve toxicity has also been reported, and a child who died receiving this drug demonstrated marked fiber loss in the posterior columns, suggesting that spinal cord penetration may be effected by this agent [11].

HEXAMETHYLMELAMINE

This agent may act as an alkylating drug or as an antimetabolite. It is predominantly used in the treatment of ovarian cancer and has both central and peripheral neurotoxic effects. In the usual doses administered (8 mg/kg/day), neurologic problems are seen in up to 20% of patients. Such involvement includes encephalopathy with hallucinations, agitation and confusion, and ataxia and tremor that may be parkinsonian or more postural in nature [29]. Peripheral neuropathy may also develop with distal sensory loss and weakness as the predominant features. This neuropathy may be enhanced in those patients having prior vincristine exposure. Such central and peripheral neurotoxicity is seen predominantly after prolonged cumulative doses, and in the case of neuropathy, pyridoxine may be beneficial in its treatment.

PROCARBAZINE

Procarbazine inhibits monoaminoxidase and is chiefly used in the treatment of Hodgkin's disease and non-Hodgkin's lymphoma, as well as in treatment of malignant glioma. Although procarbazine is technically neurotoxic, central nervous system and peripheral nervous system alterations are not prominent clinically. Formerly, procarbazine was administered at high doses by intravenous route, and somnolence was a prominent feature [8]. Lower doses (100–300 mg/daily by oral route) are not associated with somnolence, although because of the monoaminoxidase inhibition, the central nervous system effects of such drugs as barbiturates, phenothiazines and narcotics will be enhanced. The caution advised with other monoamine oxidase inhibitors regarding tyramine food such as cheese or wine has not been a clinical problem with procarbazine.

Peripheral neuropathy has been documented with procarbazine in 10%–15% of patients treated with high doses. With lower and more currently used doses, this side effect appears to be quite unusual. Nevertheless, when it occurs, general paresthesias and loss of tendon reflexes are usually seen, and ataxia may be part of the clinical syndrome. Occasionally, proximal muscle myalgia has also been seen, suggesting an associated muscle involvement. Based on work with the structurally related compound isoniazid, where neuropathy can be prevented or reversed by pyridoxine, pyridoxine therapy has been attempted when procarbazine is administered; however, there is little indication that pyridoxine in any way influences the encephalopathy or peripheral neuropathy associated with this chemotherapeutic agent.

■ STUDY QUESTIONS

True statements regarding methotrexate-induced neurotoxicity include:

1. Intrathecal administration can provoke an acute meningoencephalitis in those patients with active meningeal tumor spread, but when given prophylactically, this reaction to methotrexate is extremely rare.
2. Chronic toxicity is more common than acute toxicity and usually involves a myelopathy.

Antineoplastic Agents

3. The risk of chronic encephalopathy associated with intrathecal use of methotrexate is increased if whole-brain radiation is also given.

Answer: 3 only

The acute neurologic signs of methotrexate toxicity are meningoencephalitis and transverse myelitis. They occur in both patients with established CNS spread of tumor, and in those patients given methotrexate prophylactically. Chronic toxicity is more common than acute toxicity and the clinical picture is a progressive dementing encephalopathy, not a myelopathy. Radiation potentiates the incidence of chronic neurotoxicity.

Match the neurologic side effect with the appropriate chemotherapeutic agent.

A. Parkinsonism	1. Vincristine
B. Autonomic neuropathy	2. Cytoxan
C. Cerebellar syndrome	3. 5-FU
	4. None

Answers: A-3; B-1; C-3

5-FU is associated with both a progressive cerebellar syndrome and a reversible parkinsonian picture. Vincristine induces cranial, peripheral, and autonomic neuropathy with as little as one dose. Cytoxan is not associated with significant primary neurotoxicity, although bone marrow suppression can lead to secondary infections.

Vindesine neurotoxicity is different from vincristine effects in that the former induces:

1. More likely a distal neuropathy
2. A myopathy, not a neuropathy
3. A high incidence of seizures
4. None

Answer: 4

Vindesine and vincristine are similar, but vindesine induces a predominantly motor neuropathy that is proximal and can mimic a myopathy. On EMG examination, however, the alterations are still indicative of neuropathy.

Match the drug with the appropriate characteristic.

A. BCNU	1. When administered along with whole-brain radiation, an encephalopathy similar to the methotrexate radiation encephalopathy can be seen.
B. Cis-platinum	2. Associated with significant ototoxicity.

C. L-asparaginase

D. Cytoxan

3. The drug has not been shown to cross the blood-brain barrier and yet is associated with encephalopathy in as high as 15% of cases.

4. None

Answers: A-1; B-2; C-3; D-4

BCNU and CCNU when given in conventional doses and alone are relatively safe agents neurologically, and in fact are used with success in the management of patients with CNS tumors. However, when used with radiation, a small number of patients develop a progressive dementing process remarkably similar to that seen with methotrexate-radiation in combination. Ototoxicity, more typical of antibiotics, must always be considered in patients with cis-platinum exposure. The drug directly damages the organ of Corti and does not induce a vestibulopathy. L-asparaginase is associated with encephalopathy in spite of its inability to cross the blood-brain barrier. The mechanism has been suggested to relate to glutamate and ammonia accumulations. L-asparaginase and cis-platinum both are associated with peripheral neuropathy and hence would theoretically exacerbate the peripheral neuropathy induced by vincristine. As such, these drugs would not be used ordinarily in combination with one another.

■ REFERENCES

1. Allen JC: The effects of cancer therapy on the nervous system. J. Pediat. 93:903-909, 1978.
2. Arena PJ: Oropharyngeal sensation associated with rapid intravenous administration of cyclophosphamide. Cancer Chemother. Rep. 56:779-780, 1972.
3. Arnold H, Kuhne D, Franke H, et al: Findings in computerized axial tomography after intrathecal methotrexate and radiation. Neuroradiology 16:65-68, 1978.
4. Bethlenfalvay NC, Bergin JJ: Severe cerebral toxicity after intravenous nitrogen mustard therapy. Cancer 29:366-369, 1972.
5. Bleyer WA, Drake JC, Chabner BA: Neurotoxicity and elevated cerebrospinal fluid methotrexate concentration in meningeal leukemia. N. Engl. J. Med. 289:770-773, 1973.
6. Bradley WG: Neuropathy in vincristine in the guinea pig: an electrophysiological study. J. Neurol. Sci. 10:133-162.
7. Casey EG, Jellife AM, LeQuesne M, et al.: Vincristine neuropathy: clinical and electrophysiological observations. Brain 96:69-86, 1973.
8. Chabner BA, Sponza R, Hubbard S, et al.: High dose intermittent intravenous infusion of procarbazine (NSC-77213). Cancer Chemother. Rep. 57:361-363, 1973.
9. Cho ES: Toxic effects of adriamycin on the ganglia of the peripheral nervous system. J. Neuropath. Exp. Neurol. 36:907-915, 1977.

Antineoplastic Agents

10. Delaney P: Vincristine induced laryngeal nerve paralysis. Neurology 32: 1285-1288, 1982.
11. Fazio M, Cavellero P, Minneto E, et al. Polychemotherapy of advanced head and neck malignancies. Tumor 62:599-608, 1976.
12. French JD, West PM, VonAmerongen FK, et al.: Effects of intracarotid administration of nitrogen mustard on normal brain and brain tumors. J. Neurosurg. 9:378-389, 1952.
13. Gagliano RG, Costanzi JJ: Paraplegia following intrathecal methotrexate. Cancer 37:1663-1668, 1976.
14. Green AA, Naiman JL: Chlormabucil poisoning. Am. J. Dis. Child 116: 190-191, 1968.
15. Gustin PH, Levi JA, Wiernik PH, et al.: Treatment of malignant meningeal disease with intrathecal thiotepa: A Phase II study. Cancer Treat. Rep. 885-887, 1977.
16. Hayes DM, Cvitkovic E, Golbey RB, et al.: High dose cis-platinum diamminedichloride. Cancer 39:1371-1372, 1977.
17. Hayes FA, Green AA, Senzer N, et al.: Tetany: a complication of cis-dichlorodiammineplatinum (II) therapy. Cancer Treat. Rep. 63:547-548, 1979.
18. Ho M, Bear RA, Garvey MB: Symptomatic hypophosphatemia secondary to 5-azacytidine therapy of acute nonlymphocytic leukemia. Cancer Treat. Rep. 60:1400-1402, 1976.
19. Holland JF, Scharlan C, Gaolani S, et al.: Vincristine treatment of advanced cancer: A cooperative study of 392 cases. Cancer Res. 33:1258-1264, 1973.
20. Hay HEM, Knapton PJ, O'Sullivan JP, et al.: Encephalopathy in acute leukemia associated with methotrexate therapy. Arch. Dis. Child 47:344-354, 1972.
21. Land VJ, Sutow WW, Fernback DJ, et al.: Toxicity of L-asparaginase in children with advanced leukemia. Cancer 30:339-347, 1972.
22. Mahaley MS, Honeycutt H, Bonner H, et al.: Localization of methylbis (2-chloroethyl-C)-amine hycrochloride in nervous tissue after intravenous injection or regional cerebral perfusion in dogs. Cancer Chemother. Rep. 11:29-32, 1961.
23. Nay Smith A, Robson T: Focal fits during cyloxin therapy. Postgrad. Med. J. 55:806-807, 1979.
24. Piel IJ, Meyer D, Perlia CP, et al.: Effects of cis-platinum on hearing function in man. Cancer Chemother. Rep. 58:871-875, 1974.
25. Rall DP, Rieselbach RE, Olliverio V, et al.: Pharmacology of folic acid antagonists as related to brain and cerebrospinal fluid. Cancer Chemother. Rep. 16:187-190,1962.
26. Sandler SG, Tobin T, Henderson ES: Vincristine medical neuropathy. Neurology 19:367-374, 1969.
27. Shapiro WR, Chernik NZ, Posner JB: Necrotizing encephalopathy following instillation of methotrexate. Arch. Neurol. 28:96-102, 1973.

28. Weiss HD, Walker MD, Wiernik PH, et al.: Preclinical and Phase I clinical studies of intrathecal thio-TEPA. Proc. Am. Assoc. Can. Res. 15:65, 1974.
29. Wilson WJ, Bisel HF, Cole D, et al.: Prolonged low dosage administration of hexamethylmelamine (NSC-13875). Cancer 25:568-570, 1970.
30. Young DF: Neurologic complications of cancer chemotherapy. In A. Silverstein, ed., Neurological Complications of Therapy, pp. 57-113. Futura, Mount Kisco, New York, 1982.
31. Young DF, Posner JB: Nervous system toxicity of the chemotherapeutic agents. In PJ Vinken and GW Bruyn, eds., Handbook of Clinical Neurology, Vol. 39, pp. 91-130. Amsterdam, North-Holland Pub. Co., 1980.
32. Winkelman MD, Hines JD: Cerebellar degeneration caused by high dose cytosine arabinoside: a clinicopathological study. Ann. Neurol. 14:520-527, 1983.

CHAPTER 17

Dietary Toxins and Miscellaneous Drugs

THE first section of this chapter focuses on purposely consumed dietary substances that may provoke acute or chronic toxic signs. Reliable information on the dose of the responsible product is often difficult to determine. In the case of vitamins, people often follow the philosophy: "if one vitamin pill is good, surely one hundred will be one hundred times better."

The second section briefly covers a variety of medications that provoke significant neurotoxic signs, but for which extensive research data are usually not available. The brevity of each discussion should not suggest that the syndromes are inconsequential, but rather that the details of mechanism of action, pharmacology, and biochemistry are often not so well studied as many of the toxins in the preceding chapters.

■ DIETARY TOXINS

ALCOHOL

Alcohol is widely used product with numerous neurotoxic syndromes associated with its use. Undoubtedly, certain major clinical problems relate, not to the direct toxic effect of the alcohol, but primarily to the generalized malnutrition that often accompanies the alcoholic's life-style. Alcohol provides significant dietary calories, but is mostly metabolized directly to carbon dioxide and water and hence these "naked" calories yield little to the synthesis of amino acids, fats, and carbohydrates. Furthermore, alcohol inhibits gastric emptying and intestinal absorption of nutrients, resulting in additional poor net nutrition.

In patients with heavy alcohol intake, the inebriated state itself may leave the patient anorexic, vomiting, and disinterested in eating. As one example, the well-known Wernicke-Korsakoff syndrome appears to relate not to direct neurotoxicity from alcohol, but to thiamine deficiency often associated with alcoholism.

On the other hand, ethanol as a molecule may precipitate direct toxic damage to normal neural function. RNA and protein synthesis as well as enzyme activation can be inhibited by chronic alcohol exposure in animals [38]; these changes are most pronounced in glial tissue. Chronic alcohol exposure also alters neurotransmitter systems with increased norepinephrine turnover, possibly decreased dopamine turnover, and no change in serotonin turnover. Alcoholic inebriation and withdrawal are the only two neurologic states established to relate to alcohol itself.

Alcohol consumption is associated with toxicity to other systems and secondary neurologic dysfunction can occur. Hepatic encephalopathy, pressure palsies, and crush injury myopathy are representative examples of such secondary syndromes. Finally, a number of syndromes are well described and associated with alcohol, but lack an understood relationship to alcohol itself, general nutrition, or other systemic/traumatic causes. In Table 17.1, these four categories are summarized. Only alcohol inebriation and withdrawal are discussed here, with short mention of two entities where there is significant evidence suggesting a direct toxic effect of alcohol, fetal alcohol syndrome and cortical atrophy [49]. Neurotoxic signs may also be seen when patients are treated for their alcoholism with disulfiram (see the section on disulfiram in this chapter).

Clinical Features

Alcohol Intoxication

A commonplace disorder known to the layman as well as the physician, intoxication precipitates loquacious exhilaration and loss of inhibitions, with gradual poor coordination, drowsiness, and eventually depressed consciousness. Rarely, the patient may become acutely paranoid and destructive, termed "atypical or pathological intoxication." The pathophysiology of this paradoxically excessive stimulation is unknown. The depressive effect of ethanol is felt to relate to a general membrane depression similar to the effect of anesthetics. The anatomic site of depressant action involves cerebrum, brain stem and spinal cord. At the cellular level, the acute intoxicating effects of ethanol have been postulated to relate to alcohol intercalation within neuronal membranes with remittant conduction and transmission aberrations [53]. After chronic exposure to alcohol, brain membrane lipid content changes; these induced effects may play a significant role in the neurologic manifestation of withdrawal [21].

TABLE 17.1. Neurotoxicity Syndromes Associated with Alcohol Abuse

1. Direct effects of alcohol:
   Inebriation
   Withdrawal

2. Vitamin or other nutrient deficiencies associated with alcohol abuse:
   Wernicke-Korsakoff psychosis
   Polyneuropathy
   Toxic amblyopia
   Cerebellar anterior lobe atrophy

3. Associated with alcoholism but with unknown etiologies:
   Ventricular enlargement and enlarged cortical sulci
   Fetal alcohol syndrome
   Marchiafava-Bignami
   Central pontine myelinolysis
   Dementia

4. Associated with systemic complications of alcoholism or with trauma:
   Hepatic encephalopathy
   Subdural hematoma

The general treatment of intoxication is supportive; in the overactive, pathologically intoxicated patient, sedation with phenobarbital 200 mg subcutaneously, repeated once if needed, may control the bizarre and alarming agitation. If the patient lapses into coma, he must be treated as a potential medical emergency, since alcohol depresses medullary respiratory centers at anesthetic doses. In subjects with blood alcohol levels greater than 500 mg, hemodialysis may be required [22].

Alcohol Withdrawal [51]

Binge drinkers or chronic alcoholics who stop or significantly decrease their alcohol intake will withdraw. The most common sign of withdrawal is a coarse postural tremor that appears in the morning and abates promptly with more alcohol. If more alcohol is not available, tremor peaks 24-36 hours later and will be accompanied by progressive restlessness and agitation.

Flushed face, tachycardia, vomiting, and profuse sweating, often with dehydration, typify progressive withdrawal. Fasciculations, myoclonus, and motoric agitation accompany the rapid and irregular tremor that may become so severe that speech, eating and ambulation are compromised. When alcohol can again be located, the symptoms abate, so that if the patient is hospitalized, discharge at this time will lead to a highly motivated return to heavy drinking. Resumption of alcohol will diminish tremor (and often hallucinations, discussed below) but may aggravate dysautonomia, suggesting that alcohol must be affecting the nervous system at multiple levels simultaneously.

Hallucinations are an additional complication in alcohol withdrawal, occurring in 25%-35% of tremulous withdrawing subjects. While usually visual, hallucinations may be auditory or tactile. They may be bizarre, elaborate fantasies more typical of classic aminergic drug-induced hallucinations superimposed on a clear sensorium, or part of a severe confusional state more typical of classic anticholinergic hallucinations. The pharmacology of such hallucinations may well be varied in different states. A special form of auditory hallucinations superimposed on a clear sensorium is remarkable and is not seen in most other withdrawal states or intoxications. Voices which may be intensely personal and specific, a reprimanding parent or desperate friend, or primitive sounds like buzzes or clinks, termed "elementary hallucinations" by Bleuler, may haunt the patient. So real are these that in spite of the clear sensorium, patients will insist that the voices or sounds are actually occurring and lack the insight to accept them as hallucinations. In a rare subgroup, auditory hallucinations persist beyond the withdrawal period, although these patients' affect changes to a quiet and resigned acceptance of the sounds.

Seizures are a feared neurotoxic complication of alcohol withdrawal, occurring usually within 48 hours after alcohol cessation. These are generalized convulsions, although in a patient with prior head trauma or cerebral damage from another alcohol-related event, the seizure may start focally and rapidly spread. The seizure may be single or multiple and rarely, status epilepticus develops. The presence of withdrawal seizures identifies the patient as a high-risk candidate for full delirium tremons (DTs), since one-third of patients who seize progress to delirium tremens [52].

Delirium tremens is the profound extreme of the above symptoms with severe agitation, wild hallucinations, tremor, and autonomic dysfunction. The forced abstention from alcohol in the hospital provides a fertile environment for this medical emergency. In most cases, the syndrome spontaneously resolves after days of psychic and nervous overactivity, the patient falling into a deep sleep and awakening without significant recall of the preceding events. Because 5%-15% of DT subjects die, however, these patients must be evaluated for additional disease and monitored with caution (see below).

In spite of the frequency and morbidity of alcohol inebriation and withdrawal, the biochemical alterations that provoke these varied alterations are not clear. Animal models have always been complicated by inconsistencies in treatment protocols and in the individual neurotoxic signs investigated. Systemic alterations seen consistently in withdrawing alcoholics include hypomagnesia and alkalosis. Neuromuscular irritability, apprehension, and seizures may relate in part to these central peripheral ionic alterations. The elementary auditory hallucinations stereotypic and repetitive may, closely resemble focal seizures arising

Dietary Toxins and Miscellaneous Drugs

from primary auditory cortex. These highly organized hallucinations also seem cortical in origin, suggesting dysfunction in the accessory auditory cortex of the temporal lobes.

Because withdrawing patients are subject to prior and current head trauma, a search for extra- and intracranial disease should be made. Skull films, CT, and lumbar puncture will evaluate possible fractures, subdural hematomas, and infections. Temperature, pulse and blood pressure must be monitored with careful attention to electolyte and fluid management. Often eight liters daily of fluid will be needed to combat dehydration; because glucose can precipitate Wernicke's encephalopathy in a patient with marginal thiamine stores, much of this fluid should be given as normal saline with thiamine supplementation. A cooling mattress may be needed to combat hyperthermia, and should be readily available, since high fevers can develop over short periods. The possibility of systemic infection must also be considered. Mild sedatives can be helpful in the behavioral control, although phenothiazines should be avoided, because they may lower seizure threshold. Multiple withdrawal seizures may be treated with phenytoin or phenobarbital: long-term management of alcohol-related seizures is especially difficult with phenobarbital, however, since when the patient stops drinking, he usually stops his medications as well, inducing two simultaneous withdrawal states.

Cerebral Atrophy and Fetal Alcohol Syndrome

Enlarged ventricles and cortical sulci are features commonly seen by noninvasive scanning in alcoholics, and in patients with a known chronic history of heavy alcohol consumption [3]. Formerly diagnosed by pneumoencephalopathy or at autopsy, this finding is now readily detected by CT and NMR scanning. Such changes do not correlate directly with cognitive decline or dementia and patients may be intellectually asymptomatic. Although it has been suggested with vigor that these changes are structural and related to alcohol toxicity to the cortex, this claim is not yet substantiated. Apparent atrophy may be reversible with rehydration and return to more normal protein synthesis after alcohol cessation. Transient fluid shifts seen with Cushing's disease and anorexia nervosa can produce similar fluctuating CT findings. Although radiologists should refrain from making a clinical diagnosis from an X-ray, the presence of marked ventricular dilatation and enlarged cortical sulci in a young or middle-aged subject has led to the frequently seen CT report suggesting that the patient may likely be an undisclosed alcohol abuser. The apparent good nutritional state of many of these subjects suggests that vitamin deficiency is not the significant etiologic factor here.

In infants born of severely alcoholic mothers, a particularly pathetic clinical syndrome has been described. These neonates are small in length with a

Dietary Toxins and Miscellaneous Drugs

tiny head circumference and have distinctive facies: small palpebral fissures, cleft palate, and micrognathia. Joint deformities, cardiac abnormalities and external genital anomalies may also occur. The neurologic development may be delayed and in those who have died, Clarren and Smith found leptomeningeal thickening, agenesis of the corpus calossum, and obstructive hydrocephalus with extensive heterotopias in the brain stem [5]. Additionally, these babies withdraw from alcohol in the first days of life, developing tremors, irritability and poor sucking. It is not completely settled whether the syndrome relates to alcohol or nutrition. Support of a direct toxic effect for alcohol is provided by animal studies where embryotoxic effects are induced by chronic alcohol in the absence of nutritional deprivation. One hypothesis combining alcohol toxicity with nutritional deprivation suggests that the alcohol may disrupt the fetus's absorption of nutrients so that even if the mother is well nourished, the syndrome still relates to a fetal deficiency of folate, Vitamin A, zinc, or other essential products.

VITAMINS

These vital trace substances are generally associated with deficiency syndromes and many are not currently applicable to a text on neurotoxicology. However, since health enthusiasm has reached passionate proportions for many individuals, especially Americans, clinicians are encountering neurotoxic syndromes associated with these seemingly safe agents. Of the fat-soluble vitamins, vitamin A is directly associated with neurotoxicity, and vitamin D can alter bone and renal metabolism, causing secondary neurologic dysfunction. Of the water-soluble vitamins, only pyridoxine (B_6) is established to provoke neurologic complications. Future research may unmask other self-inflicted or iatrogenic syndromes caused by agents aimed at in fact improving health.

Vitamin A [32] clearly required for normal growth, vision, reproduction and maintenance of epithelium, in high doses accumulates and can induce the syndrome of increased intracranial pressure (pseudotumor cerebri). Foods high in vitamin A include broccoli, cabbage, and liver, although dietary hypervitaminosis A is most unusual. In artic regions, where the population ingests polar bear liver, pseudotumor cerebri due to vitamin A intoxication appears to occur without additional vitamin supplementation. Medically, vitamin A is used in the treatment of acne vulgaris and other dermatologic illnesses. Whereas the generally recommended daily allowance is 5,000 IU, individual capsules can contain 5 times that value, with subjects often ingesting 100,000 IU daily. At these doses, intoxication will develop over several months; at 200,000 IU daily, intoxication may develop within weeks. Recent publicity about vitamin A's cancer preventive properties may increase the number of people who self-expose themselves to this product.

The systemic toxicity includes erythema, pruritis, anoxia, and hepatosplenomegaly. Early signs of increased intracranial pressure include headaches, blurred vision, transient obscuration of vision, and sixth cranial nerve paresis. On fundoscopic examination, gradual papilledema develops without further signs of focal neurologic deficit. No neurologic clue exists to establish the etiology, but the skin changes, organomegaly, and history of vitamin ingestion will establish the diagnosis. Since vitamin zealots are often "antimedication," these patients must be specifically questioned about vitamins. The mechanism whereby increased intracranial pressure develops is not known, although biochemically, the vitamin stimulates the synthesis of glycoproteins and mucopolysaccharides, which may alter fluid balance centrally [7].

Vitamin D

Massive amounts of vitamin D mobilize bone calcium and phosphorus. Where there is bone demineralization and degeneration, nerve root and spinal cord compression can occur. Alterations in the calcium balance can produce generalized weakness, muscle aches, cramps, and mild metabolic encephalopathy. Meningeal symptoms and trigeminal neuralgia are two additional reported findings without clear pathogenesis. The latter may relate to bony foraminal alterations. When renal impairment occurs, progressive secondary encephalopathy, not directly related to the vitamin, develops and coma may result.

Vitamin B_6

Pyridoxine has recently been implicated in a highly selective toxic syndrome provoking a sensory ataxia and dorsal root gangliar dysfunction. Widely used, especially by women to treat premenstrual tension and edema, pyridoxine induces this neurotoxic syndrome in occasional patients consuming chronic daily doses of 2 grams or more. Gradually, the patient notes difficulty walking with lightning-like dyesthesias in the back. Numbness of the extremities occurs and importantly, facial dyesthesias, so uncommon with most toxic neuropathies other than trichloroethane, quickly develops. Areflexia, stocking/glove sensory loss, and profound sensory ataxia with preserved strength are typical. On EMG, marked slowing of the sensory nerve conduction is seen with normal motor conduction [46].

Animals treated with high doses of B_6 develop vacuolation and degeneration of dorsal root and Gasserian ganglion cells, along with a widespread degeneration of sensory nerve fibers. Treatment involves cessation of B_6 and in some cases there is dramatic, although often slow, recovery.

It is of practical importance to know that low- or moderate-dose pyridoxine, although not specifically neurotoxic, when added to the diet of a parkinsonian patient receiving levodopa will precipitiously cause an exacerbation of the Parkinson's disease. B_6 is a cofactor for dopa decarboxylase and enhances the systemic conversion of dopa to dopamine: since dopamine cannot cross the blood-brain barrier, this enhanced peripheral synthesis of dopamine in fact diminishes central delivery of dopa for effective antiparkinson therapy. When sufficient carbidopa is added to levodopa, this pyridoxine "toxicity" is probably insignificant [54].

FOOD ADDITIVES

In 1973, Feingold suggested that hyperactivity in children could largely be related to the ingestion of food additives. The outgrowth of this hypothesis, the Feingold "elimination" diet, has remained over 10 years a scientific and emotional controversy with the potential for far-reaching public health implications. Preservatives and dyes are pervasive dietary constituents in American life and are in fact difficult to avoid without enormous disruption of one's diet. Anecdotes describing hyperactive and inattentive children who dramatically improved emotionally and in their schoolwork after eliminating all such products led to extensive and costly clinical investigations. In 1982, the Nutritional Foundation Advisory Committee and the National Institutes of Health Panel concluded: "The evidence that the total Feingold diet produces improvement in the behavior of hyperactive children is equivocal. The mild and entirely subjective changes that have been reported are not in our opinion clinically important. . . . It is our opinion that the studies already completed provide sufficient evidence to refute the claim that artificial food colorings, artificial flavorings and salicylates produce hyperactivity and/or learning disability" [37].

The conclusions were based on two types of clinical tests: double-blind controlled dietary studies using the Feingold diet and another diet with additives, and "challenge" studies, where additives were given to see if hyperactivity could be precipitated. In both instances, conclusive links between disability and diet could not be established. Importantly, the dietary restrictions are so strict in the Feingold diet that its incorporation into the family regimen requires substantial modifications in multiple areas of family life. Since behavioral modification is felt to be one important aspect of helping children with attentional deficits, the diet may well have achieved success through this mechanism in many households. Certainly, the food-additive-free diet has no apparently harmful neurologic or systemic effects, hence there is no need to discourage families who choose to embark on this dietary challenge [29].

Dietary Toxins and Miscellaneous Drugs

CHINESE RESTAURANT SYNDROME: MONOSODIUM GLUTAMATE (MSG)

In 1968, Kowk, a Chinese physician, described a strange, possibly neurologic syndrome occurring when he ate at American-Chinese restaurants [26]. He suggested that MSG could be the provoking agent as this product is used widely in Chinese restaurants to enhance the flavor of food. The syndrome has three major symptoms, occurring within 15 minutes after ingestion of Chinese food and lasting approximately 1 hour: a dysesthetic facial pressure, burning dysesthesias over the trunk, and chest pain. Headache, which may be migraine in quality, is more frequently seen in patients with a prior history of headaches. Other vague symptoms like malaise and lightheadedness may accompany the triad. GI complaints also were originally included in the description but in fact do not appear to relate directly to MSG. Women appear to be more frequently afflicted than men and the general reaction rate has been estimated as high as 30% in some series. As discussed below, multiple factors appear to influence the incidence and severity of this syndrome, including subject expectation. The threshold required for the MSG syndrome has been estimated at 3 grams, the amount in a typical 200-ml serving of wonton soup [15].

It is not fully established that MSG is in fact the causative agent. In a placebo-controlled study with all subjects taking 6 grams MSG, only one patient had the typical reaction. Important contributing influences may therefore also be the vehicle, whether the subject has been fasting, and whether a protein or carbohydrate load accompanies the MSG. A significant placebo effect has been postulated since Kerr et al.'s report that 31% of subjects aware of the Chinese Restaurant Syndrome believed they themselves experienced it compared to only 2.3% of the general population [24]. Kenny reported the nonspecificity of the syndrome, with the same symptoms occurring with coffee and spiced tomato juice, without MSG [23].

The pathophysiology of the syndrome has been suggested to relate to glutamate, which may be a neurotransmitter in the central nervous system. As an excitatory agent on unidentified receptor sites, glutamate may alter synaptic transmission. Ghadimi et al. 1971 suggested that the symptoms of MSG intoxication instead relate to cholinergic overstimulation: they demonstrated a potentiated response with an anticholinergic drug if treated with physostigmine [13]. Schaumburg et al. (1969) suggested a non-neurologic vascular mechanism whereby arterial receptors are stimulated or blocked by MSG or its metabolites. Against this hypothesis, however, are the observations that pulse and blood pressure changes do not accompany the MSG syndrome [45].

IATROGENIC AND MEDICINAL TOXINS

▪ MISCELLANEOUS DRUGS

ANTIINFLAMMATORY AGENTS

Because of their ready availability in almost all households, salicylates represent a common source of intoxication, accounting for the largest yearly number of serious childhood poisonings [8]. In acute intoxication, the prominent neurologic and respiratory signs may immediately suggest the correct diagnosis and direct prompt and appropriate intervention. The neurologic manifestations of salicylate toxicity include a rapid and dramatic alteration in consciousness and global function with convulsions and coma. Confusion and restlessness are seen early, leading within a few hours to excitability, tremor, incoherent speech, and often delirium or hallucinosis. This phase has been referred to as "salicylate jag" to indicate its similarity to alcoholic inebriation, although euphoria and elation are conspicuously absent with salicylates. After this phase, a gradual depression in the level of consciousness occurs with a rapid lapse into coma. Seizures are especially common in children and are as a rule generalized [9]. The pathophysiology of the convulsions appears to relate to combined effects of metabolic and respiratory disturbances. Salicylates additionally inhibit the synthesis of gamma-aminobutyric acid (GABA), a putative neurotransmitter in the central nervous system. Since depressed levels of GABA have been suggested to relate to the lowering of seizures threshold, salicylates may induce or potentiate convulsions by this mechanism [48]. In infants, salicylate intoxication induces a marked hypoglycemia, and seizure activity is especially hazardous in this young age group [28]. Diplopia, dizziness, and decreased visual acuity can also be seen with salicylate intoxication. Involvement of the audiovestibular (eighth cranial) nerve can lead to tinnitus, vertigo, and complete deafness. This complication is more common with chronic salicylate intoxication and is seen especially in elderly patients treated for arthritic or headache conditions where aspirin or salicylate compounds are ingested daily [36].

The respiratory complications of salicylate toxicity are of paramount importance since they contribute to a severe acid-base disturbance. Salicylates stimulate respiration by three basic mechanisms: direct brain stem activation, enhanced chemosensitive response mechanisms centrally, and a compensatory hyperventilation mediated to combat metabolic increases in CO_2. In higher doses, salicylates gradually induce a depressant effect in brain stem function, so that a predominantly uncompensated respiratory acidosis may be seen. This situation merges into a combined respiratory and metabolic acidosis as three acid groups accumulate: first, salicylic acid derivatives that displace bicarbonate; second, sulfuric and phosphoric acid; and, finally, organic acids that can induce ketosis as well as acidosis [7].

This sequence from primary respiratory alkalosis to respiratory acidosis to combined respiratory-metabolic acidosis forms the hallmark of salicylate intoxication in infants and young children. In school-aged children, respiratory alkalosis and respiratory acidosis are seen, while in adults the respiratory alkalosis is the prominent feature, with depression of breathing being seen only with high levels of toxic products. Although the mechanism of this maturational resistance to metabolic acidosis remains unclear, the consistent respiratory-metabolic patterns of the different age groups assists in the acute management of these patients. Furthermore, these patterns serve especially to alert the physician to the possibility of more than one ingested toxic substance when the clinical picture deviates from the expected age sequence. These instances include adults who attempt suicide with multiple drugs and children who invade the medicine chest where more than one toxic compound is available.

Treatment of salicylate toxicity involves minimizing drug absorption, hastening drug elimination, correcting acid-base disturbance, and treating existing neurologic or medical complications [7]. Induced emesis in the awake patient is the most effective means of emptying the stomach. Enhanced elimination is effected by alkalinization of the urine or by peritoneal or hemodialysis. Careful fluid and electrolyte management are vital and depend on the age of the patient and the stage of intoxication. The complications of hypoglycemia in infants must be anticipated and thereby prevented. Seizures are usually treated with phenytoin and phenobarbital.

There is poor correlation between the serum salicylate levels and the clinical severity of intoxication [8]. Despite apparently adequate treatment and progressive lowering of toxic plasma salicylate levels, sudden and unexplained deaths are not rare. Experimental studies demonstrate that animals dying from salicylate overdose may show wide variance of plasma salicylate concentrations, but have consistent brain salicylate levels. These data suggest that brain and potentially CSF levels of salicylate may be of more critical prognostic value in the management of salicylate-intoxicated patients than plasma salicylate levels.

The salicylates were hypothesized to play a role in the pathogenesis of childhood hyperkinetic syndromes. The Feingold diet (see food additives, this chapter) included complete abstinence from all salicylates. As discussed, this diet has not, in controlled scientific studies, proved successful and salicylates do not presently appear to precipitate or exacerbate motoric hyperactivity.

Indomethacin has proven to be a very potent antiinflammatory drug but appears less efficacious than salicylates in the treatment of arthritis and rheumatoid variants. Its mode of action is still uncertain but it may act via inhibition of prostaglandin synthesis [33]. Central nervous system toxicity is one of in the most frequent dose limiting factors precluding the use of indomethacin in 30%–50% of patients. Neurotoxic effects consist of headaches, depression, agitation and, rarely, hallucinations. Ataxia, clumsiness, and impaired postural reflexes may also occur, although slow increases in dosage may prevent their development.

Phenylbutazone, used in the treatment of ankylosing spondylitis, is not associated with marked neurotoxic effects. Alteration in the sensation of taste is the most reported neurologic side effect. Phenylbutazone alters the metabolism of phenytoin and in seizure patients may be associated with anticonvulsant toxicity or increased seizure activity [33].

Naproxen has been associated with adverse neurologic reactions in approximately 8% of patients. These effects include headache, drowsiness, vertigo, inability to concentrate, and depression. Because of its protein-binding affinity, naproxen can be associated with phenytoin toxicity in seizure patients. By displacing phenytoin from proteins, naproxen causes higher levels of unbound phenytoin to circulate, so that toxic signs develop even though the total serum phenytoin level remains in the therapeutic range.

Sulindac is another recently marketed nonsteroidal antiinflammatory agent recommended for use in various types of arthritis. Its mode of action may be inhibition of prostaglandin synthesis by one of its metabolites, a sulfide. The neurotoxicity of sulindac has been estimated at between 1% and 10%, with headache and dizziness being most common complaints. Vertigo, tinnitus, and decreased hearing occur in less than 1% of reported patients. Paresthesias, peripheral neuropathy, and transient blurring of vision are quite rare, but more clincial experience is needed to confirm the true incidence of these reactions [55].

CARDIAC AGENTS

Digitalis and related cardiac glycosides are the mainstay of treatment for congestive heart failure. Neurologic complications of digitalis therapy have been recognized for almost 200 years and are characterized by nausea, vomiting, visual disturbances, seizures, and syncope. Adverse effects on the central nervous system reportedly occur in 40% to 50% of patients with clinical digitalis toxicity and may occur before, simultaneously with, or after the signs of cardiac toxicity develop [30]. Explanations for the dramatic incidence of neurotoxicity with digitalis have been inadequate and the few pathological studies compiled have not demonstrated consistent lesions.

The most frequent neurotoxic reaction and often the first sign of clinical digitalis toxicity is nausea. Nausea resulting from digitalis appears to be due to central mechanisms rather than gastrointestinal irritation. Digitalis apparently stimulates the chemoreceptor trigger zone, which lies in the floor of the fourth ventricle. Animal experiments corroborate this theory. Nausea associated with digitalis toxicity is often accompanied by vomiting and, when chronic, may lead to malnourishment, cachexia and even Wernicke's encephalopathy [43].

The incidence of digitalis-related visual disturbances has been estimated at 40%, which may occur as an isolated symptom; however, they usually occur concomitantly with other toxic signs. Blurred vision, reversible scotomas, diplopia, defects of color vision, and total amaurosis represent the spectrum of optic side effects. The pathogenesis of visual disturbances secondary to digitalis intoxication is unknown.

Seizures are known to occur as a result of digitalis toxicity and are most commonly seen in the pediatric population. The incidence of digitalis-related seizures is difficult to estimate since other seizure etiologies (i.e., arrhythmia) are so high in the cardiac patient population. The mechanism by which digitalis induces seizures has been postulated to involve inhibition of membrane ATPase and subsequent neuronal irritability.

Transient mental aberrations believed to be due to intermittent cerebral hypoperfusion resemble transient global amnesia. Syncope, probably due to conduction delay or hyperactivity of baroreceptors, has also occurred in digitalis toxicity. Other neurotoxic reactions include facial neuralgia, paresthesias, headache, weakness, and fatigue. Cerebral symptoms consisting of confusion, delirium, mania, and hallucinosis have been reported in as many as 15% of patients with digitalis toxicity. Although the mechanism for the symptoms is unknown, it is believed that they are not the result of altered cardiac function.

Quinidine is present in the cinchona bark, along with quinine and other alkaloids. It is chiefly used in treating auricular fibrillation, but, because of its quininelike antimalarial activity, it has also been employed in the tropics as a substitute in cases of quinine sensitivity. Nervous system manifestations are usually not significant, but with overdosage or in susceptible individuals, quinidine causes an intoxication similar to that of quinine. The symptoms of cinchonism are headache, nausea, vomiting, blurring of vision, and ringing of the ears. Flushing, palpitations, and even convulsions may occur. A precipitous drop in blood pressure related to vagal influences can cause syncope, vertigo, and, in rare instances, respiratory arrest.

Methyldopa has been widely prescribed since 1960, and is associated with neurotoxic side effects. The mechanism of action of methyldopa is felt to relate to inhibition of dopa decarboxylase, both centrally and peripherally. The adverse effects on the central nervous system apparently are associated with the synthesis of false catecholamine neurotransmitters, methyl-norepinephrine, and methyldopamine [50].

The most frequent side effect of methyldopa is sedation, which is usually transient in nature, but may persist in as many as 5% of patients. Mood alterations including depression are not uncommon, although most patients developing behavior changes usually have a prior history of affective illness. The depressive state is reversible upon withdrawal of the drug. Parkinsonism, resulting from dopamine depletion, has been reported several times but, considering the widespread use of this agent, is quite rare [18]. Nevertheless, patients with established Parkinson's disease should be treated with antihypertensive agents other than methyldopa and reserpine. Other minor neurological complaints associated with methyldopa include confusion, dizziness, headaches, and syncope.

Clonidine, an imidazoline derivative, is an effective drug in the treatment of hypertension. The mechanism of action of clonidine has not been fully elucidated, but it appears that this agent acts via alpha-2 adrenergic receptor stimulation. It has been suggested that this stimulation may result in an overall decrease in norepinephrine release, possibly via presynaptic inhibition. The most common adverse neurologic effect of clonidine is sedation. Other less common neurotoxic reactions include depression, irritability, nightmares, and a reversible dementia syndrome, which is felt to occur as a result of reduction in cerebral blood flow. Clonidine has been used in the pediatric population to control multifocal tics (Gilles de la Tourette's Syndrome). No large double-blind study has yet established its efficacy, but no major neurotoxic effects have been seen when the drug is used in children.

Hydralazine is the only direct-acting vasodilator generally available for the treatment of chronic hypertension. The neurologic side effects of hydralazine are few and quite uncommon in clinical practice. Peripheral neuropathy characterized by diffuse numbness and tingling is the only consistent neurotoxic reaction and is believed to be due to a direct toxic effect of hydralazine. Although hydralazine contains a nitrogen moiety also present in isoniazid, it is not clear whether this moiety is of pathophysiologic significance [42].

Propranolol is one of the multiple beta-adrenergic receptor blockers presently in clinical usage in the United States. Propranolol is mainly used in the medical management of angina pectoris, hypertension, and certain cardiac arrhythmias. It appears that propranolol promotes hypotension by reducing cardiac output, reducing renin synthesis, and possibly by central nervous system effects not yet elucidated [19].

Neuropsychiatric symptoms occur frequently during treatment with propranolol. Lassitude or insomnia and depression are the most common reactions, although vivid nightmares, hypnagogic hallucinations, and psychotic behavior have been reported with high-dose (more than 500 mg/day) propranolol therapy [12]. The nighttime behavioral problems can often be avoided by eliminating doses after 8 p.m. More recently, psychotic symptoms have been seen even with low-dose (up to 160 mg/day) therapy and especially in two classes of high-risk patients—those with prior histories of major psychiatric illness and those with hyperthyroidism. The pharmacology of propranolol-induced psychosis is unclear, although pre- and postsynaptic adrenergic inhibition has been implicated, as has serotonergic antagonism. Orthostatic lightheadedness, mild unsteadiness of gait, and dizziness may also be seen and may relate to the hypotensive effect of the drug.

Lidocaine, one of a variety of local anesthetics used widely in medical and surgical practice, is additionally a potent anti-arrhythmic agent. It is used ex-

Dietary Toxins and Miscellaneous Drugs

tensively in intensive care and coronary surveillance units and has been associated with neurotoxicity. Clearly, the CNS effects are not specific to lidocaine, and can be seen with other local anesthetics. Lidocaine-induced CNS toxicity, however, is far more common, and may relate to its rapid absorption across the blood-brain barrier. The syndrome appears to relate to a diffuse excitation of neuronal systems with an early prodrome of altered behavior. Garrulousness and loss of inhibitions may be the prominent feature, as may agitation or psychosis. Circumoral numbness, diplopia, and tinnitus may also occur, with progressive muscle twitches and tremors. Generalized myoclonic seizures and finally CNS and respiratory depression are seen with higher doses [13]. In both the cardiac and surgical patients, hypoxia and acidosis rapidly develop if the lidocaine syndrome is not reversed. Treatment focuses on adequate oxygenation and support, since the half-life of bolus lidocaine given acutely is 6-8 minutes. Since repeated injections, however, change the kinetics of lidocaine and prolong its half-life to approximately 90 minutes, more long-lasting effects can be seen [16].

CHELATING AGENTS

2,3,Dimercaptol-1-propanol (BAL) was synthesized during World War II as an antidote for arsenic-containing Lewisite gas. This compound, named British Anti-Lewisite, or BAL, has also been found to be effective against the toxic manifestations of arsenic, mercury, gold, antimony, bismuth, cobalt and nickel. The toxicity of these metals is due, at least in part, to their combination with the sulfhydryl group of the protein portion of certain enzymes; BAL counteracts this effect, presumably by supplying a sulfhydryl radical with which the toxic metallic ion preferentially unites, thus freeing the same group in the enzymes [17].

With doses of 2.5 mg/kg of body weight, toxic symptoms develop in less than 1% of individuals; with twice that dose, there is a 50%-60% increase in the occurrence of intoxication. The symptoms appear within 10 to 20 minutes after injection of the drug and subside within 50 to 90 minutes.

The usual reaction consists of headache, burning sensations in the mouth and eyes, muscular aches, paresthesias, pain in the teeth, lacrimation, salivation, rhinorrhea and profuse sweating. Restlessness, anxiety and general agitation may also develop, with progression in some instances to generalized convulsions and stupor. Abdominal pain apprehension, blepharospasm, piloerection, tachycardia, and palpitations have also been noted.

Because of the transient nature of the toxic symptoms, no treatment is needed in BAL poisoning. 25 mg of ephedrine sulfate before the injection of BAL may lessen the incidence of toxic reactions.

Penicillamine has played a role in the treatment of a wide array of disorders, including Wilson's disease, lead poisoning, cystinuria and scleroderma. Although not officially approved in the United States until quite recently for the treatment of rheumatoid arthritis, penicillamine has shown efficacy in clinical trials dating back to 1970. With the increased use of penicillamine have come increased reports of side effects. These toxic effects have been especially prominent in patients with connective tissue disorders.

The most frequently encountered neurotoxic effect of this drug is loss or abnormality of taste, which has been correlated with high doses and duration of therapy [6]. Hypogeusia occurs in 25%-30% of patients at doses of 1 gram daily within six weeks. It may be reversible with decreasing the dosage or discontinuation of the drug and may not occur at all in dosages of 500 mg or less. Zinc infiltration of taste receptors has been postulated as causing the hypogeusia induced by penicillamine.

Dermatomyositis and polymyositis characterized by typical tender proximal muscle weakness with elevation of serum aldolase and creatinine phosphokinase may occur during penicillamine therapy. This rare side effect is usually associated with serologic abnormalities resembling lupus erythematosis. Another neurologic side effect of penicillamine therapy in rheumatoid arthritis is a myasthenic reaction with ptosis, diplopia, and dysphagia [2]. Generalized weakness usually follows, especially if early signs go undetected. Edrophonium reversibility confirms the clinical diagnosis and laboratory studies demonstrate characteristic autoantibodies to acetylcholine receptor [44]. It is not known whether or not penicillamine uncovers preexisting subclinical myasthenia gravis by causing neuromuscular blockade similar to certain antibiotics. Withdrawal of the drug and treatment with cholinesterase inhibitors reverse the weakness over several months.

A final neurotoxic effect of penicillamine therapy is optic neuritis. The classic symptom of visual loss is thought to be a result of an antipyridoxine effect on the optic nerve by penicillamine. This side effect is quite rare and vitamin B_6 administration is not considered a necessary addition to penicillamine therapy.

DRUGS THAT INDUCE MYOTONIA

A number of pharmacologic agents are capable of inducing a syndrome in man that is similar if not identical to the myotonia which occurs in various disease states.

20-25-Diazacholesterol (DAG) is an azasterol that was introduced in 1960 for the treatment of hypercholesterolemia [40]. It was soon discovered that DAC could induce a myotonic syndrome where patients had difficulty relaxing their grip, percussion myotonia, EMG evidence of myotonia and weakness, as well as other features reminiscent of myotonic dystrophy, such as cataracts. Because of the high incidence of this syndrome, DAC is no longer used, although the fact that a variety of DAC congeners can also elicit myotonia suggests that this drug class should be viewed cautiously.

The pathophysiology of DAC-induced myotonia appears to relate to the accumulation in muscle membrane of a cholesterol precursor, desmosterol. Myotonia appears when about 50% of the cholesterol molecules in the sarcolemma are replaced by desmosterol. This can be brought about by either acute or chronic DAC treatment. This alteration of sarcolemma sterol content is associated with a marked decrease in membrane chloride conductance, the same physiological dysfunction which occurs in myotonia congenita. This in turn causes the repetitive muscle action potentials which account for the delayed relaxation of voluntary muscles similar to that observed in the myotonic diseases [41].

Triparanol was also used clinically for the treatment of hypercholesterolemia and, like DAC, is felt to act by selective inhibition of the reductase enzyme which results in the accumulation of desmosterol in plasma, erythrocyte, and muscle membrane [40]. Unlike DAC, prolonged treatment with triparanol is required to induce myotonia. Triparanol is no longer used clinically because of the high incidence of cataracts and skin reactions. Clomiphene, an antiestrogenic agent used clinically to induce ovulation, is chemically related to triparanol and causes the accumulation of desmosterol in various tissues, presumably due to blocking the activity of Δ-24-reductase. There is no evidence that it induces myotonia, however.

Clofibrate, an aromatic monocarboxylic acid is capable of inducing myotonia in man, or in experimental animals and is clinically significant since it is used widely to reduce serum triglyceride levels. Other agents of this class capable of causing myotonia include indoleacetic acid, indolc-cthanol (the precursor of indoleacetic acid), and the herbicide 2,4-D(2,4-dichlorophenoxyacetic acid). The mechanism by which these agents induce myotonia is not as well defined as the inhibition of Δ-24-reductase by DAC and triparanol. These agents do, however, decrease chloride conductance in a manner that is qualitatively similar to that seen in both myotonia congenita and myotonia induced by Δ-24-reductase inhibitors. The pathogenesis of this alteration is different, however. The agents may in some way bind to the sarcolemman chloride carrier or to the outer rim of the chloride conductance channel. In either case, the resulting steric influence with the conductance of chloride results in myotonia. The observation that these agents can induce myotonia in vitro further supports a direct membrane effect.

Single cases of both vincristine- and propranolol-induced myotonia have been published. In both instances a definite causal relationship is unproven. It is quite possible that subclinical myotonia may have been present in both patients prior to treatment. There are also a number of reports in the literature of either respiratory depression or abnormal musculature relaxation in myotonic patients given general anesthesia, and it has even been suggested that myotonic dystrophie patients are unusually sensitive to thiopentone. This abnormal sensitivity is not, however, clearly established and, like the reported anesthetic complications, may be primarily related not to the myotonia itself, but to weakness of respiratory musculature or cardiopulmonary disease.

METOCLOPROMIDE

Metoclopromide is a relatively new anti-emetic which is not known to have potent antipsychotic properties and is not chemically related to the phenothiazines or butyrophenones. Its use, especially in children, has been associated with the occurrence of acute dystonic reactions, which resemble those seen with acute neuroleptic administration. The most prominent manifestations include retrocollis, torticollis and oculogyric crises, which are often both quite alarming and distressing. These reactions are always self-limited and usually disappear within hours of discontinuing the drug [4]. Parenteral diphenylhydramine has been found to relieve these dystonias. Like neuroleptic-induced dystonias, these reactions are probably related to acute dopamine receptor site blockade in the basal ganglion region.

Metoclopromide-induced parkinsonism is well described after weeks of therapy and this drug should not be given to patients with Parkinson's disease [25]. As with neuroleptic-induced parkinsonism, patients develop one or more of the cardinal features of Parkinson's disease, resting tremor, cogwheel rigidity, postural reflex instability, or bradykinesia. The syndrome is self-resolving within weeks or months after the cessation of metoclopromide.

Tardive dyskinesia, seen traditionally after months or years of antipsychotic neuroleptic administration, has also been associated with chronic metoclopromide treatment. Patients develop typical lingual-facial-buccal movement and limb chorea that may become medically significant if truncal and respiratory control become compromised. The pathophysiology of tardive dyskinesia [see Chapter 12] is believed to relate to striatal dopaminergic hypersensitivity induced by long-term receptor site blockade (pharmacologic denervation hypersensitivity) by the neuroleptic. Since most patients on neuroleptics are psychotic and most neuroleptics have potent antipsychotic properties, the potential roles of nonstriatal diseases or drug effects in tardive dyskinesia have remained unclear. That metoclopromide, without antipsychotic properties and therefore not used in psychotic patients, still induces tardive dyskinesias indicates that the movement disorder is not directly related to the pathophysiology of the psychiatric disease or neurotransmitter systems and paths directly involved in its abatement.

Dietary Toxins and Miscellaneous Drugs

DISULFIRAM (ANTABUSE)

Disulfiram is used in the rehabilitation of alcoholics, since high levels of acetaldehyde accumulate when alcohol is ingested with the drug. Chronic disulfiram therapy is associated with two distinct neurotoxic syndromes, an encephalopathy and a neuropathy. The encephalopathy is usually acute or subacute in onset, characterized by delirium, paranoid and psychotic behavior, and often is confused with the diagnosis of schizophrenic reaction [20]. Generally, the behavioral response to neuroleptics or other psychotropic drugs is not marked, a finding that should suggest a toxic cause; withdrawal of disulfiram and mild sedation with supportive care but without neuroleptic therapy are recommended in the treatment of disulfiram encephalopathy. The biochemical basis for this encephalopathy is unclear, but two observations suggest that an imbalance of dopamine and norepinephrine centrally may play a role. Disulfiram inhibits aldehyde dehydrogenase, an enzyme that can covert dopamine to homovanillic acid, and inhibits dopamine beta-hydroxylase, the enzyme necessary for the conversion of dopamine to norepinephrine [35]. Inhibition of these two enzyme systems by disulfiram results in increased dopamine concentrations and decreased norepinephrine concentrations in the rat brain [14].

Disulfiram is also associated with a rare, axonal distal sensorimotor polyneuropathy [34]. The recovery after drug withdrawal both clinically and pathologically suggests a dying back or distal axonopathy rather than new degeneration secondary to the loss of nerve cells. It is not known whether disulfiram is the responsible agent or whether a toxic metabolite induces the neuropathy. It is possible that disulfiram is metabolized to carbon disulfide, a compound capable of causing an axonal neuropathy in man and animals.

In alcoholics without evidence of peripheral neuropathy before disulfiram, electrophysiologic evidence of peripheral nerve dysfunction was demonstrable after three months of therapy [39]. This observation suggests that the neuropathology may be a frequent, although subclinical complication of disulfiram therapy.

ORAL CONTRACEPTIVES

Oral contraceptives have become widely prescribed and neurotoxic syndromes have emerged in disturbing frequency. Some side effects discussed in the section on glucocorticosteroids (Chapter 11) include pseudomotor cerebri and behavioral changes. Although euphoria and psychotic behavior have been described, mental depression is the more frequent complaint. It has been suggested that altered tryptophan metabolism underlies the pathophysiology of oral-contraceptive-induced depression. Pyridoxine, 50 mg/day, has been advocated on the premise that this vitamin acts as a co-enzyme to shift tryptophan metabolism toward serotonin synthesis and away from the alternate kynurine and niacin pathways [31]. From extensive studies of cerebrovascular disease before and after the introduction of oral contraceptives, it is clear that the risk of cerebrovascular accidents in young women on oral contraceptives is markedly increased. Stroke syndromes in young women on birth control pills are 3-8 times more frequent than in those not on oral contraceptives. From Bickerstaff's report, middle cerebral artery occlusions are more frequent than in the elderly population and vertebrobasilar disease is also frequent [1]. As such, the symptoms of transient ischemic attacks and stroke syndromes may be varied. In hemispheric strokes, dominant hemispheric lesions provoke usual aphasias and right hemiparesis. Left hemiparesis with hemisensory loss in the face and body follow a right middle cerebral artery occlusion. Brain stem cerebrovascular accidents presenting with "crossed-syndrome" (e.g., decreased sensation on the right face with decreased sensation on the left body or decreased strength of the right face with decreased strength of the left body) follow vertebrobasilar disease of the brain stem circulation. Treatment of such strokes involves the removal of the oral contraceptives, and the general rehabilitation efforts used in other forms of cerebrovascular disease. Angiographic findings more typical of embolic disease are usually seen with oral-contraceptive-induced strokes, although thrombotic disease occurs as well. The factors predisposing to cerebrovascular disease in women receiving oral contraceptives include the use of high-estrogen-containing compounds, multiparity, and a change in migraine headache pattern. Of probable, but less certain importance, are previous thrombotic or embolic disease and hypertension.

Chorea is the second serious problem related to oral contraceptives. The involuntary movements appear days or weeks after starting birth control pills and may be more frequent in patients with a prior history of Sydenham's (rheumatic) chorea. The chorea usually starts abruptly and may involve only one side of the body (hemichorea). Theoretically, the early childhood chorea of rheumatic fever that relates to striatal vasculopathy and estrogens during adult life may precipitate a chemical reaction that unveils again the long quiescent lesion. A similar phenomenon occasionally occurs during pregnancy when a woman develops severe involuntary movements that terminate when the pregnancy ends (chorea gravidarum). Birth-control chorea may disappear within 48 hours of medication cessation, although the abatement can take longer.

The often rapid reversibility of the chorea suggests that the event is not a traditional vascular stroke. Other movement disorders like hemiballismus or coarse tremor have occurred when women are receiving oral contraceptives and these are usually not reversible. These latter conditions may well relate to cerebrovascular accidents.

Neuro-ophthalmologic signs also occur with patients on oral contraceptives. As discussed above, pseudomotor cerebri may occur in patients and these pa-

Dietary Toxins and Miscellaneous Drugs

tients are often not the typically obese women with pseudotumor cerebri seen in other settings. Other conditions that may cause blurring of the optic disc are papilledema, related to venous sinus obstruction, or optic neuritis. Retrobulbar neuritis also occurs in patients on birth control pills; these patients complain of prominent visual impairment without altered optic discs.

Vascular headaches (migraines) may also appear for the first time or suddenly change in pattern when oral contraceptives are started. Common migraine (without an aura) may become classic migraine with patients beginning their headache syndrome, with symptoms or signs of focal cerebral dysfunction [47]. Cases also exist where the focal deficit is not followed by headaches, suggesting the development of a vascular transient ischemic attack. In cases where migraines either appear for the first time, increase in frequency, or become focal, cessation of oral contraceptives is suggested. A final subgroup of headache patients in fact find relief of headache pain with their oral contraceptives. This patients' headaches may have a close relationship to menstruation and when on the oral contraceptives, the patient has minimal pain. Only during the week when the oral contraceptives are not ingested, will she suddenly suffer with severe headaches. These cases are rather exceptional. Treatment of traditional migraine headaches with birth control pills is unlikely to be successful and is potentially hazardous.

Various othe neurologic disorders are occasionally associated with oral contraceptive use. Seizures may change in pattern or frequency. Carpal tunnel syndrome of median nerve neuropathy or other pressure neuropathies may occur, related to the increased fluid retention associated with oral contraceptives. Drug-induced and reversible myasthenia gravis has also rarely been reported [10].

▪ STUDY QUESTIONS

Which conditions are associated with vitamin excess?
1. Clinical findings of Guillain-Barré syndrome.
2. Increased intracranial pressure and right hemiparesis.
3. Myasthenia gravis.
4. Wernicke-Korsakoff syndrome.
5. None.

Answer: 5

Excess Vitamin A and B_6 are known to cause neurotoxic syndrome. B_6 provokes a sensory neuropathy with loss of reflexes, but should not be confused with Guillain-Barré, which predominantly affects the motor system. Vitamin A causes the syndrome of pseudotumor cerebri, with increased intracranial pressure, often associated with headache and other nonfocal neurologic findings (sixth nerve paresis, unlike other cranial neuropathies is a "false-localizing" sign. Because of the long trajectory of the nerve along bony surfaces, a sixth nerve paresis does not locate the level or side of neurologic damage). Right hemiparesis, on the other hand, is highly focal and is not compatible with diffuse increased intracranial pressure alone; the clinical presentation in #2 above (increased intracranial pressure and right hemiparesis) suggests a mass lesion or tumor. Vitamin D, when given in high doses chronically, affects calcium and phosphorus balance, which may clinically provoke global weakness. The classical neuromuscular fatigue typical of myasthenia and the response to edrophonium are not seen. Wernicke-Korsakoff Syndrome is related to vitamin deprivation and not to intoxication.

True statements regarding fetal alcohol syndrome include:

1. It is seen when babies breastfeed from mothers who are alcoholics.
2. Babies are small and have cleft palates and micrognathia.
3. Alcohol withdrawal seizures may occur within 20 minutes of extrauterine life.
4. This syndrome and Marchiafava-Bignami syndrome share the same pathological finding of life-long corpus callosum agenesis.

Answer: 2 and 3

The fetal alcohol syndrome is an embryotoxic one where the fetus who has been exposed to alcohol and possibly nutritional deficiency develops abnormally. The congenital findings described in #2, above are correct and other problems include hip and joint deformities and cardiac conduction defects. These children may well withdraw from alcohol, but this event will occur 12–36 hours after severing of the umbilical circulation and not within 20 minutes of birth. Machiafava-Bignami syndrome, like fetal alcohol syndrome shows corpus callosal disease, but in infants there is agenesis and in the Machiafava-Bignami patients, the adult corpus callosum demyelinates and degenerates.

True statements regarding cortical changes in alcoholics include:

1. CT scan shows a pathognomonic finding of alcoholism: increased ventricles and enlarged cortical sulci.
2. There is poor correlation between the above CT findings and intellectual decline in alcoholics.
3. There is poor correlation between the above CT findings and cortical cell loss.
4. None of the above.

Answer: 2

Increased cortical sulci and ventricular enlargement are typically seen in alcoholics, even those who are young and middle-aged. The CT findings are suggestive of substance abuse (not always just alcohol), but not pathognomonic. Carlen [3] demonstrated poor correlation between extent of CT alterations and demonstrable intellectual impairment. Furthermore, such apparent "atrophy" is often reversible, a phenomenon that may relate to rehydration and to the return of CNS protein synthesis that occurs within weeks of stopping alcohol; as such, neuronal cell loss cannot be estimated from CT findings in these patients.

Dietary Toxins and Miscellaneous Drugs

A teenage rock star who campaigns against alcohol and drugs, advocating high dose vitamins and organic gardening, is admitted for the evaluation of progressive ataxia and dysesthesias. He has already joined a local support group for multiple sclerosis and has raised a substantial sum for artists afflicted with demyelinating disease. Evidence suggesting that the clinical picture might relate to his diet and not to primary central nervous system degeneration would include:

1. The patient ingests 150 times the daily requirement of thiamine.
2. The patient has depressed reflexes.
3. The sensory examination shows a selective loss of vibration and position sense.
4. The EMG shows marked sensory conduction slowing.

Answers: 2 and 4

Recently, a prominent sensory ataxia related to high-dose pyridoxine ingestion has been documented. Patients chronically taking 2 grams or more of vitamin B_6 have developed a progressive peripheral neuropathy affecting primarily the sensory system. From animal studies, it appears that the toxicity relates to the dorsal ganglia. Involvement of the peripheral nervous system is suggested by the findings of 2 and 4 above. In multiple sclerosis where the disease involves the myelinated fibers of the central nervous system, reflexes are increased and the EMG should be normal. When the peripheral nervous system is damaged, most sensory modalities (vibration, position, pain, temperature), are affected: with multiple sclerosis, where the heavily myelinated fibers in the central nervous system disease are affected, vibration and position sense are preferentially compromised.

Factors that contribute to the acid-base abnormality of salicylate intoxication include which of the following:

1. Salicylates initially depress medullary breathing activation.
2. Salicylates are acids which displace bicarbonate and can also lead to ketosis.
3. Myoglobinuria usually precipitates renal shutdown and metabolic acidosis.
4. All of the above.

Answer: 2

Salicylates initially activate the medullary breathing center and cause respiratory alkalosis. Later, at high doses, the medullary breathing center can be inhibited. In addition, salicylates induce and enhance the chemosensitive response and are acids as described in 2. The net response is a metabolic acidosis with either a respiratory acidosis or alkalosis. Myoglobinuria is not a feature of salicylate intoxication.

Match the drug with the prominent neurotoxic syndrome.

A. Metoclopramide   1. Myasthenia gravis
B. Clofibrate   2. Myotonia

IATROGENIC AND MEDICINAL TOXINS

C. Penicillamine
D. Digitalis

3. Visual distortions
4. Parkinsonism

Answers: A-4; B-2; C-1; D-3

Metoclopramide is associated with various extrapyramidal movement disorders, including parkinsonism, dystonia, tremor, and tardive dyskinesia. Clofibrate is among the drugs known to induce myotonia. Penicillamine is a relatively safe chelating agent used in the treatment of rheumatoid arthritis, as well as some heavy metal intoxication and Wilson's disease, but is associated with hypogeusia, myopathy, optic neuritis, and a reversible form of myasthenia gravis. Patients will suffer with the latter condition, complaining of ptosis, diplopia, dysphagia, and generalized progressive weakness. Digitalis is a widely prescribed drug that is associated with often vague visual complaints of distorted images or halo formations in the visual field. Seizures and encephalopathy may also occur.

True statements regarding birth control pills and neurologic disability include:

1. Peripheral neuropathy of the axonal type can mimic multiple sclerosis.
2. Cerebrovascular accidents usually relate to cardiac valvular vegetations.
3. Chorea often resolves within days or weeks of drug cessation and is rarely a permanent sequelae of oral contraceptive ingestion.
4. Papilledema when it occurs is due to steroid-induced hypervitaminosis A.

Answer: 2

Birth control pills are not associated with a peripheral neuropathy, but instead their toxicity relates predominantly to central nervous system function. Cerebrovascular accidents are an alarming complication of these drugs in young women and may be of embolic or thrombotic origin. They do not specifically relate to valvular vegetations. Chorea often occurs within days of the first ingestion of birth control pills and may promptly stop after drug cessation. Only in rare instances (usually a hemiballistic syndrome) will the chorea be longstanding after drug cessation. In such cases, a static cerebrovascular accident is hypothesized to underlie the chorea as opposed to the transient chorea which probably relates to a hormonally induced functional alteration in dopaminergic sensitivity at the striatum. Papilledema, when it occurs in patients on birth control pills, may be of multiple etiologies, including venous thrombosis and pseudotumor cerebri. It does not appear to relate to hypervitaminosis A, however.

■ REFERENCES

1. Bickerstaff ER: Neurological Complications of Oral Contraceptives. Clarendon Press, Oxford, 1975.
2. Brucknall RC, Dixon A, Glick EN, et al: Myasthenia gravis associated with penicillamine treatment for rheumatoid arthritis. Br. Med. J. 2:600-602, 1976.
3. Carlen PL, Wilkinson A, Wortzman G, et al: Cerebral atrophy and functional deficits in alcoholics without clinically apparent liver disease. Neurology 31: 377-385, 1981.

4. Casteels-Van Daele M, Jaeken J, Van Der Schuren P, Zimmerman A, Van Den Bon, P.: Dystonic reaction in children caused by metoclopramide. Arch. Dis. Child. 45:130-134, 1970.
5. Clarren, SK, Smith DW: The fetal alcohol syndrome. N. Engl. J. Med. 298: 1063-1067, 1978.
6. Day AT, Golding JR: Reaction of D-penicillamine in rheumatoid arthritis. Br. Med. J. 3:593, 1973.
7. DeLuca HF: Fat Soluble Vitamins. Plenum Press, New York, 1978.
8. Done AK: Salicylate, an International Symposium. Boston, Little, Brown, 1963.
9. Done AK: Treatment of salicylate intoxication. Clin Toxicol 1:451-467, 1968.
10. Fadli MF, Abdelwahabta T: Myasthenic syndromes secondary to oral contraceptives. Exerpta Med. 296:99, 1973.
11. Foles FF, Molloy R, McNall PG, Koukal LR: Comparison of toxicity of intravenously given local anesthetic agents in man. JAMA 172:1493-98, 1960.
12. Fraser HS, Carr AC: Prpranolol psychosis. Br. J. Psychiatry 129:508–509, 1976.
13. Ghadimi H, Kumar S, Abaci F: Studies of monosodium glutamate ingestion: biochemical explanation of the Chinese Restaurant Syndrome. Bioch. Med. 5:447, 1971.
14. Goldstein M, Nakajima K: Effect of disulfiram on catecholamine levels in the brain. J. Pharmacol. Exp. Ther. 157:96-102, 1967.
15. Core M: Chinese restaurant syndrome. In EFP Jelliffe and DB Jelliffe, eds., Adverse Effects of Foods. Plenum Press, New York, 1982.
16. Greenblatt DJ, Bolognini V, Koch Weser J: Pharmacokinetic approach to the clinical use of lidocaine. JAMA 236:273-277, 1976.
17. Greenhouse AH: Heavy metals and the nervous system. Clin. Neuropharmacol. 5:45-92, 1982.
18. Grodon BM: Parkinsonism occurring with mcthyldopa treatment. Br. Med. J. 1:1001, 1963.
19. Holland OB, Kaplan NM: Propranolol in the treatment of hypertension. N. Engl. J. Med. 294:930-936, 1976.
20. Hotson JR, Langston JW: Disulfiram-induced encephalopathy. Arch. Neur. 33:141-142, 1976.
21. Johnson DA, Cooke R, Loh H: Involvement of lipids in the action of ethanol and other anesthetics. Adv. Exp. Med. Biol. 126:65-68, 1980.
22. Kalant H: Absorption, diffusion, distribution, and elimination of ethanol: effects on biological membranes. In B Kissin and H Beglieter, eds., The Biology of Alcoholism, Vol. 1, pp. 1-62. Plenum Press, New York, 1971.
23. Kenny RA: Chinese restaurant syndrome. Lancet 1:311-312, 1980.
24. Kerr GR, Wu-Lee M, El-Lozy M, et al: Prevalence of the Chinese restaurant syndrome. J. Am. Diet Assoc. 75:29-33, 1979.
25. Klawans HL, Braun AR: Metoclopramide-induced parkinsonism. Neurology 33:123, 1983.

26. Kwok RHM: Chinese restaurant syndrome. New Engl. J. Med. 278:796, 1968.
27. Lely A, VanEnter CHJ: Large scale digitalis intoxication. Br. Med. J. 3: 737-740, 1970.
28. Limbeck GA, Ruvalcaba RHA, Samols E, Kelley VC: Salicylates and hypoglycemia. Am. J. Dis. Child. 109:165-167, 1965.
29. Lipton MA, Nemeroff CB, Mailman RB: Hyperkinesis and food additives. IN RJ Wurtman and JJ Wurtman, eds., Nutrition and the Brain, Vol. 4, pp. 1-28. Raven Press, New York 1979.
30. Lyon AF, DeGraff AC: The neurotoxic effects of digitalis. Amer. Heart J. 65:839-840, 1963.
31. Malek-Ahmadi P, Behrmann PJ: Depressive syndrome induced with oral contraceptives. Dis. Nerv. Sys. 37:406-408, 1976.
32. Miller DR, Hayes KC: Vitamin excess and toxicity. In H. Hathcock, ed., Toxicology, Vol. 1. Academic Press, New York, 1982.
33. Mills JA: Non-steroidal anti-inflammatory drugs (Part I). N. Engl. J. Med. 290:781-784, 1974.
34. Moddel G, Bilbao JM, Payne D, Ashby P: Disulfiram neuropathy. Arch. Neur. 35:658-660, 1978.
35. Mussachio J, Goldstein M, Anagnoste B: Inhibition of dopamine beta hydroxylase with disulfiram. J. Pharmacol. Exp. Ther. 152:52-61, 1965.
36. Myers EN, Bernstein JM, Fostiropolous G: Salicylate ototoxicity, a clinical study. N. Engl. J. Med. 273:587-590, 1965.
37. National Advisory Committee on Hyperkinesis and Food Additives. Final report, Nutritional Foundation, New York, 1980.
38. Noble EP, Tewari S: Ethanol and brain ribosomes. Fed. Proc. 34:1942-1945, 1975.
39. Palliyath S, Schwartz B: Disulfiram neuropathy. Neurology 34:170, 1984.
40. Peter JB, Campion DS, Dromgoole SH, Nagatoma T, Andiaman RM: Similarities and differences between human myotonia and drug-induced myotonia in rats. In WG Bradley, D Gardner-Medwin, and JN Walton, eds., Recent Advances in Myology, pp. 434-440. Amsterdam, Excerpta Medica, 1975.
41. Peter JB, Fiehn W: Diazacholesterol myotonia accumulation of desmosteral and increased adenosine triphosphate activity of sarcolemma. Science 179: 910-912, 1973.
42. Pfeifer HJ, Greenblott DJ, Koch-Weser J: Clinical toxicity of reserpine in hospitalized patients. Prog. Am. J. Med. Sci. 271:269-276, 1976.
43. Richmond J: Wernicke's encephalopathy associated with digitalis poisoning. Lancet 1:344-345, 1959.
44. Russell AS, Lindstrom JM: Penicillamine-induced myasthenia gravis associated with antibodies to acetylcholine receptor. Neurology 28:847-849, 1978.
45. Schaumburg HH, Byck R, Gerstyl R, et al: Monosodium glutamate. Science 163:826-828, 1969.

46. Schaumburg MD, Kaplan J, Weindbank MD, et al: Sensory neuropathy from pyridoxine abuse: a new megavitamin syndrome. N. Engl. J. Med. 309: 445-448, 1983.
47. Shafey S, Scheinberg P: Vascular headaches and oral contraceptives. Ann. Intern. Med. 65:863-865, 1966.
48. Symonds C: Excitation and inhibition in epilepsy. Brain 82:133-146, 1959.
49. Tabakoff B, Noble EP, Warren KR: Alcohol, nutrition, and the brain. In RJ Wurtman and JJ Wurtman, eds., Nutrition and the Brain, Vol. 4, pp. 159-213. Raven Press, New York, 1979.
50. Uretsky NJ: Effect of alpha-methyldopa on the metabolism of dopamine in the striatum of the rat. J. Pharmacol. Exp. Ther. 189:359-369, 1975.
51. Victor M: The alcohol withdrawal syndrome. Ann. NY. Acad. Med. 215: 210, 1973.
52. Victor M: The pathophysiology of alcoholic epilepsy. Res. Publ. Assoc. Res. Nerv. Ment. Dis. 46:431-434, 1968.
53. Wallgren H: Effect of ethanol on intracellular respiration and cerebral function. In B Kissin and H Begleiter, The Biology of Alcoholism, Vol. 1, pp. 103-125. Plenum Press, New York, 1971.
54. Weiner WJ: Vitamin B6 in the pathogenesis and treatment of diseases of the central nervous system. In HL Klawans, ed., Clinical Neuropharmacology, Vol. 1, Raven Press, New York, 1976.
55. Woodbury DM, Fingl E: Analgesic antipyretics, anti-inflammatory agents and drugs employed in gout. In LS Goodman and AG Gilman, eds., The Pharmacological Basis of Therapeutics, pp. 325-358. Macmillan, New York, 1975.

Index

Acetone, 78
Acetylcholine, 150, 193-194, 215, 216, 263, 269 (*see also* Anticholinergic effects of drugs and toxins, Cholinergic drugs, and Cholinergic toxicity)
Acetylcholinesterase, 107-109
Ackee, 167
Acrylamide, 125-126
Acrodynia, 23
Actinomycin D, 305
Adriamycin, 305
Akathisia, 216-217
Alcohol
  biochemistry, 313-314
  barbiturates, and, 242
  clinical features of intoxication and withdrawal, 314-318, 334
  Coprinus mushrooms and, 163
  hypnosedatives and, 244
  isoniazid and, 285
  marijuana and, 268
  mercury and, 23
  methyl chloride and, 100
  treatment of intoxication or withdrawal, 315, 317
  tricyclic antidepressants and, 221
Aldehyde dehydrogenase, 331
Aldrin, 118
Algae, 156
Alkylating agents, 294-297
Aluminum, 45-48, 58

Amanita mushrooms, 162-163, 164, 166
Amantadine, 194-203, 271 (*see also* Dopaminergic drugs)
Amatoxin, 166
Aminoglycosides, 276, 277-280, 289
Aminolevulinic acid, 6-7, 12, 14-15, 22
Aminophylline, 227, 261
Amphetamine
  autonomic stimulation, 253
  biochemistry, 254-256, 271
  clinical features of intoxication, 253-254, 272
  metabolism, 257
  monoamine oxidase inhibitors with, 225
  practical management of intoxication, 256-257
  stereotypy, 235
Amphotericin B, 276
Amyl alcohol, 77-78
Anencephaly, 47, 57
Anesthesia, 278-279
Anesthetics, halothane, 100, 103-104
Aniline, 83-84
Antianxiety drugs, 219-221
Anticholinergic effects of drugs and toxins
  aminoglycosides, 279
  antidepressants, 222, 223
  atropine, 107-112, 161-166, 204
  botanical, 166-167, 170
  carbamazepine, 190
  curare, 176-177

341

[Anticholinergic effects of drugs and toxins]
  hallucinogens, 263
  lincomycin, 284
  mushrooms, 161-166
  neuroleptics, 213-217
  organophosphates, 108-110
  Parkinson's disease, 193-194, 204
  phencyclidine, 269
  tetanus, 137
  ticks, 149
  snake venoms, 150
Anticonvulsants, 185-194, 207-208 (see also individual drugs)
Antidepressants, 221-227
  biochemistry, 224
  carbamazepine and, 190
  clinical features of intoxication, 221-227
  lithium carbonate, 226-227, 228
  monoamine oxidase inhibitors, 221, 225-226, 229
  newer generation antidepressants, 223-225
  tricyclic antidepressants, 221-223, 228, 245
Antifungal drugs, 287-288 (see also individual drugs)
Antiinflammatory agents, 322-324
Antimalarial drugs, 288-289
Antimony, 46, 47, 49
Antineoplastic drugs, 293-312 (see also individual drug names)
Antiparkinson drugs, 192-203
Antipsychotic drugs see Neuroleptics, Lithium carbamate
Antituberculous drugs, 285-287
Antivenenes, 151
Anxiolytics, 219-221
Ara-C, see Cytarabine
Arsenic, 36-44
  alcohol effects, 37, 40
  biochemical effects, 36-37, 40
  cancer and, 39
  clinical features of intoxication, 38-40, 42, 177-178
  diagnosis of intoxication, 40-41, 103
  levels in intoxication, 40-41
  lines, 32, 39
  occupations associated with toxicity, 36-37, 42
  pathology, 36-38
  pregnancy and, 42

[Arsenic]
  safety limits, 40-41
  sources, 36-37, 42
  threshold limit values, 36
Arthritis, 51-52
Asparaginase, 304, 305-306, 310
Aspirin, 278, 335
Ataxia, see Cerebellar dysfunction
Atropine, 107-112, 161-166, 204
Attentional deficit disorder, 241, 253, 258, 320
Automatisms, 242
Autonomic nervous system and dysfunction
  alcohol, 315
  anxiolytics, 220
  botulism, 141
  bromides, 50-51
  caffeine, 254
  central stimulants, 256
  cocaine, 259
  fish toxins, 154, 156
  hallucinogens, 264
  hypnosedatives, 244
  marijuana, 268
  narcotics, 236
  neuroleptics, 212, 213-214, 219
  nicotine, 262
  scorpion toxins, 152
  tricyclic antidepressants, 221
  vinca alkaloids, 295

Baclofen, 198, 206
BAL, 13, 14, 30, 56, 327
Barbiturates
  biochemistry, 239-240
  clinical features of intoxication, 208, 238, 241-244
  drug-drug interactions, 189, 192, 220, 236, 239, 282, 330
  effects on babies, 243
  management of intoxication, 243
  substitution with, 244, 246, 248
Barium, 46, 47, 49
BCNU, 306-307, 309
Bees, 149, 157
Benzene, 79-80
Benzodiazepines, 219-220
  central stimulant intoxication and, 257
  methyl chloride and, 100
  phencyclidine intoxication and, 270

INDEX

Birth control pills *see* Oral contraceptives
Bismuth, 46, 47, 49
Bleomycin, 304-305
Botanical toxins, 161-181 (*see also* individual plants)
Botulism
  aminoglycosides and, 280, 289
  biochemistry, 140-141, 143
  clinical features of intoxication, 141-143
  sudden infant death syndrome (SIDS), 143-144
  treatment of intoxication, 143-144
Bromides, 46, 47, 50-51, 59
  effect of halothane, 100
Bromocriptine, 195-203, 214 (*see also* Dopaminergic drugs, Ergots)
Butyrophenones, 211-219

Caffeine, 251, 261-263
  amphetamine, relationship to, 254
  biochemistry, 251, 262
  clinical features of intoxication, 261-263
  methyl chloride, effects on, 100
  structural relationships, 251, 252
Calcium
  aminoglycosides and, 279
  black widow spider and, 154
  fish toxins and, 156
  halothane and, 101
Calcium disodium edetate (EDTA), 13, 14, 30
Calcium oxalate, 76-77
Calycanthine, 169
Camphor, 124
Cancer, 39 (*see also* Antineoplastic drugs)
Cannabinoids, 267-268
Carbamazepine, 189-190, 192, 208
  erythromycin effects, 283
Carbidopa, 198-199
Carbon disulfide, 97-98, 331
Carbon monoxide
  biochemistry, 92
  carboxyhemoglobin and, 92
  clinical features, 91-95, 102-103
  sources, 91-92
  treatment, 94-95
Carbon tetrachloride, 85-86
Cardiac drugs, 324-327
CCNU, 306-307

Central stimulants, *see* Stimulants
Cerebellar dysfunction, *see* chart, p. xvi
Cerebrovascular disease and accidents, *see* chart, p. xvi
Chelation, 12-16, 30, 56, 327-329
Chemotherapy, *see* Antineoplastic drugs
Chickpea, 168
Chinese restaurant syndrome, 321
Chloral hydrate, 247
Chlorambucil, 294, 297
Chloramphenicol, 276, 282
  phenobarbital and, 193
Chlordane, 118
Chlordecone, 119-120, 127
Chloroquine, 276- 288
Chlorpromazine, *see* Neuroleptics
Cholinergic drugs
  choline chloride, 196
  lecithin, 196
  organophosphates, 107-112
  physostigmine, 166, 170, 196, 201, 203
  neostigmine and peripheral cholinesterase inhibitors, 203-204
  use in treating anticholinergic intoxication
    anticholinergic plants, 166-167
    antidepressant overdose, 222
    tardive dyskinesia, 218
Cholinergic toxicity
  cholinesterase inhibitors, 203-204
  scorpion, 149
  snake venoms, 150
  spiders, 153
  tetanus, 137
Chorea, *see* chart, p. xix (Extrapyramidal and Involuntary Movement Disorders)
Cicutoxin, 169
Ciguatoxin, 156
Cis-platinum, 307, 309
Citrovorum factor, 300
Clindamycin, 276, 284
Clitocybe mushrooms, 162, 165
Clofibrate, 328, 336
Clonidine, 326
Cobalt, 20
Cocaine
  autonomic system stimulation, 259
  biochemistry, 251-252, 258-260
  clinical features of intoxication, 259
  practical management, 260
Colostomies, 49-50

343

Convulsant plants, 169-170
Coprinus mushrooms, 162, 163
Coproporphyrins, 12, 14-15, 22
Cortical blindness, see chart p. xxii
Corticosteroids, see Steroids
Cranial neuropathies, see chart, p. xvii
  (see also specific ocular abnormalities)
Curare, 176-177 (see also Anticholinergic effects of drugs and toxins)
Cyanides, 173
Cyclophosphamide, 296, 309, 310
Cycloserine, 276
Cyproheptadine, 265
Cytarabine, 301-302
Cytochrome oxidase activity, 97, 174
Cytosine arabinoside, see Cytarabine

Dantrolene, 214
DDT, 115-116
Delirium tremens, 316
Dementia, see Encephalopathy
Dentists, 103
Depressant plants, 169
Dermatitis, 23, 39, 51, 55
Desmosterol, 329
Dialysis dementia, 47-48
Diabetes mellitus, 121
20-25-Diazacholesterol (DAC), 328
Diazepam, see Benzodiazepines
Dieldrin, 118
Dietary toxins, 313-321
Digitalis, 324, 336
Dihydrolipoate, 37
Dimercaprol (BAL), 13, 14, 30, 56
Dioxin, 121-122, 127
Diphtheria, 135-137, 289
Disulfiram, 331
Dopamine, 172, 190, 211, 215-216, 218, 219, 223, 253, 260, 261, 265, 269, 314
Dopaminergic drugs, 172, 195-203, 239
Dopaminergic antagonists, 206, 211-219
Drug holiday, 202-203, 207
Dystonia, see chart p. xix

EDTA, 13-14, 16, 30
Encephalopathy, see chart, p. xviii
Endorphins, 237
Endosulfan, 118

Endrin, 118
Ergots, 171-173, 194-203, 264
Erythromycin, 276, 283
Estrogens, see Oral contraceptives
Ethambutol, 276, 286
Ethanol, see Alcohol
Ethchlorvynol, 244
Ethionamide, 276, 287
Ethylene glycol, 76-77, 86, 87
Ethylene oxide, 98-99, 104
Extraocular muscle paresis, see chart, p. xxii
Extrapyramidal disorders, see chart, p. xix, text references listed under individual movement disorders

Feingold diet, 320-322
Ferroxidase, 48
Ferrosamine, 48
Fetal toxicity
  alcohol, 317-318, 334
  lead, 5, 6
  mercury, 25
  zinc, 57
Fish toxins, 154
5-Fluorouracil, 301, 308
Folate, 187, 296
Food additives, 320

Gamma-aminobutyric acid (GABA), 114, 124-125, 137-139, 145, 191, 205, 285, 322
Gasoline, 70-71
Gila monsters, 153-154
Gold, 51-52, 58, 59
Glutamate, 321
Glutethimide, 247
Glyceraldehyde phosphate dehydrogenase, 6
Glycine, 114, 167
Guanidine, 143
Guillain-Barré syndrome, 43, 52, 55, 157, 238 (see also Peripheral neuropathy)
Gyromitra mushrooms, 166

Hallucinations, see Encephalopathy
Hallucinogens, 251, 263-267 (see also Mushrooms)
  biochemistry, 263-265
  clinical features of intoxication, 266
  treatment of intoxication, 267
Haloperidol, 211-219 (see also Neuroleptics)

INDEX

Halothane, 100-101
Heatstroke, 214, 228
Heroin, *see* Narcotics
Hexachlorocyclohexane, 117
Hexachlorophene, 123, 127
n-Hexane, 81-82, 86
Huffer's neuropathy, 67, 69
Huntington's chorea, 254
Hydralazine, 326
Hydrazine, 124-125
Hydrogen sulfide, 96-97, 104
Hydrocarbons, 115-121
Hydrocyanic acid, 173
Hymenoptera, 148-149
Hyperactivity, 241, 320 (*see also* Attentional deficit disorder)
Hypertension, *see* Autonomic nervous system
Hyperthyroidism, 254
Hypnosedatives, 239-247
Hypoglycemia, 167, 322
Hypoglycin A, 167
Hypotension, *see* Autonomic nervous system

Ibotenic acid, 162, 165
Increased intracranial pressure, 9
Indomethacin, 323
Insecticides, 107-131
Isobenzan, 118
Isoniazid, 276, 285-286, 290, 304
Isopropyl alcohol, 78

Jamaican Vomiting Sickness, 167

Khat, 168-169

Lathyrism, 168
Latrotoxin, 153
Lead
  biochemical effects, 3-5, 6-7, 12, 14-15
  calcium deficiency, 14, 15
  children, 3, 5-6, 9, 11, 14, 15
  clinical features of intoxication, 9-11
  diagnosis of intoxication, 11, 12, 14-15
  iron deficiency effects, 6, 15
  levels, 3-4, 11-12
  lines, 11, 32
  pathology, 8
  pica, 3
  porphyria, differentiation from lead toxicity, 6

[Lead]
  protoporphyrin, erythrocyte, 12, 14-15
  safety limits, 5
  sources, 4-5
Lecithin, 196 (*see also* Cholinergic drugs)
Levodopa
  biochemistry, 194
  clinical features of intoxication, 194-203
  neuroleptic malignant syndrome, 214
  treatment of intoxication, 195-203
Lidocaine, 326-327
Lincomycin, 276-284
Lithium carbonate, 204, 226-228
Lysergic acid diethylamide (LSD), 251, 252, 264-265

Magnesium, 168, 279, 316
Malignant hyperthermia, 101, 103-104, 177, 213, 279
Mania, 211, 213
Manganese, 52-54
Marijuana, 267-268
Mees lines, 39
Melphalan, 295
Meningitis
  cytarabine, 295
  methotrexate, 295
Mental retardation, 10, 27
Meperidine, 225 (*see also* Narcotics)
Meprobamate, 221
Mercury
  alcohol, effect on toxicity, 23
  biochemical effects, 20, 21-22, 25-26, 30-32
  clinical features of intoxication, 22-24, 26-29, 32-33, 172
  cobalt and, 20
  diagnosis of intoxication, 29, 103
  fetal intoxication, 25
  inorganic, 20-24, 29-32
  organic, 24-32
  pathology, 21-22, 26
  recovery from intoxication, 31-32
  renal damage, 21, 22
  selenium and, 20, 54
  sources, 19-20, 25, 26
  storage, 20, 21, 24, 26
  treatment of intoxication, 33-34
  vitamin deficiency and, 20, 31
  vitamin E, 31
Mescaline, 251, 252, 263-264, 266
Methanol, 74-76, 86, 87

Methaqualone, 236, 245
Methemoglobin, 91-95, 174
Methionine, effect of nitrous oxide on, 96
Methotrexate
  biochemistry, 297-298
  citrovorum factor, 300
  clinical features of intoxication, 298-299, 308
  treatment of intoxication, 299
Methyl bromide, 121
Methyl-n-butyl ketone (MBK), 82-83
Methyl chloride, 99-100, 103-104
Methylene blue, 174
Methylphenidate, 251, 252, 258, 260 (see also Stimulants)
Methysergide, 197, 265
Metoclopramide, 320, 336
Metronidazole, 276
Migraine headaches, 219, 332-333
Minocycline, 283
Moelsch–Woltman syndrome, 138
Monoamine oxidase inhibitors, 221, 225, 229, 245, 308
Monosodium glutamate, 321
Motor neuron disease, see chart, p. xx
Mushrooms, 161-167, 264
Myalgia, muscle spasms, and trismus, see chart, p. xx
Myasthenia gravis, 177, 192, 203-205, 207, 280, 289
Myelopathy, see chart, p. xxi
Myoclonus, see chart, p. xix
Myopathy, see chart, p. xxi
Myotonia, 328-330 (see also chart, p. xxi)

Nalidixic acid, 276, 284
Naloxone, 234-235, 236
Naproxen, 324
Narcotics
  biochemistry, 232-233
  clinical features of intoxication, 232-239, 247-248
  heroin abuse, 233-236
  MPTP, 238
  treatment of intoxication, 232-239
  Ts and Blues, 238
Neuroleptics
  biochemistry, 211-212
  clinical features of intoxication, 213-219, 227-228

[Neuroleptics]
  MAO inhibitors and, 225
  neuroleptic malignant syndrome, 213, 214
  Parkinson's disease, 193, 202
  stimulants and, 257
  treatment of intoxication, 196-197
Neuromuscular blockade, see chart, p. xxi
Neuropathy, see Peripheral neuropathy
Nicotinamide, 120
Nitrite therapy, 96
Nitrofurantoin, 276, 281-282
Nitrogen mustard, 294-295
Nitrosoureas, 295, 306-307
Norepinephrine, 218-225, 253, 314 (see also Autonomic nervous system)
Notexin, 150, 151
Nutmeg, 264

Ocular abnormalities, see chart, p. xxii
On-off, 197
Opiates, see Narcotics, Endorphins
Optic neuritis, see chart, p. xxii
Oral contraceptives, 331-333
Organic solvents, 65-90 (individual solvents listed by name)
  absorption and clearance, 65
  occupations associated with exposure, 66-68
  sources, 66-68
  threshold limit values, see Threshold limit values
Organophosphates, 107-112, 126-127
  biochemistry, 108, 111
  sources, 108
  clinical features of toxicity, 109-111
  diagnosis, 111-112
Ototoxicity, 276, 278, 282, 283 (see also chart, p. xvii, Cranial Neuropathy)

Papilledema, see chart, p. xxii
Paraldehyde, 275
Parathion, see Organophosphates
Parkinson's disease, 192-203, 207, 319-320
Parkinsonism, see chart, p. xix
Pemoline, 251, 252 (see also Stimulants)
Penicillamine, 13, 14, 30, 327-328
Penicillins, 275-277, 289
Pentazocine, 238
Periodic paralysis, 49

INDEX

Peripheral neuropathy, *see* chart, p. xxiii
Periwinkle, 302
Pesticides, 107-131
Phallotoxin, 166
Phencyclidine, 251, 252, 269-271, 272
Phenobarbital
  biochemistry, 239
  clinical features of intoxication, 208, 241-243
  drug-drug interactions, 189, 192, 244, 282
  substitution with, 244, 246, 248, 315
  treatment of intoxication, 243
  use in treating other intoxications, 317
Phenols, 122-123
Phenothiazines
  biochemistry, 213
  clinical features of intoxication, 213-219
  infants and, 213
  neuroleptic malignant syndrome, 213
  treatment of intoxication, 213-219
Phenylbutazone, 324
Phenylethyl malanic acid (PEMA), 189
Phenylethylamine, 251, 252, 264
Phenylpropenolamine, 262
Phenytoin
  biochemistry, 185-186
  blood levels, 185-186
  clinical features of intoxication, 186-188, 208
  drug-drug interactions, 192, 219, 282, 286, 324
  management of intoxication, 188
  use in treating other toxic syndromes, 270, 317
Pica, 3, 5
Picrotoxin, 113-115
Plant toxins, 161-181
Plexopathy, *see* Peripheral neuropathy
Polychlorinated biphenyls (PCBs), 122
PNU, 120-121
Poliomyelitis, 43
Polymixins, 276
Porphyrins and porphyrea, 12, 14-15, 55, 71, 80, 244
Pralidoxine, 112-113
Primidone, 189, 192 (*see also* Phenobarbital)
Procainamide, 137
Procaine, 289
Procarbazine, 308
Propranolol, 226, 260, 326-327, 339
Protoporphyrins, 12, 14-15
Prussian blue, 56
Pseudocholinesterase, 107
Pseudotumor cerebri, *see* chart, p. xxii
Psilocybe, 163, 264, 266
Psychiatric drugs, 211-231
Punding, 255
Pupillary changes, *see* chart, p. xxii
Pyridoxine, *see* Vitamin B6
Pyridylmethynitrophenyl urea (PNU), 120
Pyrimethamine, 280

Quinidine, 137, 278

Reserpine, 216-218, 219, 228, 260
Retrobulbar neuritis
  benzene, 79
  trichlorethylene, 84
Risus sardonicus, *see* Trismus
Rodenticides, 120-121, 127-128

Salicylates, 335
Schizophrenia, 211, 223
Scorpions, 149, 152
Sea food, 24
Selenium, 54
Seizures, *see* chart, p. xxiv
Serotonin, 154, 264-265, 171-173, 218-225, 314
Silicon, 57-58
Solvent mixtures
  clinical features, 70-72
  gasoline, 72-73
  pathology, 69-70
  treatment of toxicity, 72-74
Snakes, 149-152
Spiders, 153
Spina bifida, 57
Spironolactone, 31
Steroids, 151, 204-205, 258
Stiff-person syndrome, 138
Stimulants
  biochemistry, 251-253, 258, 261-262
  clinical features of intoxication, 253-256, 258, 259-260, 262-263
  drug-drug interactions, 225-226
  management of intoxication, 256-258, 260-261, 262

Sudden infant death syndrome (SIDS), 143-144
Sulfonamides, 276, 280
Sulindac, 324
Strychnine, 113-115, 127, 169
Sydenham's chorea, 254, 332
Systemic lupus erythematosus, 254
Styrene, 123-124
Sulfhydral groups and enzymes, 6, 21, 22, 26, 37, 57

Taipoxin, 150-151
Tarantulas, 153
Tardive dyskinesia, 218-219
Tetanus
  biochemistry, 137
  clinical features of intoxication, 138-140
  sources, 137-138
  treatment of intoxication, 139-140
Tetrachlorethane, 118-119
Tetracyclines, 276, 283
Tetraethyl lead, *see* Gasoline
Tetrahydrocannabinol, 267
Tetrahydrofolinic acid, 280
Tetrodotoxin, 155-156
Thallium, 54-57
Thiamine, 37
Thioacetamide, 31
Thioctic acid, 166
Thiotepa, 294, 297
Threshold limit values, 5, 29, 30, 36, 67, 92, 99, 108
Ticks, 149, 152
Toluene, 80-81
Toxaphene, 118

Tranquilizers, 211-231
Tremor, *see* chart, p. xix, *also* chart, p. xvi (Cerebellar Dysfunction) (*see also* Parkinsonism and Cerebellar dysfunction)
Trichlorethylene, 84-85, 86-87
Tricyclic antidepressants, *see* Antidepressants
Triorthocresylphosphate, 113, 127
Triparanol, 329
Tripelennamine, 238
Trismus, *see* chart, p. xx
Tryptamine, 251, 252, 264
Tryptophan, 331
Tubocurarine, 177

Vacor, 120
Valproate, 190-192, 208
Venoms, 146-160
Vestibular toxicity, 276, 278-279, 282-283
Vinca alkaloids, 302-304, 309, 329
Vitamin A, 318
Vitamin B-1, 37
Vitamin B-6, 285, 287, 290, 308, 319, 332, 333-334, 335
Vitamin B-12, 96
Vitamin D, 319
Vitamin deficiency, 20, 31, 96
Vitamin E, 31

Wernicke encephalopathy, 317, 324
Wernicke–Korsakoff syndrome, 317

Xanthines, 261-263

Zinc, 56-57